Study Guide

Pharmacology for Nursing Care

Ninth Edition

RICHARD A. LEHNE, PhD

Prepared by

Jennifer J. Yeager, PhD, RN
Assistant Professor
Department of Nursing
Tarleton State University
Stephenville, Texas

ELSEVIER

ELSEVIER

3251 Riverport Lane
St. Louis, Missouri 63043

STUDY GUIDE FOR LEHNE'S PHARMACOLOGY FOR
NURSING CARE, NINTH EDITION

ISBN: 978-0-323-32259-1

Notices

Knowledge and best practice in this field are constantly changing. As new research and experience broaden our understanding, changes in research methods, professional practices, or medical treatment may become necessary.

Practitioners and researchers must always rely on their own experience and knowledge in evaluating and using any information, methods, compounds, or experiments described herein. In using such information or methods they should be mindful of their own safety and the safety of others, including parties for whom they have a professional responsibility.

With respect to any drug or pharmaceutical products identified, readers are advised to check the most current information provided (i) on procedures featured or (ii) by the manufacturer of each product to be administered, to verify the recommended dose or formula, the method and duration of administration, and contraindications. It is the responsibility of practitioners, relying on their own experience and knowledge of their patients, to make diagnoses, to determine dosages and the best treatment for each individual patient, and to take all appropriate safety precautions.

To the fullest extent of the law, neither the Publisher nor the authors, contributors, or editors, assume any liability for any injury and/or damage to persons or property as a matter of products liability, negligence or otherwise, or from any use or operation of any methods, products, instructions, or ideas contained in the material herein.

ISBN: 978-0-323-32259-1

Content Strategist: Jamie Randall
Content Development Specialist: Samantha Taylor
Publishing Services Manager: Hemamalini Rajendrababu
Project Manager: Saravanan Thavamani

Printed in the United States of America
Last digit is the print number: 9 8 7 6 5 4 3 2 1

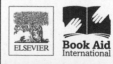

Working together
to grow libraries in
developing countries

www.elsevier.com • www.bookaid.org

Introduction

The critical thinking and study questions in this *Study Guide* include review of knowledge, application of knowledge to nursing care, analysis of nursing situations that require clinical decision-making, and prioritization of nursing actions. When this book is used as a study guide, the questions that do not have a ➤ or ✳ before them are excellent tools to augment the initial reading of the textbook before attending class and to use for review after classroom activities. Knowledge of drug action, interactions, administration directives, and adverse effects is required before the nurse can engage in clinical decision-making.

The questions that have a ➤ or ✳ before them require more than repetition of the information in the textbook. Questions preceded by ➤ require application and analysis of information; whereas those preceded by ✳ require prioritization, including selecting the most important information or action. Identifying the correct answer to these questions requires careful examination of the data and reflection on the patient in a holistic manner. The student will have to integrate other nursing knowledge, such as developmental considerations and laboratory values, as well as timing and prioritization of actions. These ➤ and ✳ critical thinking questions reflect the reasoning that students and new graduate nurses must be able to perform to safely administer pharmacotherapy. They are an excellent source of review when preparing for the NCLEX® examination.

A useful strategy when presented with the case studies in this workbook is to read the last sentence first. Knowing the question that is being asked guides identification of pertinent information in the case. When reading the rest of the information in the case, identify key words and data. Identify assessment findings and laboratory values that are normal or abnormal. Think about the situation to identify if it is a normal part of nursing care or if it requires collaboration with the prescriber.

Critical thinking by the nursing student requires assimilating classroom learning and clinical experience. No two experiences are the same. Be careful not to add information into the question based on your experience with patients when answering questions in this *Study Guide*. But *do* engage in discussion about similar patient experiences with faculty and peers. Be prepared to explain your thinking. It will enrich your learning experience.

The author and Elsevier welcome any feedback you have about the content of the *Study Guide*.

Answers to the Case Studies can be reviewed online at http://evolve.elsevier.com/Lehne/.

Contents

1

Orientation to Pharmacology

STUDY QUESTIONS

Matching

Match the term with its definition.

1. ___ Any chemical that can affect living processes.
2. ___ The medical use of drugs.
3. ___ The study of drugs and their interactions with living systems.
4. ___ The study of drugs in humans.

    a. Clinical pharmacology
    b. Drug
    c. Pharmacology
    d. Therapeutics

Completion

Fill in the blank with the property of an ideal drug that the nurse considers in the following situations.

5. The nurse teaches a patient to avoid engaging in hazardous activities when taking an antihistamine for allergy symptoms.

_____

6. The nurse explains that a generic form of a newly prescribed drug is available to a patient who has limited insurance coverage for drugs.

_____

7. The nurse researches if an antidote is available when administering drugs that have the potential to cause significant harm or death.

_____

8. The nurse administers ciprofloxacin (Cipro) through a second intravenous line separate from all other drugs.

_____

9. The nurse explains that quinapril and Accupril are names for the same drug.

_____

10. The nurse reassesses the patient 20-30 minutes after administering an opiate analgesic.

_____

11. During discharge teaching, the nurse assesses if the patient will be able to take a prescribed drug 4 times a day as ordered.

_____

12. When a patient is or could be pregnant, the nurse researches the pregnancy category of every drug administered.

_____

13. The nurse teaches patients that the medicine cabinet is a bad place to store medications because the heat and humidity can damage the drug.

_____

14. The nurse is aware that African Americans often do not respond as well as Caucasians to angiotensin-converting enzyme inhibitors (ACE I) prescribed for hypertension.

_____

CRITICAL THINKING, PRIORITIZATION, AND DELEGATION QUESTIONS

15. Which patient would be the highest priority when providing nursing care to multiple patients?
    a. A patient who would like to know if a newly prescribed drug is available in generic form
    b. A patient who has requested a laxative because he has not had a bowel movement in 2 days
    c. A patient who received oral drugs 1 hour ago and has complained of tingling around his mouth
    d. A patient who is prescribed a drug, the name of which the nurse does not recognize

16. Which *nursing* action would best meet the therapeutic objective of drug therapy?
    a. Assessing the patient for adverse effects of drug therapy
    b. Prescribing a drug with the fewest adverse effects
    c. Prescribing a drug with the fewest serious adverse effects
    d. Recommending that a patient avoid taking drugs because there are possible adverse effects

CASE STUDY

A patient returned to the nursing unit after an esophago-gastroduodenoscopy (EGD) at 1200. She did not receive her 0900 oral drugs before the procedure because of an order for nothing by mouth (NPO).

1. What factors must the nurse consider when deciding which of the 0900 oral drugs should be administered at this time?

2

Application of Pharmacology in Nursing Practice

STUDY QUESTIONS

Matching

Match the nursing action with the seven aspects of drug therapy.

1. ____ Knowing the major adverse reactions of a drug, when they are likely to occur, early signs of development, and interventions to minimize discomfort and harm
2. ____ The rights of drug administration coupled with the knowledge of pharmacology
3. ____ Knowing the reason for drug use and being able to assess the patient's medication needs
4. ____ Knowing the early signs of toxicity and the proper intervention when it occurs
5. ____ Collecting baseline data, identifying high-risk patients, and determining the patient's capacity for self-care
6. ____ Taking a thorough drug history, advising the patient to avoid drugs that may interact with prescribed medication, and monitoring for adverse interactions
7. ____ The process to determine if a drug is beneficial or causes harm

    a. Preadministration assessment
    b. Dosage and administration
    c. Evaluating and promoting therapeutic effects
    d. Minimizing adverse effects
    e. Minimizing adverse interactions
    f. Making as-needed (PRN) decisions
    g. Managing toxicity

CRITICAL THINKING, PRIORITIZATION, AND DELEGATION QUESTIONS

8. The nurse is preparing to administer an antihypertensive drug (medication that lowers the blood pressure). The nurse assesses the patient's blood pressure at 110/70 mm Hg. What action should the nurse take at this time?
    a. Administer the medication because the antihypertensive medication is prescribed.
    b. Assess the patient's baseline blood pressure and the blood pressure before and after the last dose of this medication to determine if the medication should be administered.
    c. Call the prescriber, report the current blood pressure, and ask if the medication should be administered.
    d. Withhold the medication because the patient's blood pressure is too low to administer an antihypertensive drug.

✳ 9. The nurse should withhold a drug and contact the prescriber if the patient reported an allergy to the drug with which symptom occurring shortly after the last time the drug was taken?
    a. Constipation
    b. Dry mouth
    c. Vesicular rash
    d. Wheezing

10. Which postoperative patient assessment would warrant withholding an opiate analgesic that depresses the central nervous system (CNS)?
    a. BP 150/92 mm Hg
    b. Pulse 110 beats/min
    c. Respirations 9/min
    d. Temperature 102.2° F (39° C)

11. Which nursing diagnosis would be most appropriate for a patient who is receiving an opiate analgesic that depresses the central nervous system (CNS)?
    a. Fatigue
    b. Impaired physical mobility
    c. Risk for activity intolerance
    d. Risk for injury

＊12. A patient who is admitted to the nursing unit from the postanesthesia care unit (PACU) is moaning in pain. The patient is due for another dose of pain medication. What is the nursing priority at this time?
    a. Administer prescribed pain-relieving drugs.
    b. Assess the patient's vital signs, tubes, and surgical site.
    c. Obtain the patient's pain rating on a scale of 1-10.
    d. Review the patient's allergy history.

13. The nurse is preparing to administer insulin based on the patient's metered blood glucose level. Which action could be delegated to a licensed practical/vocational nurse (LPN/LVN)?
    a. Documenting the insulin that the RN administered
    b. Drawing up the insulin in the syringe
    c. Identifying the patient for medication administration
    d. Obtaining the metered blood glucose level

CASE STUDY

A 52-year-old man is admitted with uncontrolled hypertension. He has been prescribed three medications: benazepril maleate (Lotensin) 40 mg twice a day; hydrochlorothiazide 25 mg four times a day; and verapamil (Calan) 80 mg three times a day. The patient admits that he does not take the drugs as prescribed. The nurse identifies that the patient does not think he needs the drugs because he cannot "feel" his high blood pressure and he does not have insurance for drugs.

1. What are possible interventions to overcome these factors that are interfering with the patient's ability to perform self-care with this medication regimen?

2. How does the nurse determine if administered antihypertensive drugs are effective?

3. The nurse is preparing to administer hydrochlorothiazide, a diuretic drug that lowers blood pressure by increasing the excretion of water and electrolytes—sodium and potassium—via the kidneys. What laboratory tests should the nurse review before administering this drug?

4. What should be included when providing teaching about a newly prescribed drug?

3

Drug Regulation, Development, Names, and Information

STUDY QUESTIONS

Matching

Match the drug with its type of name.

1. ___ acetaminophen
2. ___ N-(4-hydroxyphenyl) acetamide
3. ___ Tylenol

    a. Chemical name
    b. Generic name
    c. Brand name

Completion

Fill in the blank with type of drug name.

4. The _____ name is never used for more than one medication.

5. The _____ name tells the nurse the active ingredients of the drug.

6. The _____ name of a drug will be the same, no matter which company produces the drug.

7. The _____ name may suggest the action of the drug such as PhosLo which lowers phosphorus.

8. _____ names of drugs in the same therapeutic class often have a similar suffix, making them easy to identify.

9. Nursing drug reference books are usually organized by _____ names.

10. Fosinopril, lisinopril, moexipril, quinapril, and ramipril are examples of _____ names.

CRITICAL THINKING, PRIORITIZATION, AND DELEGATION QUESTIONS

11. When preparing discharge instructions for a patient, what should the nurse do?
    a. Ask the patient which name he or she uses for the drug and use only that name in discharge teaching.
    b. Explain the generic name only so the patient does not become confused.
    c. Explain the trade name only because it is easier for the patient to remember.
    d. Review the prescriptions written for discharge and include the stated trade name and generic name in discharge teaching.

12. A patient has been taking a brand-name drug for a chronic condition for several years. Recent changes in his insurance plan require the use of generic drugs whenever they are available. The patient asks the nurse if he should pay out of pocket to continue receiving the brand-name drug. The nurse's response should be based on which fact(s)? (Select all that apply.)
    a. That continuing to use the brand-name drug will prevent confusion.
    b. That drugs requiring monitoring of blood levels should have levels checked when changing from brand-name to generic drugs.
    c. That generic drugs contain the same active ingredients as their brand-name counterparts.
    d. That generic drugs usually are not absorbed at the same rate as brand-name drugs.
    e. That brand-name drugs contain different active ingredients than generic drugs.

13. The nurse is teaching a patient about tamsulosin (Flomax), which has been prescribed for difficulty voiding due to an enlarged prostate. Because the patient travels extensively and not all countries require prescriptions to get drugs, what it is important for the nurse to teach the patient?
    a. That a drug labeled Flomax may have different active ingredients in different countries.
    b. That drugs purchased in countries other than the United States and Canada are usually unsafe.
    c. That Flomax is not available anywhere except the United States and Canada.
    d. That doses of Flomax in countries that use the metric system are different than doses of drugs in the United States.

14. Which resource(s) most likely provide(s) current, complete positive and negative information about a drug? (Select all that apply.)
    a. Drug sales representatives
    b. Drug Facts and Comparisons
    c. Internet search
    d. Pharmacists

CASE STUDY

The nurse is caring for a patient who has high blood cholesterol (hyperlipidemia). The patient states that she became worried about her high cholesterol when her sister had a "heart attack." She went to a health food store to see if they had any natural products that could help lower her cholesterol. She noticed a sign on the counter asking for volunteers to enter a study. Volunteers are to submit a copy of their blood cholesterol results and again at the end of a year after taking the product as directed for a full year. Explain why the results of this study may not be reliable based on these factors.

1. Control

2. Randomization

3. Blinding

4
Pharmacokinetics

STUDY QUESTIONS

Matching

Match the terms and definitions relating to drug change and movement.

1. ___ Absorption
2. ___ Distribution
3. ___ Elimination
4. ___ Excretion
5. ___ Metabolism
6. ___ Pharmacokinetics

   a. Change in drug structure
   b. Change in drug structure and movement out of the body
   c. Movement from blood into tissue and cells
   d. Movement into and out of body
   e. Movement into the blood
   f. Movement out of the body

Match the method of movement with characteristics for that method of movement.

7. ___ May require energy or pores
8. ___ Requires small size
9. ___ Requires lipid solubility

   a. Passage through channels
   b. Direct penetration of the membrane
   c. Passage with the aid of a transport system

True or False

For each of the following statements, enter T *for true or* F *for false.*

10. ___ Cell membranes are composed of fat with phosphate.
11. ___ Most drugs enter cells through channels or pores.
12. ___ P-glycoprotein transports many drugs out of cells.
13. ___ A transport mechanism is needed for a water-soluble drug to enter a cell.
14. ___ Ionization is a process that allows a drug to enter a cell.
15. ___ If a quaternary ammonium compound drug is injected into a vein it will produce effects, but it will not if taken orally.
16. ___ Polar drugs can enter fetal circulation and breast milk.
17. ___ Acetylsalicylic acid (aspirin), like most drugs, is primarily absorbed in the small intestine.
18. ___ Enteric drugs should not be crushed because crushing these preparations can cause stomach distress or cause the acid in the stomach to alter the drug.
19. ___ A depot intramuscular (IM) injection of an antibiotic to treat syphilis will be completely effective within 24 hours after administration.
20. ___ The protein-bound portion of a drug in circulation is not able to exert its action.
21. ___ *First-pass effect* means most of the drug is activated by the liver, so it must be administered orally.
22. ___ A drug with extensive first-pass effect may be given sublingually to allow the drug to be absorbed directly into the systemic circulation.
23. ___ Adding a drug to a patient's drug regimen can cause the other drugs to be metabolized more slowly or more rapidly.
24. ___ Intestinal enzymes can release drugs from bile in the duodenum, causing the drug to be reabsorbed.
25. ___ The nurse would expect that an IV antibiotic prescribed for bacterial meningitis would most likely get to the site of infection if the drug is water-soluble.
26. ___ Chemotherapy is administered through a central intravenous line because chemotherapy is caustic to the vein and a large central vein has rapid blood flow, which dilutes and moves the medication quickly.

CRITICAL THINKING, PRIORITIZATION, AND DELEGATION QUESTIONS

✳27. The nurse is administering an intravenous push dose of an opiate analgesic (morphine sulphate). After administering half of the dose, the nurse notes that patient's respirations have decreased from 15/minute to 11/minute. What is the priority nursing action at this time?
   a. Assess the patient's current pain.
   b. Call the prescriber.
   c. Stimulate the patient.
   d. Stop administration of the rest of the drug.

✳28. The nurse inadvertently administers heparin 100 units/mL subcutaneously, which is available on the nursing unit as part of an intravenous flush protocol, instead of the heparin 5000 units/mL that was prescribed to prevent postoperative deep vein thrombosis (DVT). What is the priority nursing concern?
   a. Assessing the patient for DVT.
   b. Consulting the prescriber for direction.
   c. Filling out an incident report.
   d. Preventing excessive bleeding.

29. The nurse realizes that when injecting insulin, which lowers blood glucose, into the subcutaneous fat above the deltoid muscle in a very thin child, the drug may have been inadvertently administered into the muscle. What is the patient at risk for?
   a. Blood glucose dropping too rapidly
   b. Blood glucose not dropping rapidly enough

30. Which laboratory test result suggests that a patient's excretion of a drug may be impaired?
   a. AST: 72 international units
   b. INR: 4.2
   c. eGFR: 30 mL/min
   d. WBC: 13,000/mm^3

✳31. What is a priority nursing action in PACU to promote excretion of most anesthetics?
   a. Encourage deep-breathing.
   b. Maintain a patent IV line.
   c. Monitor urine output.
   d. Prevent constipation.

32. Digoxin (Lanoxin) is a drug that has a narrow therapeutic range. When administering this drug, what does the nurse need to do? (Select all that apply.)
    a. Administer the medication only on an as-needed (PRN) basis.
    b. Carefully monitor the patient for therapeutic and toxic effects.
    c. Be diligent about the timing of administering the medication.
    d. Monitor blood levels of the drug to assess if it is in the therapeutic range.
    e. Teach the patient that the drug takes several weeks to reach full effectiveness.

33. Grapefruit juice inhibits the cytochrome P450 CYP3A4 drug-metabolizing enzyme and inhibits P-glycoprotein in the intestines for days after ingestion. This especially affects calcium channel blockers, benzodiazepines, cyclosporine, and -statin drugs. The nurse should teach a patient who is prescribed any of these drugs that drinking grapefruit juice can cause what problem?
    a. Excessive first-pass effect
    b. Excess levels of drug in the blood
    c. Lack of therapeutic effect of the drug
    d. Rapid excretion of the drug

34. A patient stopped taking levothyroxine (Synthroid) 3 days ago. This drug has a half-life of 7 days. He tells the nurse that the drug must not have been necessary because he does not feel any different. What is the basis of the nurse's explanation of why the patient has not noticed any change in how he feels?
    a. The patient's dose was probably too high, so the drug is still working.
    b. The patient could not have been taking the drug as prescribed.
    c. The drug probably was not needed if the patient has not experienced any symptoms.
    d. The drug's previous doses have not been completely eliminated from the body.

CASE STUDY

The nurse is caring for a hospitalized patient who has been prescribed the following medications: 0800 glyburide (DiaBeta) 10 mg; 0900 quinapril HCl (Accupril) 20 mg. Breakfast is served at 0810. Hospital policy states that medications may be administered 30 minutes before or after the designated time. To save time, the nurse plans to administer both of these medications at 0830.

1. Research the onset of these medications and explain why this is not a good plan.

5
Pharmacodynamics

STUDY QUESTIONS

True or False

For each of the following statements, enter T *for true or* F *for false.*

1. ____ Pharmacodynamics includes the study of how drugs work.
2. ____ Phase 2 of the dose-response relationship starts at the point when the therapeutic effect does not increase with increasing the dose.
3. ____ *Maximal efficacy* is defined as the largest effect that a drug can produce.
4. ____ *Potency* is defined as the dose of drug needed to get the desired effect.
5. ____ Two drugs in the same therapeutic class with different recommended doses (2 mg vs. 200 mg) can have equal effects.
6. ____ A drug that stimulates the transcription factor receptors may not reach a peak therapeutic effect until taken regularly for days to weeks.
7. ____ A drug that is selective for specific receptors will produce more unintended effects than a nonselective drug.
8. ____ If a drug is selective for specific receptors, it is safe.

9. ___ *Affinity* is the strength of attraction between a drug and its receptor.

10. ___ Drugs with high intrinsic activity cause an intense response.

11. ___ An agonist drug blocks the stimulation of a receptor.

12. ___ If a receptor is constantly bombarded by a drug, the cell can down-regulate and decrease the response to the drug.

13. ___ A patient who suddenly stops taking an antagonist drug may experience hypersensitivity of the receptor and overstimulation.

14. ___ The ED_{50} is usually the recommended dose for the drug.

CRITICAL THINKING, PRIORITIZATION, AND DELEGATION QUESTIONS

15. The nurse is reading research about a drug. The literature states that the drug is *potent*. What does this mean?
    a. The drug produces its effects at low doses.
    b. The drug produces strong effects at any dose.
    c. The drug requires high doses to produce its effects.
    d. The drug is very likely to cause adverse effects.

16. Except for gene therapy, which statements are true about drug-receptor interactions? (Select all that apply.)
    a. Drugs can mimic the actions of endogenous molecules.
    b. Receptors for drugs do not respond to hormones and neurotransmitters produced by the body.
    c. The binding of a drug to its receptor is usually irreversible.
    d. Drugs can block the actions of endogenous molecules.
    e. Drugs can give the cell new functions.

17. The nurse is administering morphine sulphate for moderate to severe postoperative pain. Based on the other regulating effects of morphine, what should the nurse do? (Select all that apply.)
    a. Assess respirations and hold the medication if adventitious breath sounds are present.
    b. Assess respiratory rate and hold the medication if respirations are weak or fewer than 12/min.
    c. Maintain the patient on complete bedrest with all four side rails elevated to prevent injury.
    d. Assist the patient when ambulating to prevent injury.
    e. Encourage ambulation if not contraindicated to promote bowel motility.

18. Which assessment finding suggests hypersensitivity of receptors when a patient suddenly stops taking atenolol (Tenormin), a beta$_2$ receptor antagonist that slows the heart rate?
    a. BP 80/56 mm Hg
    b. Pulse 118 beats/min
    c. Respirations 26/minute
    d. Temperature 104° F (40° C)

✳19. An unresponsive patient who has overdosed on methadone HCl (Metadol), an opiate, is brought into the emergency department with severely depressed respirations. The patient receives intravenous naloxone HCl (Narcan), a narcotic antagonist, with a dramatic improvement in the level of consciousness and respiratory rate and effort within minutes. Which is a priority nursing action 45-60 minutes after the naloxone HCl is administered?
    a. Assess for return of pain because the effect of the naloxone HCl should be peaking.
    b. Assess for the need to administer another dose of naloxone HCl as the naloxone HCl effect is ending.
    c. Prepare to administer the drug intramuscularly if the drug has not taken effect.
    d. Prepare to counteract the effects of opiate withdrawal.

20. When the therapeutic index of a drug is narrow, what should the nurse expect?
    a. Blood levels of the drug would be monitored throughout therapy.
    b. The drug would produce the desired effect at low doses.
    c. The drug would produce many adverse effects at low doses.
    d. The drug would only be used in an emergency.

6
Drug Interactions

STUDY QUESTIONS

True or False

For each of the following statements, enter T *for true or* F *for false.*

1. ___ A prescriber may prescribe a drug solely because of its interaction with another drug.

2. ___ Powdered drugs can be mixed once they are dissolved in a liquid.

3. ___ Alcohol, bananas, cigarette smoking, chewing tobacco, chocolate candy, garlic, and grapefruit juice can interact with drugs and cause adverse effects.

4. ___ Antacids increase urinary excretion of alkaline drugs.

5. ___ Adding potassium clavulanate to amoxicillin (Augmentin) prevents the body's beta-lactamase enzyme from destroying the amoxicillin.

6. ___ The nurse should consult with the prescriber regarding adequate blood levels of oral drugs when a patient has persistent diarrhea.

CRITICAL THINKING, PRIORITIZATION, AND DELEGATION QUESTIONS

✳ 7. The nurse is providing discharge teaching for a patient who will be taking metronidazole (Flagyl) after discharge. The drug information states to caution the patient that a reaction similar to the action of disulfiram (Antabuse) can occur. It is a priority to teach the patient to avoid which food or drink?
   a. Beer
   b. Chocolate
   c. High-fat food
   d. Sugar

8. It is the nurse's responsibility at an institution to decide what time a drug will be administered. Cholestyramine (Questran) has been prescribed for a patient who takes many drugs for diabetes and hypertension. The patient takes the other drugs at 0900 and 1700. At this institution, drugs can be given up to 1 hour before or after the assigned time. Based on proper timing of administration of this drug, when should the cholestyramine be administered?
   a. 0800
   b. 0900
   c. 1000
   d. 1100

9. Patients receiving certain drugs that are metabolized by the CYP3A4 enzyme should not drink grapefruit juice because grapefruit juice inhibits the CYP3A4 enzyme and the drug transporter P-glycoprotein. The patient asks what might happen if she drinks grapefruit juice and takes the medication. The nurse's response is based on knowledge that the effect could be what?
   a. Lack of response because the drug will not be absorbed
   b. Lack of response because it does not get to the site of action
   c. Impaired metabolism and excretion of the drug
   d. Liver damage because the CYP3A4 enzyme destroys the liver

✳ 10. A male patient is prescribed clopidogrel (Plavix) to prevent blood clots after experiencing a myocardial infarction (MI). He self-prescribes omeprazole (Prilosec OTC) for heartburn. Because omeprazole can inhibit the efficacy of clopidogrel (Plavix), it is a priority for the nurse to teach the patient to report which effect?
   a. Dizziness
   b. Nausea and vomiting
   c. Joint pain
   d. Sudden shortness of breath or chest pain

▶11. A patient has been taking phenytoin (Dilantin), a drug with a narrow therapeutic index, to control seizures. If fenofibrate (Tricor) is prescribed to lower triglycerides, drug interaction puts the patient at risk for which effect?
   a. Excessively low triglycerides
   b. Seizures
   c. Toxicity from the fenofibrate (Tricor)
   d. Toxicity from the phenytoin (Dilantin)

12. Tobacco induces the CYP1A2 liver enzyme. Methadone is metabolized by the CYP1A2 liver enzyme. If a drug-addicted patient was treated with methadone and smoked cigarettes, what would this tobacco use be expected to do?
   a. Diminish the effect of methadone
   b. Make the effect of methadone more intense
   c. Speed the elimination of methadone
   d. Slow the elimination of methadone

▶13. A patient has been prescribed sildenafil (Viagra) for erectile dysfunction. The nurse teaches the patient that metabolism of this drug may be increased, possibly decreasing the effect, if the patient uses which dietary supplement?
   a. Fish oil
   b. Iron
   c. Garlic
   d. Multivitamin

14. A patient who drinks grapefruit juice and does not inform the prescriber may experience muscle pain from the adverse effect of rhabdomyolysis, which is possible if the patient is prescribed which drug?
   a. Lovastatin (Mevacor) for high cholesterol
   b. Nifedipine (Procardia) for hypertension
   c. Triazolam (Halcion) for insomnia
   d. Verapamil (Calan) for atrial fibrillation

CASE STUDY

The nurse is caring for a 92-year-old patient who was admitted yesterday with pneumonia. The patient's history includes hypertension and heart failure. The patient is exhibiting signs of experiencing hallucinations.

1. What information does the nurse need to provide to the prescriber to help determine if this behavior is related to a drug interaction?

7

Adverse Drug Reactions and Medication Errors

STUDY QUESTIONS

Matching

Match the term with its description.

1. ____ Clay-colored stool with nausea and vomiting
2. ____ eGFR 50 mL/min and urinary output 750 mL/day; fluid intake 1500 mL/day
3. ____ Fatigue and hemoglobin/hematocrit 9.2%/28 mg/dL
4. ____ Frequent infections or infection with rare microbe and WBC count fewer than 5,000/mm^3
5. ____ Numbness and tingling around the mouth and respiratory distress
6. ____ Pulse 52 beats/min and unexplained fainting

   a. Anaphylaxis
   b. Hemolytic anemia
   c. Hepatotoxicity
   d. QT prolongation
   e. Nephrotoxicity
   f. Neutropenia

Completion

7. Withdrawal syndrome occurs when a drug is stopped when a person is _____ _____ on the drug.

8. A(n) _____ reaction is an immune response.

9. _____ means cancer-causing.

10. Drugs that are _____ can harm a fetus if the patient takes the drug while she is pregnant.

11. Effects that are nearly unavoidable secondary drug effects at therapeutic doses are called _____ _____.

12. Genetic differences can cause uncommon drug responses. These are called _____ reactions.

13. _____ disease is when a drug causes symptoms closely resembling a disease.

14. _____ is the detrimental physiologic effects caused by excessive drug dosing.

CRITICAL THINKING, PRIORITIZATION, AND DELEGATION QUESTIONS

15. Which is not an adverse effect of a drug as defined by the World Health Organization (WHO)?
    a. Constipation from codeine for pain
    b. Nausea and vomiting from chemotherapy
    c. Reflex tachycardia from calcium channel blocker vasodilators to lower blood pressure
    d. Respiratory depression from overdose of benzodiazepine sleeping pills

16. When do adverse drug reactions occur more often? (Select all that apply.)
    a. When patients take multiple drugs
    b. When patients take potent drugs
    c. When a drug error occurs
    d. When patients are younger than 1 year old
    e. When patients have multiple chronic illnesses

✳17. The nurse has administered quinapril (Accupril). One hour after administration, the patient reports a tingling sensation of the lips. The nurse notes that the patient has perioral edema. Which action is of greatest priority?
    a. Document the finding.
    b. Hold the next dose of the medication.
    c. Notify the prescriber.
    d. Withhold all food and water.

18. Which symptom suggests an ototoxic reaction to a drug?
    a. Dizziness
    b. Headache
    c. Nausea
    d. Tinnitus

19. Before administering lovastatin (Mevacor), a -statin drug known to be toxic to the liver, the nurse reviews the patient's laboratory tests. Test results include alanine aminotransferase (ALT) 134 international units/L, and aspartate aminotransferase (AST) 97 units/L. Which action is most appropriate at this time?
    a. Administer the drug.
    b. Assess the vital signs, and if stable, administer the drug.
    c. Hold the drug and report the results to the prescriber ASAP.
    d. Hold the drug.

20. The nurse is mentoring a nursing student. The student complains that it is unfair that the nursing program requires 100% proficiency in dose calculation on a dose calculation examination during the last semester because it is stressful for students. What is the basis of the nurse's response to the student?
    a. Explain that students must be able to calculate drug doses under stress and dosing errors can be fatal.
    b. Share with the student the policy that existed when the nurse was in school.
    c. Support the student's efforts to overturn the policy because it is unrealistic.
    d. Support the school policy because 100% proficiency on dose calculations is required on the state board National Council Licensure Examination (NCLEX) examination.

21. The nurse is caring for a patient who is experiencing severe pain. Morphine sulfate 10 mg intramuscular (IM) is ordered every 4 hours as needed. The patient asks the nurse to administer the medication via an existing intravenous (IV) cap because the patient dislikes the pain of an IM injection. What should the nurse do in this situation?
    a. Administer the medication IM because that is the way that it is ordered.
    b. Administer the medication via the intravenous cap.
    c. Determine if the dose is safe for IV administration and administer it via the IV cap if it is safe.
    d. Explain to the patient that the nurse cannot change the route of a medication without a prescriber's order and that paging the prescriber may take some time.

✳22. A nurse has incorrectly administered an excessive dose of a prescribed drug to a patient. Which intervention would be least likely to be beneficial in this situation?
a. Assess the patient for effects of the drug.
b. Place the nurse on unpaid leave.
c. Report the error to the institution's safety coordinator.
d. Require the nurse to identify possible strategies to prevent this type of error in the future.

23. When should the nurse report possible adverse effects of new drugs to www.fda.gov/medwatch?
a. Every time a patient experiences an adverse effect
b. Never; this is the prescriber's job
c. When the nurse notes an adverse symptom when administering a newly released drug
d. When the nurse is sure that a drug is causing an adverse effect

24. What is not required on FDA-approved MedGuides for patients?
a. The name of drug
b. What the drug is supposed to do
c. The safe dose range of the drug
d. What to do if a dose is missed
e. Who should not take the drug

25. Which is the criterion for a black box warning in the drug literature?
a. There is potential for serious adverse effects.
b. A MedGuide is not required.
c. Benefits of the drug do not compensate for adverse effects.
d. The drug is provided as a sample from the prescriber.

26. What is the reason for the iPLEDGE component of the Risk Evaluation and Mitigation Strategy (REMS) for isotretinoin?
a. The drug can cause dysrhythmias.
b. The drug must be taken as directed to be effective.
c. The drug is sedating and could lead to injury if taken when driving.
d. The drug can cause fetal harm if taken during pregnancy.

8

Individual Variation in Drug Responses

STUDY QUESTIONS

Completion

1. Dose requirements for drugs with a narrow therapeutic range are most accurately calculated based on the patient's _____ _____ _____ .

2. When a patient takes a drug for a long time and becomes tolerant, the nurse would expect the prescriber to _____ the dose to achieve the desired effect.

3. _____ is the ability of a drug to reach the systemic circulation from its site of administration.

4. _____ is a reduction in drug responsiveness brought on by repeated dosing over a short time.

5. If the nurse is administering warfarin to a malnourished patient with a serum protein level of 2.9 g/dL, the nurse would expect the patient to be at increased risk for _____ .

6. Based on differences in metabolism of alcohol, if both a man and woman consume the same amount of alcohol (on a weight-adjusted basis) and take the drug metronidazole (Flagyl), the disulfiram-like reaction between alcohol and the drug in the woman should be more _____ and last _____ than for the man.

CRITICAL THINKING, PRIORITIZATION, AND DELEGATION QUESTIONS

7. A terminal cancer patient has been receiving narcotic analgesics for severe pain for more than 6 months. The prescriber has increased the dose of the long-acting opiate and added an "as-needed" opiate for breakthrough pain. What should the nurse do?
   a. Question the higher dose of medication because the patient is at risk for narcotic addiction.
   b. Question why the medication is being prescribed on a regular and an as-needed basis.
   c. Recognize that the higher dose is needed because the patient would have undergone down-regulation of opiate receptors.
   d. Recognize that the additional medication is needed because cancer causes an up-regulation of opiate receptors.

8. A nitroglycerin transdermal patch is ordered to be applied at 0900 and removed at 2100. The patch from the previous day is still in place when the nurse is preparing to administer the 0900 patch. What is the best action by the nurse?
   a. Leave the old patch on and apply the new one in a different site.
   b. Remove the old patch and apply the new one in a different site.
   c. Remove the old patch and do not apply a new patch until tomorrow.
   d. Remove the old patch and consult with the prescriber for further directions.

✳ 9. The nurse is caring for a 57-year-old African-American man who has been prescribed sulfamethoxazole and trimethoprim (Septra IV) and whose history includes a G-6-PD deficiency. It would be a priority to report which laboratory test result for this patient to the prescriber?
   a. ALT 278 IU/L
   b. BUN 2.2 mg/dL
   c. Hemoglobin 8 mg/dL
   d. INR 1.2

10. A patient is completely dependent on a respirator to initiate respirations. Recent laboratory values include pH 7.48, pco_2 32 mm Hg, and HCO_3 20 mEq/L, indicating respiratory alkalosis. What would be the effect of this acid-base imbalance on acidic drugs?
    a. Ionization of the drug in the blood, increasing the blood level of the drug
    b. Trapping of the drug in the cells, decreasing the blood level of the drug

11. Which symptom of an electrolyte imbalance would be of most concern to the nurse when a patient is prescribed digoxin (Lanoxin)?
    a. Fatigue
    b. Perioral tingling
    c. Arrhythmia
    d. Muscle weakness and spasms

9

Drug Therapy During Pregnancy and Breast-Feeding

STUDY QUESTIONS

True or False

For each of the following statements, enter T *for true or* F *for false.*

1. ____ Drugs are not a common cause of birth defects.
2. ____ The health of the fetus supersedes the health of the mother when drugs are prescribed to pregnant patients.
3. ____ The health of the fetus depends on the health of the pregnant patient.
4. ____ Pregnant women should not take any drugs.
5. ____ The goal of the Medication Exposure in Pregnancy Risk Evaluation Program is to identify drugs that have adverse effects on birth outcomes.
6. ____ Hepatic metabolism decreases during pregnancy.
7. ____ Glomerular filtration increases during pregnancy.

8. ____ All drugs can cross the placenta to some extent.

9. ____ Drugs are most likely to pass into fetal circulation if they are water-soluble.

10. ____ Angiotensin-converting enzyme inhibitor drugs for hypertension are prohibited during the second and third trimesters of pregnancy.

Matching

Match the drug with its potential teratogenic effect(s).

11. ____ Alcohol
12. ____ Ibuprofen
13. ____ Isotretinoin
14. ____ Lisinopril
15. ____ Methotrexate
16. ____ Phenytoin
17. ____ Tetracycline
18. ____ Valproic acid

    a. CNS, craniofacial, and cardiovascular defects
    b. CNS and limb malformations
    c. Growth retardation and CNS defects
    d. Low birth weight and mental retardation
    e. Neural tube defects
    f. Premature closure of the ductus arteriosus
    g. Renal failure and malformed skull
    h. Tooth and bone anomalies

CRITICAL THINKING, PRIORITIZATION, AND DELEGATION QUESTIONS

19. Based on pharmacokinetics, drugs are most likely to pass into fetal circulation if they are
    a. highly polar.
    b. ionized.
    c. protein bound.
    d. lipid-soluble.

20. A patient with a history of heroin addiction has delivered a full-term infant. Which signs and symptoms suggest the infant is experiencing withdrawal symptoms?
    a. Shrill cry and irritability
    b. Respiratory depression and lethargy
    c. Peripheral cyanosis and hypotension
    d. Apgar score of 3 at 1 minute and 4 at 5 minutes

21. A pregnant patient with a history of controlled hypertension asks the nurse why the prescriber changed her high blood pressure medication from quinapril (Accupril) to methyldopa (Aldomet). The nurse's response should be based on what knowledge?
    a. Methyldopa is more effective for treating hypertension during pregnancy.
    b. Methyldopa is pregnancy category B and quinapril is pregnancy category C in the first trimester and category D in the second and third trimesters.
    c. The dose of quinapril is more potent than the dose of methyldopa.
    d. Quinapril crosses the placenta, but methyldopa does not.

22. What is an important role of the nurse when a pregnant patient has a known exposure to a known teratogen during week 4 of the pregnancy?
    a. Ordering an ultrasound
    b. Providing the diagnosis from the ultrasound to the parents
    c. Providing information and emotional support
    d. Recommending termination of pregnancy if a severe malformation is detected

23. Which instruction should be included in patient teaching regarding breast-feeding and drug therapy?
    a. Avoid taking any drugs.
    b. Avoid drugs that have a long half-life.
    c. The best time to take a needed drug to minimize transfer to the infant is just after breast-feeding.
    d. Use sustained-release formulas of drugs.

CASE STUDY

A patient with a history of heroin addiction has delivered a full-term infant.

1. What should be included in the nursing care to address possible drug withdrawal in the neonate?

2. Exposure to teratogens during the embryonic period can produce gross malformation in the fetus. What nursing actions can help decrease teratogenesis during this period?

10

Drug Therapy in Pediatric Patients

STUDY QUESTIONS

True or False

For each of the following statements, enter T *for true or* F *for false.*

1. ____ All drugs that are considered safe to administer to adults are safe for administration to pediatric patients if the dose is adjusted appropriately for size.

2. ____ For drug purposes, *infancy* is defined as from the end of 4 weeks to 1 year of age.

3. ____ The majority of drugs used in pediatrics have never been tested on children.

4. ____ Intramuscular absorption of drugs is slower in the infant than in the adult.

5. ____ Toddlers often need higher doses per body weight than preschool children.

6. ____ Approximating safe doses of drugs for children is most accurate when calculated based on weight.

CRITICAL THINKING, PRIORITIZATION, AND DELEGATION QUESTIONS

7. Premature infants are at risk for what kind of response to drugs?
   a. Inadequate and short-lived response
   b. Intense and prolonged response
   c. Inadequate but prolonged response
   d. Intense but short-lived response

8. An infant is diagnosed with scurvy caused by vitamin C deficiency. Based on the principles of pH-dependent ionization and ion trapping and the differences in gastrointestinal physiology in the infant, the nurse would expect that the prescribed dose of vitamin C (ascorbic acid) adjusted for weight would be what?
   a. Less than an adult dose
   b. Equal to an adult dose
   c. More than an adult dose
   d. None; vitamin C should not be given to infants.

9. A pregnant patient received morphine sulfate late in labor. The neonate was born 22 minutes later. Because the drug crosses the placenta and the characteristics of the blood-brain barrier of the neonate, which neonatal assessment finding would be of most concern to the nurse?
   a. Abdominal breathing
   b. Pulse 160 beats/min
   c. Respirations 22/min
   d. Temperature 98.1° F (36.7° C)

10. The nurse is preparing to administer 4.5 mL of medication to a shy 6-year-old child. Which nursing intervention is most likely to gain cooperation from the child with taking the drug?
    a. Use a syringe to accurately measure the medication and ask the parents if they have any special technique for administering medication that has been effective with this child.
    b. Mix the medication in a 6-ounce glass of juice to mask the taste.
    c. Place the medication in a large empty glass so that the child can see that there is only a small amount of medication.
    d. Use a syringe to accurately measure the medication and squirt the medication into the child's mouth.

11. Which drugs are recommended by the American Academy of Pediatrics (AAP) as safe and effective for relieving cold symptoms in a 4-year-old child? (Select all that apply.)
    a. Acetaminophen (Tylenol)
    b. Dextromethorphan ("DM" cough suppressants)
    c. Ibuprofen (Motrin)
    d. Ibuprofen and pseudoephedrine (Children's Motrin Cold)
    e. Phenylephrine (PediaCare decongestant)

12. Which is the recommendation by the Centers for Disease Control and Prevention (CDC) for over-the-counter (OTC) cough and cold drug use in children younger than 2 years?
    a. Do not give any OTC drugs to a child younger than 2 years.
    b. Do not give any OTC cough and cold preparations to a child younger than 2 years.
    c. OTC cough and cold drugs are safe and effective if the preparation is specifically made for children and is properly measured.
    d. Use accurate measuring devices specifically designed for pediatric use when administering OTC cough and cold drugs to children younger than 2 years.

13. The safe dose of a liquid drug for a 6-month-old is 0.75 mL. Which would be best used to accurately administer the drug?
    a. 1-mL syringe without the needle
    b. 3-mL syringe without the needle
    c. 5-mL syringe without the needle
    d. Calibrated plastic medicine cup

DOSE CALCULATION QUESTIONS

14. The prescriber has prescribed 225 mg of a drug twice a day for a 7-year-old child who is 43 inches tall and weighs 45 lb. The recommended adult dose of this drug is 500 mg twice a day. Based on body surface area, is this dose safe?

15. The drug is available in an elixir of 250 mg/5 mL. How much medication will the nurse administer?

CASE STUDY

New parents tell the nurse that it is impossible to get their infant to take an oral suspension of an antibiotic. They tell the nurse that they have been putting the medicine into the baby's formula.

1. What can the nurse do to increase adherence to the drug regimen?

11

Drug Therapy in Geriatric Patients

STUDY QUESTIONS

True or False

For each of the following statements, enter T *for true or* F *for false.*

1. ___ The goal of therapy for the older adult is to cure the disease.
2. ___ There is a wider individual variation in drug response in the older adult.
3. ___ Older adults are less sensitive to drugs.
4. ___ Older adults absorb less of the dose of medication than young adults.
5. ___ Absorption of many drugs slows with aging.
6. ___ Changes in body fat and lean body mass that occur with aging can cause lipid-soluble drugs to have a decrease in effect and water-soluble drugs to have a more intense effect.
7. ___ Liver enzyme activity often is increased in the older adult.
8. ___ Drug accumulation secondary to decreased renal excretion is the most common cause of adverse reactions in older adults.
9. ___ A reduction in the number of receptors and/or decreased affinity for receptors in the older adult may decrease the response to drugs that work by receptor interactions.

CRITICAL THINKING, PRIORITIZATION, AND DELEGATION QUESTIONS

*10. When evaluating kidney function in the older debilitated adult, it is a priority for the nurse to review the results if which test?
   a. Serum blood urea nitrogen (BUN)
   b. Serum creatinine
   c. Creatinine clearance
   d. Renal ultrasound

11. An older adult with liver disease is receiving several drugs that are normally highly protein bound. The patient's serum albumin is 2.8 mg/dL (normal 3.5 to 5 mg/dL). The nurse needs to assess the patient for symptoms of
   a. excessive action of the drugs.
   b. inadequate action of the drugs.

►12. The nurse is preparing to administer the NSAID ketorolac (Toradol) to a debilitated 83-year-old woman who has joint pain. Which symptom would warrant withholding the drug and contacting the prescriber?
   a. Constipation
   b. Difficulty waking up in the morning
   c. Dizziness when changing from a prone to upright position
   d. Tarry stools

*13. Which assessment is a priority before administering methyldopa (Aldomet) to a geriatric patient?
   a. Alertness and orientation
   b. BP and pulse
   c. Bowel and bladder elimination
   d. Intake and output

*14. The nurse is aware that anticholinergic adverse effects of drugs commonly cause more problems in older adults than in younger adults. Which anticholinergic effect would be a priority to report to the prescriber?
   a. Blurred vision
   b. Dry mouth
   c. Has not voided in 16 hours
   d. No bowel movement for 48 hours

15. The nurse is aware that an older adult patient is at risk for which problem when prescribed tolterodine (Detrol)?
   a. Diarrhea
   b. Disturbed sensory perception
   c. Fluid volume deficit
   d. Impaired skin integrity

CASE STUDIES

Case Study 1

The nurse knows that adverse drug reactions and drug-drug interactions in the older adult patient can have many different causes. How can the nurse decrease the incidence of adverse drug reactions and drug-drug interactions in the older adult based on the following factors?

1. Altered pharmacokinetics

2. Multiple severe illnesses and multiple-drug therapy

3. Poor adherence

Case Study 2

A 76-year-old patient who has mild arthritis and a cataract of the left eye has been prescribed four medications with varied time intervals.

4. Identify the steps that the nurse could use to overcome obstacles and promote adherence to the prescribed drug regimen.

12

Basic Principles of Neuropharmacology

STUDY QUESTIONS

Matching

Match the term with its definition.

1. ____ Areas on the axon where neurotransmitters are stored.
2. ____ Areas on the postsynaptic cells that can be stimulated or blocked by drugs.
3. ____ Drugs that activate receptor activity.
4. ____ Drugs that prevent receptor activity.
5. ____ Moving the axon potential down the neuron.
6. ____ Arrival of this at an axon terminal triggers release of a transmitter.
7. ____ Molecules from the axon terminal that bind to receptors on the postsynaptic cell.
8. ____ The process by which information is carried across the synaptic gap.
9. ____ The process by which the parts of neurotransmitters are recycled back to the neuron from which they were released.

   a. Action potential
   b. Agonist
   c. Antagonist
   d. Axonal conduction
   e. Neurotransmitter (transmitter)
   f. Receptor
   g. Reuptake
   h. Synaptic transmission
   i. Vesicle

True or False

For each of the following statements, enter T for true or F for false.

10. ____ The impact of a drug on a neuronally regulated process is dependent on the ability of that drug to influence receptor activity.
11. ____ Activation of a receptor always results in speeding up a physiologic process.
12. ____ Drugs can cause an increase in the formation of neurotransmitters.

13. ____ Drugs can promote but cannot prevent transmitter release.
14. ____ Selective serotonin reuptake inhibitors increase the release of serotonin from the vesicles into the synapse.
15. ____ Selectivity is one of the most desirable qualities that a drug can have.

CRITICAL THINKING, PRIORITIZATION, AND DELEGATION QUESTIONS

▶ 16. The nurse would be especially cautious when administering a nonselective blocker of alpha$_1$, beta$_1$, and beta$_2$ receptors to patients with which chronic disorder(s)? (Select all that apply.)
    a. Asthma
    b. Benign prostatic hyperplasia
    c. Diabetes mellitus
    d. HIV infection
    e. Rheumatoid arthritis

17. Selective serotonin reuptake inhibitors are a class of antidepressant drugs. What is their mechanism of action?
    a. Decrease the synthesis of serotonin in the axon
    b. Decrease the pumping of serotonin back into the axon from which it was released
    c. Increase the release of serotonin from the vesicles into the synapse
    d. Stimulate receptors for serotonin

18. A cholinergic drug that mimics the action of acetylcholine would cause the heart rate to slow because the drug does what?
    a. Blocks receptors for acetylcholine
    b. Causes an increased release of acetylcholine
    c. Causes a decreased release of acetylcholine
    d. Stimulates cardiac receptors for acetylcholine

19. What characteristics allow naloxone (Narcan) to take the place of an opiate at opiate receptors and reverse respiratory depression caused by an opiate (narcotic) analgesic? (Select all that apply.)
    a. Binding of naloxone and opiates to opiate receptors is reversible.
    b. Naloxone has a longer half-life than opiates.
    c. Naloxone has a stronger affinity for the receptor.
    d. Naloxone is selective for opiate receptors.
    e. The dose of naloxone is larger than the dose of the opiate.

20. Drugs that block transmitter reuptake have what effect on receptor activation?
    a. They decrease receptor activation.
    b. They increase receptor activation.
    c. They have no effect on receptor activation.
    d. They have an unknown effect on receptor activation.

13

Physiology of the Peripheral Nervous System

STUDY QUESTIONS

Matching

Match the divisions of the nervous system to functions that can be influenced by drugs.

1. ___ Regulation of smooth muscle
2. ___ Thinking, emotion, and processing data
3. ___ The somatic and autonomic nervous systems
4. ___ Heart, secretory glands, and smooth muscle
5. ___ Performs "housekeeping" chores of the body

    a. Autonomic
    b. Central
    c. Parasympathetic
    d. Peripheral
    e. Somatic

Completion

6. Stimulation of the somatic nervous system causes contraction of _____ _____.

7. Parasympathetic stimulation of the eye causes _____ _____ and _____ _____.

8. Sympathetic stimulation of the lungs causes _____ and increased _____ _____.

9. Parasympathetic stimulation of the heart causes _____ of the heart rate.

10. Sympathetic stimulation of the gastrointestinal tract causes slowing of gastrointestinal _____ and _____.

11. Parasympathetic stimulation of the urinary bladder causes urinary _____.

12. Sympathetic stimulation shunts blood from organs to _____ _____.

CRITICAL THINKING, PRIORITIZATION, AND DELEGATION QUESTIONS

▶ 13. A patient with a blood pressure (BP) of 188/104 mm Hg takes a potent vasodilating drug to lower the blood pressure. One hour after administration, the BP has dropped to 135/78 mm Hg in response to the drug. Which additional assessment finding is an expected response to this rapid change in BP?
    a. Capillary refill of 2 seconds
    b. Rubor when legs dangling
    c. Pulse increase of 20-30 beats/min
    d. Urine output increase of 15 additional mL/hr

14. Why do most drugs that affect muscarinic receptors of the parasympathetic nervous system produce adverse effects?
    a. High doses are needed to get therapeutic effects.
    b. Most drugs that affect muscarinic receptors are nonselective.
    c. Muscarinic receptors are stimulated by epinephrine, which is secreted by the adrenal gland.
    d. Muscarinic receptors are present on all postganglionic neurons.

✳15. A military nurse receives a soldier from a combat zone who may have been exposed to nerve gas. Because nerve gas inhibits the enzyme cholinesterase, which normally breaks down the neurotransmitter acetylcholine, it is a priority for the nurse to assess for what?
    a. Bradycardia
    b. Fever
    c. Headache
    d. Yellowing of skin

▶16. The nurse would consult with the prescriber if an anticholinergic drug was prescribed for a patient with which health issue?
    a. Diarrhea
    b. Gastroesophageal reflux disease (GERD)
    c. Hypotension
    d. Urinary retention

✳17. Doxazosin (Cardura), an alpha$_1$ adrenergic blocking drug, is prescribed for a patient with benign prostatic hyperplasia (BPH) to promote urine flow and manage hypertension. A priority nursing concern for this patient is assessing for what?
    a. Cardiac output—bradycardia
    b. Safety—dizziness with position changes
    c. Skin—poor skin turgor
    d. Self-care—weak hand grasps

18. Which is the only neurotransmitter that activates beta$_2$ adrenergic receptors?
    a. Acetylcholine
    b. Dopamine
    c. Epinephrine
    d. Norepinephrine

19. Tamsulosin (Flomax) is a drug that selectively blocks alpha$_{1A}$ receptors in the bladder neck and iris. It would be a priority to report current or past use of this drug to a surgeon who is planning to do which type of surgery?
    a. Cataract removal
    b. Colon resection
    c. Herniorrhaphy
    d. Valvuloplasty

20. A decrease in inactivation of norepinephrine occurs with administration of monoamine oxidase (MAO) inhibitor drugs. What is a priority assessment when administering these drugs?
    a. Alertness and orientation
    b. BP and pulse
    c. Bowel sounds and abdominal distention
    d. Muscle strength and reflexes

CASE STUDY

A patient receives a nonselective drug administered to slow the heart rate and acts by blocking stimulation of beta$_1$ and beta$_2$ sympathetic nervous system receptors. (Think of the opposite of "fight or flight.") What would be the possible related adverse effects on the following organs or processes? What are the appropriate nursing actions for these adverse effects?

1. Eyes

2. Respiratory rate

3. Airway

4. Gastrointestinal motility

5. Production of glucose by the liver and release into the blood

6. Heart

14

Muscarinic Agonists and Antagonists

STUDY QUESTIONS

Administration and Consultation

1. The nurse is preparing to administer a muscarinic agonist. If the following preadministration assessment findings were present, indicate if it would it be safe to administer the drug (administer) or if consultation with the prescriber would be indicated (consult).

   a. Pulse 110 beats/min _____

   b. BP 100/60 mm Hg _____

   c. Wheezing _____

   d. Drooling _____

   e. Postoperative abdominal distention

   _____

   f. Recent bowel resection _____

   g. Recent vaginal delivery of a 7-lb neonate

   _____

   h. Postvoid residual of 350 mL of urine, without obstruction _____

   i. Positive hemoccult of stool _____

   j. TSH 0.2 microunits/mL; T$_4$ 18 mcg/dL

   _____

CRITICAL THINKING, PRIORITIZATION, AND DELEGATION QUESTIONS

2. A young camper finds some wild mushrooms and eats them. Which symptoms suggest to the camp nurse that the camper is experiencing muscarinic poisoning? (Select all that apply.)
   a. Tachycardia
   b. Hypertension
   c. Profuse salivation and lacrimation
   d. Dilated pupils that do not respond to light
   e. Wheezing

✻ 3. The emergency department nurse receives a patient brought in by an ambulance with suspected poisoning from exposure to muscarinic insecticide. The priority nursing action is to prepare
   a. to relieve the pain of muscle spasms.
   b. for possible respiratory arrest.
   c. to place the patient in a side-lying position because the patient is likely to vomit.
   d. to administer intravenous fluids.

4. The nurse has administered atropine as a preoperative medication. The patient complains of a sudden feeling of warmth. Her skin is warm and dry, and her face is flushed. What should the nurse do?
   a. Notify the surgeon STAT.
   b. Assess the patient's vital signs and notify the surgeon.
   c. Assess the patient's vital signs and mental status and notify the operating room that surgery must be postponed.
   d. Assess the patient's vital signs and mental status and, if within normal limits, document the findings and continue the preoperative protocol.

5. What form of antidote would the nurse expect to be prescribed for a person who is at risk of exposure to toxic levels of insecticide or nerve gas?
   a. Extended-release tablet
   b. Enteric-coated tablet
   c. Liquid
   d. Self-injectable pen

6. Oxybutynin (Ditropan) is a prescribed anticholinergic drug that is available in four formulations. A patient has experienced many adverse effects when taking oxybutynin immediate-release tablets (Ditropan IR) for overactive bladder (OAB). She asks the nurse how the transdermal patch could cause fewer adverse effects if it is essentially the same drug. The nurse's response should be based on what knowledge?
   a. Transdermal absorption bypasses metabolism in the intestinal wall.
   b. The transdermal form is water-soluble and poorly absorbed.
   c. The transdermal form is a different drug than oral oxybutynin.
   d. The transdermal form is less effective than the extended-release oral form.

✳ 7. The nurse is administering trospium (Sanctura XR) to a 78-year-old patient who has a history of OAB, diabetes, osteoarthritis, and osteoporosis. As the nurse explains the drug action, the patient asks how this drug is different from oxybutynin (Detrol LA), which is less expensive. The nurse should explain that the priority reason for the prescriber's choosing trospium instead of oxybutynin, based on age and chronic conditions, is prevention of what effect?
   a. Blood sugar spikes
   b. Constipation
   c. Dry mouth
   d. CNS side effects

8. Emergency department prescriber's orders for a patient with advanced HIV admitted with a mycobacterium infection include clarithromycin (Biaxin) 500 mg PO twice a day and continuing all home medications. The patient's regimen includes darifenacin (Enablex) ER 15 mg once a day, delavirdine 400 mg three times daily, nevirapine 200 mg twice a day, and ritonavir 600 mg twice a day. Based on possible drug interactions with darifenacin, the nurse should do what?
   a. Give the medications with food to prevent GI distress.
   b. Administer the medications so that there is at least 1 hour between each medication.
   c. Review the home medications and the medication order with the prescriber.
   d. Hold all of the medications.

9. The nurse should review the patient's history for unexplained fainting or long-QT syndrome before administering which medication? (Select all that apply.)
   a. Darifenacin (Enablex)
   b. Fesoterodine (Toviaz)
   c. Solifenacin (VESIcare)
   d. Tolterodine (Detrol)
   e. Trospium (Sanctura)

10. What response to tolterodine (Detrol) and fesoterodine (Toviaz) would the nurse expect if a patient lacks the P450 cytochrome CYP2D6 isoenzyme? (Select all that apply.)
   a. More adverse effects
   b. Lack of therapeutic response
   c. Prolonged drug action
   d. Need to take the drug on an empty stomach

11. Trospium (Sanctura) 20 mg once a day is prescribed for an older adult patient with OAB. The nurse instructs the patient to take the medication at what time of day?
   a. One hour before breakfast
   b. One hour after breakfast
   c. With the first bite of breakfast
   d. Any time during the day as long as it is at the same time each day

12. The nurse is caring for a patient who has taken an overdose of a tricyclic antidepressant drug that has pronounced antimuscarinic properties. The nurse should prepare to do what? (Select all that apply.)
   a. Support breathing.
   b. Administer atropine.
   c. Administer drugs for hypotension.
   d. Administer phenothiazine antipsychotic drugs to treat delirium.
   e. Administer physostigmine.

13. Which intervention for dry mouth caused by anticholinergic drugs would be least likely to produce adverse effects?
   a. Cough drops
   b. Listerine original mouthwash
   c. Water
   d. Sugar-free candy made with sorbitol

∗14. A patient who is prescribed oxybutynin (Gelnique) has been experiencing dry mouth. It is a priority for the nurse to assess for which action that can possibly cause inadvertent excessive dosing of this drug?
    a. Not drinking a full glass of water with the drug
    b. Not washing hands after administering the drug
    c. Taking the drug at the same time as other drugs
    d. Taking on an empty stomach

DOSE CALCULATION QUESTIONS

15. A patient is prescribed 5 mg of oxybutynin syrup every 12 hours. Oxybutynin syrup is available as 5 mg/5 mL. How much syrup should the nurse administer per dose?

16. The recommended subcutaneous dose of atropine for a child is 0.01 mg/kg, not to exceed 0.4 mg.
    a. What is the recommended dose for a child who is 32 inches long and weighs 24 lb?

    b. Based on the recommended dose, what amount of drug should the nurse draw into the syringe if atropine is available as 0.5 mg/mL?

CASE STUDY

A 66-year-old woman with a history of type 2 diabetes mellitus, hypertension, depression, and OAB is admitted to a medical unit with the diagnosis of altered mental status. Assessment findings include BP 182/110 mm Hg, P 118, R 14, and T 102.4° F. The patient is becoming confused and is exhibiting symptoms that suggest she is hallucinating. The patient resists efforts to open her eyes for pupil assessment. Skin is flushed and warm; mucous membranes are dry. Bowel sounds are hypoactive, and there are multiple areas of dullness when percussing the abdomen. The bladder is palpable above the pubic symphysis, with bladder scan reading 650 mL. Admission laboratory test results include BUN 32 mg/dL; creatinine 2.3 mg/dL; glucose 178 mg/dL; WBC 12,400/mm³. Creatinine clearance has been ordered, and the collection was started at 0600. The nurse is preparing the patient's 0900 medications including tolterodine (Detrol).

1. What do laboratory test results suggest?

2. What concern does the nurse have about administering tolterodine?

3. What symptoms suggest antimuscarinic toxicity?

4. What should the nurse do?

5. The prescriber discontinues the tolterodine. The patient's condition improves. The patient is concerned about bladder control. What teaching can the nurse provide to assist a patient with OAB to attain bladder control?

15

Cholinesterase Inhibitors and Their Use in Myasthenia Gravis

STUDY QUESTIONS

Matching

Match the medication to its use.

1. ___ Used to diagnose myasthenia gravis
2. ___ Antidote for poisoning by organophosphate insecticides
3. ___ Used to treat drug-induced muscarinic blockade
4. ___ Irreversible cholinesterase inhibitor used to treat glaucoma
5. ___ Irreversible cholinesterase inhibitor nerve gas that can be used in bioterrorism
6. ___ Antidote for cholinergic crisis
7. ___ Short-acting reversible cholinesterase inhibitor that does not cross blood-brain barrier
8. ___ Organophosphate insecticide

    a. Atropine
    b. Echothiophate
    c. Edrophonium
    d. Malathion
    e. Neostigmine
    f. Physostigmine
    g. Pralidoxime
    h. Tabun

CRITICAL THINKING, PRIORITIZATION, AND DELEGATION QUESTIONS

9. What can cholinesterase inhibitors do?
   a. Intensify transmission at neuromuscular junctions
   b. Intensify transmission at muscarinic, ganglionic, and neuromuscular junctions
   c. Prevent transmission at neuromuscular junctions
   d. Prevent transmission at muscarinic, ganglionic, and neuromuscular junctions

10. Therapeutic doses of cholinesterase inhibitors have which effect(s)? (Select all that apply.)
    a. Constrict pupils
    b. Constipate
    c. Relieve wheezing
    d. Slow respirations
    e. Strengthen skeletal muscle contraction

11. Toxic levels of cholinesterase inhibitors can do what? (Select all that apply.)
    a. Blur vision
    b. Cause respiratory depression
    c. Cause tetany
    d. Constipate
    e. Increase heart rate

＊12. What is a priority nursing concern when neostigmine is used to reverse neuromuscular blockade in postoperative patients?
    a. Aspiration of secretions
    b. Diaphoresis
    c. Flatus
    d. Urinary incontinence

13. A 66-year-old man has been taking ambenonium (Mytelase) for myasthenia gravis for 4 years. He is admitted to the hospital for a prostate biopsy. The ambenonium is scheduled to be administered. What should the nurse do?
    a. Administer the drug.
    b. Hold the drug.
    c. Assess for urine retention before and after administering the drug.
    d. Consult with the urologist before administering the drug.

14. The nurse is caring for a male patient who is prescribed pyridostigmine (Mestinon) 240 mg, three times daily for myasthenia gravis. The patient states that he is experiencing an extreme increase in muscle weakness and that he needs the nurse to administer 300-mg doses. What should the nurse do?
    a. Administer 240 mg because that is the dose ordered by the prescriber.
    b. Administer 300-mg doses because myasthenia gravis patients often need to adjust the dose of medication according to symptoms.
    c. Call the prescriber and request an order for the increased dose.
    d. Immediately assess the patient for other symptoms including excessive muscarinic stimulation, and contact prescriber with patient's request and assessment findings.

DOSE CALCULATION QUESTIONS

15. Ambenonium (Mytelase) 25 mg is ordered by mouth 3 times a day. The pharmacy stocks 10-mg tablets. How many tablets should the nurse administer for one dose?

16. Neostigmine (Prostigmin) is to be administered as test for myasthenia gravis as a single dose of 0.02 mg/kg. The patient weighs 154 lb. Neostigmine (Prostigmin) is available as an injectable solution of 0.5 mg/mL. How much neostigmine should be administered to this patient?

CASE STUDIES

Case Study 1

A patient who is receiving a reversible cholinesterase inhibitor for myasthenia gravis is brought into the emergency department by his family because of extreme muscle weakness and difficulty breathing.

1. In this situation, why is it important to determine if the cause of the weakness is myasthenic crisis versus cholinergic crisis?

2. What assessments should the nurse perform? What questions should the nurse ask the patient and family? Why?

3. The prescriber is unsure, by history, if the patient is experiencing myasthenic crisis or cholinergic crisis. She orders administration of edrophonium to differentiate. What should the nurse do, along with preparing to administer the edrophonium?

4. The nurse is doing discharge teaching for this patient. What teaching should the nurse do to help the patient monitor the response to medication for his myasthenia gravis?

Case Study 2

The nurse has been asked to speak to a 4H group in a farming community on preventing poisoning by organophosphate insecticides. The nurse has stressed the importance of following all directions provided and seeking clarification if any directions are unclear.

5. What information should the nurse include to prevent
   a. exposure through the skin or eyes when using insecticides?
   b. exposure through the respiratory tract when using insecticides?
   c. oral exposure?

6. What would the nurse include in an explanation of why insecticides have such potential for poisoning humans?

7. What information would the nurse include when explaining which symptoms warrant seeking immediate medical attention when using pesticides?

8. What information should be provided regarding the treatment for pesticide poisoning?

16

Drugs that Block Nicotinic Cholinergic Transmission: Neuromuscular Blocking Agents and Ganglionic Blocking Agents

STUDY QUESTIONS

Matching

Match the term with its definition.

1. ____ Muscle twitching
2. ____ Process that leads to muscle contraction
3. ____ Pumping positively charged ions from inside to outside the cell membrane
4. ____ Uneven distribution of electrical charges across the inner and outer cell membrane
5. ____ Positive charges move inward, making the inside of a membrane more positively charged than the outside of the membrane

    a. Depolarization
    b. Excitation-contraction coupling
    c. Fasciculations
    d. Polarization
    e. Repolarization

CRITICAL THINKING, PRIORITIZATION, AND DELEGATION QUESTIONS

6. A patient who is 8 weeks pregnant must have surgery. The anesthesiologist administers vecuronium (Norcuron) to achieve muscle relaxation. Because this is a quaternary ammonium compound, what is the most likely effect of this medication on the developing fetus?
    a. Unknown
    b. Respiratory depression
    c. Bradycardia
    d. Teratogenesis

✳ 7. Which preoperative laboratory test result would be a priority to report to the anesthesiologist when a patient is scheduled to have a competitive neuromuscular blocking agent because this condition increases the risk of respiratory arrest when turbocaine is administered?
    a. ALT 30 IU/L
    b. BUN 14 mg/dL
    c. Fasting blood glucose 175 mg/dL
    d. Potassium 3.1 mEq/L

8. The patient is at greater risk for enhanced neuromuscular blockade when which antibiotics are used? (Select all that apply.)
    a. Penicillins
    b. Tetracyclines
    c. Quinolones
    d. Aminoglycosides

9. Which drug would decrease the risk of hypotension when atracurium is administered?
    a. Acetaminophen (Tylenol)
    b. Acetylsalicylic acid (aspirin)
    c. Diphenhydramine (Benadryl)
    d. Ibuprofen (Motrin)

10. The nurse should assess for and plan interventions to relieve muscle pain 12-24 hours after surgery for patients who have received which drug?
    a. Atracurium
    b. Pancuronium
    c. Succinylcholine
    d. Tubocurarine

11. An anesthesia resident is supervising the reversal of the neuromuscular blockade for a patient who has received succinylcholine. The resident directs the nurse to administer 0.5 mg of neostigmine (Prostigmin) intravenously. What should the nurse do? (Select all that apply.)
    a. Administer the medication slowly and monitor respirations.
    b. Question the resident, because neostigmine intensifies the neuromuscular blockade caused by succinylcholine, a depolarizing neuromuscular blocker.
    c. Administer the medication only if mechanical assistance for ventilation is available.
    d. Question the resident as to whether atropine should also be administered.

＊12. A patient will be receiving succinylcholine before electroconvulsive therapy. What is the nursing priority?
  a. Administering the succinylcholine
  b. Administering atropine if toxicity occurs
  c. Performing the electroconvulsive therapy
  d. Preparing for possible respiratory arrest

DOSE CALCULATION QUESTION

13. Dantrolene (Dantrium) 2.5 mg/kg is prescribed STAT by rapid IV infusion for a 220-lb patient who is experiencing malignant hyperthermia after anesthesia with succinylcholine. How many mg should the nurse administer?

CASE STUDIES

Case Study 1

The postanesthesia care unit (PACU) nurse is caring for a patient who received a competitive neuromuscular blocking agent during surgery to remove a cancerous section of the bowel. The patient is admitted to the PACU with mechanical ventilation and a nasogastric (NG) tube to low-intermittent suction.

1. What are the priority assessments that the PACU nurse must monitor while the patient is still under the effects of the competitive neuromuscular blocking agent?

2. The nasogastric tube is draining a large amount of bile-colored liquid. How does this affect potassium levels and nursing care?

3. As the patient regains neuromuscular functioning, the nurse instructs the patient to take deep breaths. How does deep-breathing counteract the adverse effects of histamine release stimulated by the competitive neuromuscular blocking agent?

Case Study 2

A patient is receiving a neuromuscular blocker for prolonged paralysis during mechanical ventilation.

4. Describe measures that should be included in nursing care and their rationale.

5. The patient spikes a temperature of 102° F within an hour after the neuromuscular agent infusion is begun. The infusion of the neuromuscular blocking agent is stopped, the patient receives a dose of dantrolene (Dantrium), and the patient's temperature begins to drop. Why was dantrolene administered to lower this patient's temperature instead of an antipyretic such as acetaminophen?

17
Adrenergic Agonists

STUDY QUESTIONS

Matching

Match the receptor with main therapeutic uses for stimulation of the receptor.

1. ____ Vasoconstriction
2. ____ Increased force of myocardial contraction
3. ____ Relief of severe pain
4. ____ Promotes bronchodilation

a. $Alpha_1$
b. $Alpha_2$
c. $Beta_1$
d. $Beta_2$

True or False

For each of the following statements, enter T for true or F for false.

5. ___ Catecholamines are inactivated before reaching systemic circulation if administered orally.
6. ___ Catecholamines cross the blood-brain barrier, activating the central nervous system.
7. ___ Catecholamines include the drugs epinephrine, norepinephrine, isoproterenol, dopamine, and dobutamine.
8. ___ Catecholamines are effective when administered by any parenteral route.
9. ___ Catecholamines are polar molecules.
10. ___ Catecholamines are destroyed by monoamine oxidase (MAO) and catechol-O-methyltransferase (COMT) enzymes in the liver and intestinal wall.

CRITICAL THINKING, PRIORITIZATION, AND DELEGATION QUESTIONS

11. Direct-acting adrenergic drugs mimic the action of what? (Select all that apply.)
    a. Acetylcholine (ACh)
    b. Dopamine
    c. Epinephrine (epi)
    d. Norepinephrine (NE)

12. The nurse is caring for a patient who is receiving a dopamine intravenous (IV) drip. The nurse has been assessing her patient's vital signs every 15 minutes. The nurse notes that since the last assessment, the IV dopamine solution has turned pink. What should the nurse do?
    a. Stop the IV infusion, assess the patient for adverse effects, and notify the prescriber.
    b. Stop the infusion, notify the pharmacy for an immediate replacement, and assess the patient.
    c. Continue to assess the patient and infuse the solution as prescribed.
    d. Continue to assess the patient and infuse the solution as prescribed for up to 24 hours after hanging.

13. Patients with which chronic diseases would be at most risk for adverse effects from adrenergic agonists? (Select all that apply.)
    a. Chronic obstructive pulmonary disease (COPD)
    b. Gastroesophageal reflux disease (GERD)
    c. Hypertension
    d. Diabetes
    e. Osteoarthritis

14. The nurse is working in the emergency department. A local anesthetic combined with epinephrine is often used when suturing wounds that need a small area of anesthesia and are likely to bleed. Assessment findings that would warrant consultation with the prescriber before administering a drug containing epinephrine include what? (Select all that apply.)
    a. Blood pressure 86/50 mm Hg
    b. History of AV heart block
    c. History of angina pectoris
    d. Poor capillary refill
    e. Pulse 50 beats/min

*15. The nurse has administered epinephrine IM to a patient with a history of asthma and type 1 diabetes mellitus (T1DM). It is a priority to assess for which possible effect of this drug?
    a. Hot, dry, flushed skin
    b. Dizziness with position changes
    c. Sensitivity to light
    d. Tremor

16. A patient has a history of depression. Treatment with which antidepressant is most likely to decrease the inactivation of dopamine and increase the risk of toxicity? (Select all that apply.)
    a. Bupropion
    b. Nortriptyline
    c. Sertraline
    d. Tranylcypromine

17. Phenylephrine (Neo-Synephrine) is available over the counter (OTC) as a nasal decongestant. A patient states that she understands why the label says it should not be used if she has high blood pressure, but she does not understand why it should not be used by diabetics. The nurse's response is based on knowledge that phenylephrine can cause what? (Select all that apply.)
    a. Anorexia
    b. Diaphoresis
    c. Hypoglycemia in the diabetic patient
    d. Hyperglycemia in the diabetic patient
    e. Tremor, which the patient may interpret as hypoglycemia

18. The nurse is administering an IV dopamine infusion. The nurse assesses the large antecubital vein and notes that the site is swollen, cold, and extremely pale. What is the basis of the nurse's next action?
    a. A clot has formed and can break off and become an embolus.
    b. Extravasation of dopamine may have caused tissue necrosis.
    c. The nurse should infuse dopamine only through a central vein.
    d. The IV infusion must continue at this site until another IV is successfully started.

DOSE CALCULATION QUESTIONS

19. A woman in cardiogenic shock is ordered an IV infusion of dopamine at a rate of 300 mcg/min. The patient weighs 154 lb. The dopamine infusion is available in a dilution of 100 mg/250 mL. The infusion pump is calculated in mL/hr. What is the flow rate that the nurse will program into the infusion pump?

20. Dobutamine HCl (Dobutrex) is available in a vial of 250 mg/20 mL. The prescribed dose for a patient weighing 110 lb is 250 mcg/min. What is the recommended dilution and administration rate?

CASE STUDY

A 4-year-old child comes to the emergency department with angioedema, wheezing, and hypotension after eating a peanut butter cookie. Epinephrine is administered.

1. Describe how epinephrine treats the symptoms of anaphylactic shock.

2. The child is prescribed an epinephrine auto-injector (EpiPen Jr). What should the nurse teach the parents and the child about administering the medication?

3. How can the parents ensure that their young child has the EpiPen Jr. available at all times?

18
Adrenergic Antagonists

STUDY QUESTIONS

Matching

Match the disorder treated with adrenergic antagonist drugs with the most specific outcome for the disorder.

1. ____ Blood pressure (BP) 90/60 mm Hg to 120/80 mm Hg
2. ____ Brisk capillary refill
3. ____ Postvoid residual less than 75 mL

a. Benign prostatic hyperplasia (BPH)
b. Pheochromocytoma
c. Raynaud's disease

True or False

For each of the following statements, enter T for true or F for false.

The nurse would consult the prescriber before administering the drug if a patient was just prescribed alfuzosin (Uroxatral) and the nurse just learned that the patient has a history of

4. ____ Angina pectoris
5. ____ Advanced HIV infection
6. ____ Diabetes mellitus type 2
7. ____ Erectile dysfunction
8. ____ Frequent urinary tract infections
9. ____ Hepatitis B
10. ____ Hypertension
11. ____ Ventricular dysrhythmia

CRITICAL THINKING, PRIORITIZATION, AND DELEGATION QUESTIONS

12. The generic names of alpha$_1$ receptor antagonists share what common suffix?
    a. -azole
    b. -lol
    c. -osin
    d. -sartan

*13. It is a priority for the nurse to evaluate which laboratory test result before administering alfuzosin (Uroxatral) to a patient?
    a. AST/ALT
    b. BUN/creatinine
    c. FBS/A1c
    d. Na$^+$/K$^+$

14. A patient has just been prescribed prazosin (Minipress). Which statement from the patient would indicate a need for further teaching?
    a. "I should avoid driving and other hazardous activities for 12-24 hours after I first take this medication or have a dose increase."
    b. "I should take the medication first thing in the morning."
    c. "I should sit on the edge of the bed for a few minutes before standing up when I get up in the morning."
    d. "I should be sitting or lying 30-60 minutes after I take the first dose of this medication."

*15. A patient with coronary artery disease is receiving terazosin for hypertension. It would be a priority for the nurse to report to the prescriber which effect of the drug?
    a. Drop of 15 mm Hg in systolic BP with position changes
    b. Headache
    c. Increase in pulse of 20 beats/min
    d. Nasal congestion

*16. A patient who is prescribed an alpha$_1$-adrenergic antagonist for high blood pressure is brought into the emergency department after taking sildenafil (Viagra) supplied by a friend. The priority for the nurse is to assess for and follow orders to prevent what effects?
    a. Atrial fibrillation and palpitations
    b. Migraine headache and photophobia
    c. Prolonged erection and discomfort
    d. Severe hypotension and vascular collapse

17. When administering tamsulosin (Flomax), which assessment would indicate that therapy has achieved the desired effect?
    a. Voiding 250 mL every 2-3 hours while awake
    b. Position changes without dizziness
    c. Absence of dysuria when voiding
    d. Postvoid residual less than 300 mL

18. How should tamsulosin (Flomax) be administered?
    a. With food at any time of day
    b. 1 hour before or 2 hours after the same meal each day
    c. 30 minutes after the same meal each day
    d. With a full glass of water and remain upright for 30 minutes

19. A patient who is receiving phenoxybenzamine (Dibenzyline) to treat pheochromocytoma faints. BP is 75/40 mm Hg, P 135 beats/min. The nurse contacts the prescriber and prepares to administer what?
    a. Epinephrine
    b. Norepinephrine
    c. Intravenous fluids
    d. Metoprolol

20. The generic names of beta$_1$ and beta$_2$ receptor antagonists share what common suffix?
    a. -azole
    b. -lol
    c. -osin
    d. -sartan

21. What assessment finding would warrant withholding a beta blocker and consulting the prescriber?
    a. Apical pulse 48 beats/min
    b. BP 110/70 mm Hg
    c. 2+ ankle edema
    d. Capillary blood sugar 90 mg/dL

22. The nurse is caring for a full-term neonate whose mother took the drug betaxolol throughout pregnancy. Which assessment finding would be a priority to report to the pediatrician?
    a. Apical pulse 80 beats/min
    b. BP 65/45 mm Hg
    c. Plasma glucose 48 mg/dL
    d. Respirations 35/min
    e. Temperature 37.2° C (99° F)

*23. Which of these new assessment findings, if identified 1 hour after administering metoprolol (Lopressor), would be a priority to report to the prescriber?
    a. Drop in apical pulse from 80 to 65 beats/min
    b. Warm, flushed, dry skin
    c. Crackles throughout lung fields
    d. Headache

24. Which of these conditions, if identified in the history of a patient receiving a drug classified as a first-generation beta blocker, would be a concern to the nurse? (Select all that apply.)
    a. AV heart block
    b. Chronic obstructive pulmonary disease
    c. Depression
    d. Diabetes mellitus
    e. Severe allergic reaction to bee stings

*25. It is a nursing priority to report which of these laboratory test results, if identified in a patient who is prescribed metoprolol (Lopressor), to the prescriber?
    a. Creatinine 1.2 mg/dL
    b. Ejection fraction on echocardiogram of 20%
    c. Hemoglobin A_{1c} (glycosylated hemoglobin) 5.5%
    d. Sinus rhythm on electrocardiogram (ECG)

►26. Which of these findings would be of most concern to the nurse if a patient is prescribed propranolol (Inderal)?
    a. Apical pulse 94 beats/min
    b. BP 157/88 mm Hg
    c. Urinary urgency
    d. Wheezing

27. Which adrenergic antagonists block $alpha_1$, $beta_1$, and $beta_2$ receptors?
    a. Atenolol and bisoprolol
    b. Acebutolol and pindolol
    c. Carvedilol and labetalol
    d. Propranolol and timolol

*28. It is a priority for the nurse to monitor for excessive cardiosuppression when a patient is prescribed metoprolol and what other drug?
    a. Atorvastatin (Lipitor)
    b. Hydrochlorothiazide (HydroDIURIL)
    c. Terazosin (Hytrin)
    d. Verapamil (Calan)

DOSE CALCULATION QUESTIONS

29. Phentolamine is reconstituted to 5 mg/mL. Intravenous push directions state to administer over at least 1 minute. The nurse will administer each 0.1 mL over what minimum time period in seconds?

30. Labetalol is prescribed by continuous intravenous infusion at 2 mg/min, to be adjusted by patient response. It is supplied at a concentration of 2 mg/3 mL. The intravenous pump is calibrated in mL/hr. What rate will the nurse initially program into the pump?

CASE STUDIES

Case Study 1

A 58-year-old man has just been prescribed prazosin (Minipress) for hypertension.

1. Explain the common adverse effects and nursing teaching needed to provide both comfort and safety for this patient.

2. What assessments should be performed before the nurse administers an $alpha_1$-adrenergic antagonist for hypertension, and what assessment findings would warrant not administering the medication and notifying the prescriber?

3. The patient's BP is not controlled by his prescribed alpha$_1$ antagonist. The prescriber has added a loop diuretic and a beta$_1$ blocker. The patient asks, "Why do I have to take three different medications for my blood pressure? Can't I just have a higher dose of one medication?" How should the nurse explain the rationale for this drug regimen?

4. Why is it very important to address ejaculation problems and other adverse effects with this patient?

Case Study 2

A 45-year-old man is being treated for hypertension. Several types of antihypertensive medications have been tried without success. He also has been taking glargine insulin (Lantus) 22 units every morning and aspart insulin (NovoLog) on a sliding scale according to blood sugar for diabetes. His prescriber orders metoprolol 50 mg once a day. When the patient tries to fill the prescription using his insurance, the pharmacist notifies him that his insurance covers only the less expensive beta blocker, propranolol, unless the patient experiences adverse effects or has an absolute contraindication for the use of propranolol. The prescriber can appeal to the insurance company and justify the use of the more expensive decision. The prescriber asks the office nurse to initiate the insurance appeal form.

5. Describe and explain the adverse effects that this patient might experience relating to his diabetes diagnosis and propranolol.

6. The insurance appeal is approved, and the patient receives metoprolol, a beta$_1$-selective adrenergic antagonist. The patient states, "I'm glad I do not have to take propranolol. I have had frequent episodes of hypoglycemia because with my job I cannot always eat when I should." What should the nurse do and why?

7. The nurse discovers that this patient has a history of poor adherence to medication regimens. Why are beta-adrenergic blockers poor choices for this patient?

19
Indirect-Acting Antiadrenergic Agents

STUDY QUESTIONS

Completion

1. Indirect-acting antiadrenergic drugs' net effect is to reduce activation of _____ _____ receptors.

2. _____ is the primary use for centrally acting alpha$_2$ agonists.

3. The effect of centrally acting alpha$_2$ agonists is like that of _____ _____ _____ _____ _____.

4. The most common adverse effects of clonidine are _____, _____, and _____.

5. The principal mechanism of blood pressure reduction with methyldopa is _____.

CRITICAL THINKING, PRIORITIZATION, AND DELEGATION QUESTIONS

6. The nurse is teaching a 56-year-old truck driver about taking clonidine. It is very important to explain that the patient should take the medication in what way?
   a. As two doses 12 hours apart
   b. With a larger dose at bedtime
   c. With food
   d. On an empty stomach

✳ 7. It would be a priority to withhold clonidine and report which laboratory test result?
   a. ALT 55 IU/L
   b. Creatinine 1.4 mg/dL
   c. hCG 900 IU/mL
   d. WBC 10,500/mm³

8. The nurse is teaching a patient who has been prescribed clonidine for hypertension. Which statement suggests a need for additional teaching?
   a. "Effects like drowsiness should get better after I take the drug for several weeks."
   b. "I should stop taking the drug if I experience weird dreams."
   c. "I should inform all of my health care providers that I am taking this drug."
   d. "Increasing fiber and fluid in my diet can decrease the risk of constipation."

✳ 9. Depletion of the neurotransmitters norepinephrine and serotonin by reserpine makes it a priority for the nurse to assess the patient's
   a. blood count.
   b. bowel sounds.
   c. mental status.
   d. stool for blood.

▶ 10. The nurse is caring for a patient who is receiving reserpine for hypertension. The patient is passive, has poor eye contact and appetite, and is difficult to engage in conversation. The nurse is concerned that the patient is experiencing a drug-induced depression. The nurse should share her concern with the
   a. patient.
   b. patient and the prescriber.
   c. prescriber and the patient's family.
   d. patient, the prescriber, and the patient's family.

11. A patient is receiving methyldopa. Which laboratory tests should be monitored throughout therapy? (Select all that apply.)
   a. Bilirubin and Coombs' test
   b. Hematocrit and hemoglobin
   c. Potassium and sodium
   d. Self-metered blood glucose and A1c
   e. Troponin T and electrocardiogram

12. A patient is receiving methyldopa 250 mg twice a day. Vital signs are BP 170/90 mm Hg, P 92, and R 20. The nurse is reviewing new laboratory test results, which include ALT 35 international units/L, creatinine 0.8 mg/dL, BUN 20 mg/dL, Coombs' test positive, sodium 145 mEq/L, and potassium 4.8 mEq/L. The nurse should do what?
   a. Administer the medication and continue to assess the patient.
   b. Administer the medication and notify the prescriber of the vital signs and laboratory results.
   c. Hold the medication and notify the prescriber of the vital signs and laboratory results.
   d. Hold the medication and page the prescriber STAT.

13. A patient was started on reserpine 0.5 mg once a day 4 days ago for hypertension unresponsive to other antihypertensive agents. The nurse assesses the patient's BP, which is 155/72 mm Hg. The patient is discouraged. What is the nurse's best response?
   a. "At first, reserpine promotes norepinephrine release, which can elevate BP temporarily."
   b. "The medication must be taken on an empty stomach."
   c. "It takes 1-2 weeks for norepinephrine depletion to occur."
   d. "Reserpine primarily affects systolic blood pressure."

DOSE CALCULATION QUESTIONS

14. Reserpine, 500 mcg once a day, is prescribed. Available are 0.25-mg tablets. How many tablets should be administered?

15. Methyldopate for intravenous infusion 10 mg/mL is prepared in 5% dextrose in water. The 100-mL bag is to be infused in 30 minutes. What rate should the nurse program into the intravenous pump if it is calibrated in mL/hr?

CASE STUDY

A 68-year-old woman who plays tennis regularly has been prescribed guanfacine 10 mg once a day for hypertension not controlled by other agents. The prescriber asks the office nurse to provide teaching regarding this medication.

1. What should the nurse teach about side effects?

2. What should the nurse teach about drug-herb/supplement interactions and drug-food interactions?

3. What serious reactions can occur if this drug is stopped abruptly?

20

Introduction to Central Nervous System Pharmacology

CRITICAL THINKING, PRIORITIZATION, AND DELEGATION QUESTIONS

1. The evidence supporting which of the following as neurotransmitters in the CNS is completely convincing? (Select all that apply.)
   a. Dopamine
   b. Adenosine
   c. Glutamate
   d. Serotonin

2. Which of the following neurotransmitters are present in both the CNS and PNS? (Select all that apply.)
   a. GABA
   b. Norepinephrine
   c. Acetylcholine
   d. Oxytocin

3. Which are characteristics of drugs that are able to cross the blood-brain barrier? (Select all that apply.)
   a. Lipid-soluble
   b. Highly ionized
   c. Move via transport systems
   d. Protein-bound
   e. Water-soluble

4. A patient who has been taking an opiate analgesic for chronic pain due to terminal cancer needs higher doses to produce the same pain relief as when originally prescribed. This may be an example of what?
   a. Addiction
   b. Physical dependence
   c. Tolerance
   d. Withdrawal syndrome

CASE STUDY

A patient has recently been diagnosed with major depression. Medication has just been prescribed that alters CNS neurotransmission. The patient verbalizes concerns to the nurse because the medication is "not working." She is also experiencing some daytime sedation.

1. How should the nurse respond?

2. The patient asks why drug companies have not been able to develop new psychotherapeutic drugs that do not have adverse effects. What would be the basis of the nurse's response?

3. There are many psychotherapeutic drugs that are effective in treating patients' symptoms. What factors decrease patient adherence with these medications?

21

Drugs for Parkinson's Disease

STUDY QUESTIONS

Completion

Name the class of drugs by action.

1. _____ _____ activate dopamine receptors.

2. _____ enhances effect of dopamine by blocking degradation.

3. _____ _____ block muscarinic receptors in the striatum.

4. _____ _____ _____ _____ prevent dopamine breakdown.

5. _____ promotes dopamine synthesis.

6. _____ promotes dopamine release and may block dopamine reuptake.

CRITICAL THINKING, PRIORITIZATION, AND DELEGATION QUESTIONS

7. What is a realistic outcome for a patient receiving drug therapy for Parkinson's disease (PD)?
   a. Absence of tremor
   b. A normal gait
   c. Improved ability to perform activities of daily living
   d. Reversal of neurodegeneration

8. How do selegiline (Eldepryl, Zelapar) and rasagiline (Azilect) improve mild PD symptoms?
   a. Block acetylcholine stimulation of GABA release
   b. Prevent dopamine breakdown
   c. Block the effect of GABA on skeletal muscles
   d. Increase dopamine secretion

9. A PD patient who is receiving levodopa displays slow, involuntary, writhing movements of the extremities. The nurse holds the medications and notifies the prescriber. What terminology should the nurse use when documenting this movement?
   a. Ballismus
   b. Choreoathetosis
   c. Fasciculation
   d. Tremor

✳10. Which finding would be of most concern if the nurse is preparing to administer levodopa?
   a. Ataxia
   b. Dark-colored urine
   c. Dizziness with position changes
   d. Tics

11. Dietary teaching that may help the "on-off" phenomenon of PD includes avoiding which foods?
   a. Foods with a high glycemic index
   b. High-fat meals
   c. High-protein foods
   d. Processed foods

12. Which drug would not be a concern if prescribed for the psychological effects of PD and the adverse effects of treatment with levodopa/carbidopa?
   a. Chlorpromazine (Novo-Chlorpromazine)
   b. Clozapine (Clozaril)
   c. Haloperidol (Haldol)
   d. Tranylcypromine (Parnate)

＊13. Which is the most appropriate nursing action when the nurse notes an asymmetric, irregular, darkly pigmented mole on the back of a patient who is receiving levodopa for PD?
   a. Notify the prescriber of the mole characteristics.
   b. Continue to assess the patient.
   c. Tell the patient that he should consult a dermatologist.
   d. Stop administering the levodopa.

14. Sinemet and Parcopa are levodopa-carbidopa combinations prescribed. What is the effect of the addition of carbidopa to the regimen? (Select all that apply.)
   a. It adds to the therapeutic effect because carbidopa more readily crosses the blood-brain barrier than levodopa.
   b. It allows for an increase in levodopa dosage without significant adverse effects.
   c. It decreases adverse effects such as nausea and vomiting.
   d. It decreases the risk of adverse effects of abnormal movements and psychiatric symptoms.
   e. It inhibits the conversion of levodopa to dopamine in the intestines and in tissue outside the CNS.

15. It is important for the nurse to teach the patient who is prescribed pramipexole (Mirapex) to avoid use of which OTC medication for heartburn?
   a. Nizatidine (Axid)
   b. Famotidine (Pepcid)
   c. Cimetidine (Tagamet)
   d. Ranitidine (Zantac)

16. It would be a priority to report which laboratory test finding when a patient is receiving ropinirole (Requip)?
   a. ALT 285 international units/L
   b. BUN 22 mg/dL
   c. eGFR 55 mL/min
   d. Hgb 11.8 g/dL

17. The medication administration record (MAR) for a patient with PD lists apomorphine (Apokyn) 1 mg subcutaneous with trimethobenzamide (Tigan) 300 mg, up to three doses per day as needed. Which situation warrants the nurse administering this medication?
   a. A sleep attack
   b. An "off" episode
   c. Nausea
   d. Psychotic symptoms

18. It would be of greatest priority to consult the prescriber if which new finding was noted when assessing a patient who is prescribed bromocriptine (Parlodel)?
   a. Abnormal movements
   b. Confusion
   c. Red, swollen, hot hands
   d. Heart murmur

19. A patient who is receiving tolcapone (Tasmar) complains of nausea and abdominal pain. His urine is dark amber. Which laboratory test results would be most significant when the nurse reports these symptoms to the prescriber?
   a. ALT 175 international units/L; AST 159 international units/L
   b. BUN 22 mg/dL; creatinine 1.1 mg/dL
   c. Hgb 12 g/dL; Hct 39%
   d. Na$^+$ 142 mEq/L; K$^+$ 4.8 mEq/L

20. The nurse notes an orange color to the urine of a PD patient who is scheduled to receive a dose of entacapone (Comtan). What should the nurse do in this situation?
   a. Assess for symptoms of liver failure.
   b. Consult with the prescriber.
   c. Continue nursing care, including administration of the medication.
   d. Hold the medication and contact the prescriber immediately.

21. Which drug(s) should not be prescribed when a patient is prescribed selegiline (Eldepryl)? (Select all that apply.)
   a. Butorphanol (Stadol)
   b. Fluoxetine (Prozac)
   c. Hydromorphone (Dilaudid)
   d. Meperidine (Demerol)
   e. Sertraline (Zoloft)

DOSE CALCULATION QUESTIONS

22. Pramipexole (Mirapex) 1.5 mg by mouth is prescribed. The hospital pharmacy stocks pramipexole 0.25 mg. How many tablets should the nurse administer?

23. Orally disintegrating selegiline (Zelapar) 2.5 mg once a day is prescribed. Available is selegiline (Zelapar) 1.25 mg. How many tablets will the nurse administer?

CASE STUDY

A 54-year-old male patient who works as a welder has recently been diagnosed with PD. He is married, and has two adult children and one college-age child.

1. What assessments does the nurse need to make to aid the prescriber in determining the needed therapy for this patient?

2. The patient is prescribed selegiline. Why is it important to assess the patient's mood and teach the patient to use the same pharmacy for all prescriptions?

3. What teaching should the nurse provide about the possible adverse effects of selegiline?

4. The patient's symptoms progress, and his medication regimen is changed to carbidopa/levodopa (Sinemet). The patient asks why this combination drug has been prescribed. What information can the nurse provide?

5. The patient is admitted to a medical unit for a 10-day "drug holiday" because of significant adverse effects. It is anticipated that the patient will have a severe return of symptoms, including rigidity and postural instability. What are probable nursing issues, and what interventions will the nurse employ to address these problems?

22
Alzheimer's Disease

STUDY QUESTIONS

True or False

For each of the following statements, enter T *for true or* F *for false.*

1. ____ A blood test can confirm the diagnosis of Alzheimer's disease (AD).
2. ____ An early symptom of AD is loss of appetite.
3. ____ Current drug therapy for AD is not highly effective for relieving symptoms.
4. ____ Effects of drugs for AD are long-lasting.
5. ____ High levels of the neurotransmitter acetylcholine are found in patients with AD.
6. ____ Neuritic plaques are found in the hippocampus and cerebral cortex of patients with AD.
7. ____ Production of an abnormal form of a protein (tau) results in neurofibrillary tangles of AD.
8. ____ Apolipoprotein E4 (apoE4) is protective for AD.
9. ____ Research suggests that many AD patients experience more intense symptoms on arising in the morning.
10. ____ Research suggests cholinesterase inhibitors enhance transmission by central cholinergic neurons.
11. ____ The American College of Physicians recommends trying a cholinesterase inhibitor in all patients with mild to moderate AD.
12. ____ The neuronal damage occurring with AD is irreversible.
13. ____ Drugs can be helpful in treating secondary effects of AD such as depression and incontinence.

CRITICAL THINKING, PRIORITIZATION, AND DELEGATION QUESTIONS

14. High levels of homocysteine are associated with an increased risk of AD and other disorders. The nurse can teach patients to lower their homocysteine levels by eating a diet high in vitamins B_6 and folate found in what foods?
    a. Citrus fruits and meat
    b. Fruits and vegetables
    c. Dairy products and eggs
    d. Green, leafy vegetables and legumes

✳15. The nurse is caring for a patient who is receiving rivastigmine (Exelon) for AD. What is the nursing priority relating to the most common adverse effects of the drug?
    a. Ensuring adequate fluids and nutrition
    b. Monitoring liver function tests
    c. Preventing unusual bruising or bleeding
    d. Reviewing other prescribed drugs for drug interactions

16. Adverse effects of cholinesterase inhibitors come from parasympathetic stimulation. What is a nursing intervention to prevent a common adverse effect?
    a. Assess for symptoms of hyperglycemia.
    b. Assist with activities of daily living because of tremors.
    c. Include adequate fiber and fluids to prevent dehydration from diarrhea.
    d. Provide mouth moisturizers for dry mouth.

17. The nurse should be particularly cautious when administering a cholinesterase inhibitor drug to any patient with a history of which condition? (Select all that apply.)
    a. Asthma
    b. Chronic obstructive pulmonary disease (COPD)
    c. Heart failure (HF)
    d. Hypertension
    e. Peptic ulcer disease

18. Which treatment for dyspepsia could potentially decrease the renal excretion of memantine (Namenda) and cause toxicity?
    a. Calcium carbonate (TUMS)
    b. Lansoprazole (Prevacid)
    c. Ranitidine (Zantac)
    d. Sodium bicarbonate (baking soda)

19. Which result would warrant withholding administration of memantine (Namenda) and notifying the prescriber?
    a. ALT 112 international units/L
    b. BUN 18 mg/dL
    c. eGFR 45 mL/min
    d. Potassium 4.7 mEq/L

20. What is a benefit of use of risperidone (Risperdal) and olanzapine (Zyprexa) for AD patients?
    a. Amplified effects of other drugs
    b. Decreased neuropsychiatric symptoms
    c. Improved appetite
    d. Improved memory

21. Research suggests that which treatment decreases the risk of or slows the symptoms of AD? (Select all that apply.)
    a. Omega-3 fatty acids
    b. Ginkgo biloba
    c. Vitamin C
    d. Postmenopausal hormone therapy
    e. None of the above

DOSE CALCULATION QUESTIONS

22. Galantamine (Razadyne) IR 8 mg orally twice a day is prescribed. Available is galantamine (Razadyne) ER 8 mg. How many capsules should the nurse administer?

23. Memantine (Namenda) is prescribed as 5 mg by mouth in the morning (0800) and 10 mg by mouth in evening (1800). The nurse is preparing to administer the 0800 dose. Available is memantine (Namenda) 2 mg/mL. How much memantine (Namenda) should the nurse administer, and how should the nurse measure this dose?

CASE STUDY

A 77-year-old man who has a history of AD, diabetes mellitus (DM), hypertension, and seasonal allergies has been admitted with a hip fracture that occurred when wandering around the house at night. He is scheduled for an open reduction and internal fixation of the fracture the next morning. On admission the nurse discovers that the patient's spouse had been administering ginkgo biloba for the past 8 months in hope that it would improve his memory.

1. Why is it important for the nurse to report this to the orthopedic surgeon?

2. The patient's spouse is concerned that the patient's confusion, memory loss, and wandering have not improved much and that he seems to have gotten worse since the weather got warm. The patient's spouse has provided a list of all of the patient's prescribed medications, which include hydrochlorothiazide (HydroDIURIL), metformin (Glucophage), and galantamine (Razadyne). Based on the patient's history, what class of over-the-counter (OTC) medication does the nurse need to report to the prescriber because it could be contributing to the patient's sudden decline in functioning?

3. What assessments (including reviewing laboratory tests) should the nurse perform before administering the galantamine (Razadyne), and what findings would warrant consulting the prescriber?

4. The patient's ALT is 178 international units/L, and his bilirubin is 3.2 mg/mL. The prescriber instructs the patient's spouse and the patient to discontinue the galantamine (Razadyne), not take any OTC antihistamines, and start taking rivastigmine (Exelon). The patient's spouse asks the nurse why the prescriber changed the medication to one in the same class if the galantamine is not working well and is hurting the patient's liver.

5. The nurse should teach the patient's spouse what information regarding adverse effects of rivastigmine (Exelon)?

6. The patient's spouse heard from friends of something sold in the health food store to cure AD. The friend said that the store provided results of research that states that the supplement is effective in improving memory in AD patients. The patient's spouse is on a limited budget and asks the opinion of the nurse. How should the nurse respond?

23

Drugs for Multiple Sclerosis

STUDY QUESTIONS

True or False

For each of the following statements, enter T *for true or* F *for false.*

1. ____ Research suggests initiation of the disease process is linked to genetic, environmental, and microbial factors.
2. ____ Current drug therapy repairs the myelin sheath on peripheral nerves.
3. ____ Current drug therapy for MS can cure the disease.
4. ____ Current drug therapy for MS can decrease the formation of lesions.
5. ____ Current drug therapy for MS can decrease symptoms during a relapse.
6. ____ Current drug therapy for MS can improve mobility and safety.
7. ____ Current drug therapy for MS can produce remissions in all types of MS.
8. ____ Current drug therapy for MS can slow the disease process.
9. ____ All patients with relapsing-remitting MS should receive an immunomodulator.
10. ____ Interferon beta, glatiramer, and fingolimod are more effective than natalizumab.
11. ____ Current drug therapy is most effective if the patient has primary progressive MS.

CRITICAL THINKING, PRIORITIZATION, AND DELEGATION QUESTIONS

12. A 26-year-old patient seeks medical care for blurred vision and severe muscle weakness. Which information from her history suggests possible risk factors for multiple sclerosis (MS)? (Select all that apply.)
    a. She is a smoker.
    b. She is taller than average.
    c. She has had mononucleosis twice while in college.
    d. Her father has had a cerebrovascular accident ([CVA], stroke).
    e. Her maternal and paternal grandparents were Norwegian immigrants.

13. Which of the following best describes treatment of relapsing-remitting MS with immunomodulators?
    a. They should always be administered orally.
    b. They should be used only if attacks last more than 1 week.
    c. They should continue indefinitely unless it is totally ineffective or toxic.
    d. They should only be used during periods of relapse.

14. The nurse is administering high-dose intravenous (IV) methylprednisolone to a patient who is experiencing an acute relapse of MS. Which chronic condition, if also present, could be adversely affected by this treatment?
    a. Asthma
    b. Diabetes mellitus (DM)
    c. Hypertension
    d. Rheumatoid arthritis

＊15. A patient with MS who is hospitalized with pneumonia is receiving the immunomodulator interferon beta-1a (Avonex) IM 30 mcg once a week. It would be of greatest priority for the nurse to report which laboratory test result to the prescriber?
    a. ALT 45 international units/L
    b. Hemoglobin A1c 5.2%
    c. RBC 4.9 million cells per microliter
    d. WBC 12,000/mm³

16. The nurse is administering mitoxantrone (Novantrone) to a patient who was unresponsive to other immunomodulating drugs for MS. The nurse should hold the medication and contact the prescriber if the patient exhibits which symptoms?
    a. Diaphoresis and low blood sugar
    b. Dizziness and orthostatic hypotension
    c. Headache and elevated blood pressure
    d. Weight gain of 3 lb in 24 hours and shortness of breath

17. A patient is scheduled to receive mitoxantrone (Novantrone). What would be a reason to withhold the medication and contact the prescriber? (Select all that apply.)
    a. Amenorrhea
    b. Blue-green colored urine
    c. LVEF 60%
    d. hCG 350 international units/L
    e. Neutrophils 1000 cells/mm³

18. A patient who is receiving mitoxantrone (Novantrone) should not receive which immunization(s)? (Select all that apply.)
    a. Hepatitis B vaccine
    b. Influenza vaccine
    c. Measles, mumps, and rubella (MMR)
    d. Tetanus, diphtheria toxoids, and acellular pertussis (Tdap)
    e. Varicella virus vaccine

19. A patient with MS experiences nausea, vomiting, tea-colored urine, clay-colored stools, and right upper quadrant (RUQ) tenderness. ALT results are 200 international units/L. The nurse would consult with the prescriber if the patient was prescribed which drug? (Select all that apply.)
    a. Betaseron
    b. Copaxone
    c. Mitoxantrone
    d. Dimethyl fumerate

20. Which symptom suggests a complication of detrusor-sphincter dyssynergia in an MS patient?
    a. Dysuria
    b. Difficulty initiating urination
    c. Nocturia
    d. Urinary urgency

21. Which teaching is most effective in preventing constipation when bulk-forming products are used for fecal incontinence?
    a. Administer the product after meals.
    b. Administer the product before meals.
    c. Administer the product in the morning and a stimulant laxative at night.
    d. Administer the product with at least 240 mL of fluid.

22. An MS patient complains that she is still depressed and fatigued despite being prescribed fluoxetine (Prozac) for 3 months. What action by the nurse would be most appropriate at this point?
    a. Encourage the patient to increase her intake of caffeine.
    b. Explain that the effects of antidepressants take many months to occur.
    c. Plan for the patient to discuss this problem with the prescriber.
    d. Start 1:1 suicide precautions.

DOSE CALCULATION QUESTIONS

23. A patient is prescribed an initial subcutaneous dose of 8.8 mcg of interferon 1a (Rebif) for the first 2 weeks of therapy. The drug is supplied as 22 mcg/0.5 mL. How much drug should the patient administer with each dose?

24. The nurse prepares natalizumab (Tysabri) 300 mg/15 mL in 100 mL of normal saline solution for IV infusion. The drug is to be administered over 1 hour. How much solution should infuse during each 10 minutes of the hour?

CASE STUDY

A 36-year-old college professor has been diagnosed with relapsing-remitting MS after the birth of her first child.

1. What assessments are important for the nurse to include when caring for this patient?

2. Her symptoms have significantly resolved. What are the primary factors of the pathophysiologic process of MS that explain how the symptoms can abate but the disease is still present?

3. What are some possible nursing diagnoses for this patient throughout the disease process?

4. When the nurse is administering medications, the patient refuses the drug, stating, "What's the use? My mom had MS and the drugs didn't help. She died in 1990. She was only 57 years old." What should be the basis of the nurse's response?

5. The patient with MS is started on the immunomodulator interferon beta-1a (Avonex) IM 30 mcg once a week. What should the nurse include in teaching regarding this drug?

6. The patient and the prescriber have tried treatment with the immunomodulators without success. They have agreed to try the immunosuppressant mitoxantrone (Novantrone). What teaching should the nurse provide this patient?

7. What steps does the nurse need to take before administering the mitoxantrone (Novantrone) by IV infusion?

8. The patient is experiencing urinary incontinence. What pharmacologic and nonpharmacologic measures can be employed to prevent this problem?

24

Drugs for Epilepsy

STUDY QUESTIONS

Matching

Match the term with its definition.

1. ___ Abnormal motor phenomena associated with epilepsy
2. ___ Any seizure activity that lasts longer than 30 minutes
3. ___ Brief loss of consciousness with or without mild, symmetric motor activity
4. ___ General term that includes alteration in consciousness, motor, sensory, autonomic, and psychoillusionary symptoms that occur with epilepsy
5. ___ Group of hyperexcitable neurons that start seizure activity
6. ___ Muscle rigidity followed by muscle jerks usually lasting ≤ 90 seconds and followed by a period when patient is difficult to arouse
7. ___ Partial seizure that transitions to generalized seizure activity
8. ___ Repetitive movements that lack purpose such as lip smacking
9. ___ Seizure activity in young children associated with an elevated temperature
10. ___ Severe form of epilepsy with developmental delay and a mixture of partial and generalized seizures
11. ___ Sudden, very brief, local *or* generalized muscle contraction
12. ___ Sudden loss of muscle tone
13. ___ Symptoms reflect the area of the brain being stimulated, last a minute or less, and patient does not become unconscious at any point during the seizure
14. ___ Trance-like state for 45-90 seconds followed by automatism

   a. Absence seizure (petit mal)
   b. Atonic seizure
   c. Automatism
   d. Complex partial seizure
   e. Convulsions
   f. Febrile seizure
   g. Focus

   h. Lennox-Gastaut syndrome (LGS)
   i. Myoclonic seizure
   j. Secondary generalized seizure
   k. Seizure
   l. Simple partial seizure
   m. Status epilepticus
   n. Tonic-clonic (grand mal) seizure

CRITICAL THINKING, PRIORITIZATION, AND DELEGATION QUESTIONS

15. What is a mechanism of action of an antiepileptic drug (AED)? (Select all that apply.)
   a. Bind to sodium channels when they are in the inactive state
   b. Block the actions of glutamate at NMDA and AMPA receptors
   c. Impair influx of calcium in axon terminals to prevent transmitter release
   d. Inhibit the action of the neurotransmitter GABA

16. Developmentally, what would be the most likely reason an 18-year-old male patient may refuse to seek treatment for possible seizure activity?
   a. Concern that he may lose his driver's license if diagnosed with epilepsy
   b. Drugs are not likely to be helpful
   c. Fear of injury when performing hazardous activities
   d. Refusal to maintain a seizure frequency chart

17. What should be included in teaching when a patient who has been taking valproic acid (Depakene) and carbamazepine (Tegretol) is to begin attempting drug withdrawal?
   a. Dose of both drugs should be gradually decreased.
   b. Dose of one drug should be gradually decreased while maintaining the usual dose of the second drug.
   c. Carbamazepine should be stopped and the valproic acid continued for at least a week.
   d. Valproic acid should be stopped and the carbamazepine continued for at least a week.

18. Research suggests that there is a statistically significant increased risk of thoughts of suicide when a patient is prescribed which AED? (Select all that apply.)
    a. Carbamazepine (Tegretol)
    b. Depakene (Depakote)
    c. Lamotrigine (Lamictal)
    d. Phenytoin (Dilantin)
    e. Topiramate (Topamax)

19. Which statement is true regarding newer AEDs versus traditional AEDs?
    a. Birth defects are more common when a pregnant woman takes newer AEDs.
    b. None of the newer AEDs induces drug-metabolizing enzymes.
    c. Research suggests newer AEDs are more effective.
    d. There is less clinical experience with newer AEDs.

✱20. Which action is of greatest priority to address phenytoin's (Dilantin's) narrow therapeutic index?
    a. Check plasma levels of the drug as prescribed.
    b. Increase intake of dairy products.
    c. Have regular dental checkups.
    d. Use two reliable forms of birth control.

21. Which laboratory test result would be of most concern to the nurse when a 27-year-old female patient admitted after injuries sustained in an MVA is prescribed phenytoin (Dilantin), cimetidine (Tagamet), diazepam (Valium), and warfarin (Coumadin)?
    a. ALT 35 IU/L
    b. hCG 3270 mIU/mL
    c. INR 2.1
    d. Phenytoin 15 mcg/mL

✱22. When caring for a patient who is receiving phenytoin (Dilantin), which assessment finding is a priority to report to the prescriber?
    a. Morbilliform-like rash
    b. Continuous back-and-forth movements of the eyes
    c. Excessive growth of gum tissue
    d. Inadequate consumption of foods rich in calcium and vitamin D

23. Parents have received instructions regarding administration of 5 mL twice a day of phenytoin (Dilantin suspension) to their child. Which statement made by the parents suggests a need for further teaching?
    a. "We must be sure to shake the medication thoroughly before measuring the dose."
    b. "We should give him a teaspoonful of the drug at each dose."
    c. "We should give him the medication with breakfast and with a snack before bedtime."
    d. "It is important that we space the drug doses as we have been instructed."

24. Which problem is most likely to occur with carbamazepine (Tegretol) therapy, but not phenytoin (Dilantin)?
    a. Sedation
    b. Reduced osmolarity of blood
    c. Swelling and discoloration of the hands and arms
    d. Swollen gums

✱25. Which nursing action would be of greatest priority when the patient who is prescribed carbamazepine (Tegretol) has an absolute neutrophil count (ANC) of 500/mm³?
    a. Handwashing
    b. Limited visitors
    c. No fresh fruit or vegetables
    d. Protective isolation

✱26. What is the priority nursing action when a patient who is prescribed carbamazepine (Tegretol) complains of vertigo?
    a. Ensuring patient safety
    b. Paging the prescriber STAT
    c. Reviewing most recent lab results of CBC, BUN, and electrolytes
    d. Withholding the medication

27. The nurse is teaching a patient about adverse effects that occur with carbamazepine (Tegretol). Which instruction should not be included in this teaching?
    a. Avoid situations where you are likely to be exposed to people with contagious infections.
    b. Plan your day to allow for rest periods.
    c. Stop taking the drug if you experience double vision.
    d. Use an electric razor instead of a standard razor because you may bleed easily.

*28. To prevent a life-threatening skin reaction, it would be a priority to review which laboratory test results if administering carbamazepine (Tegretol) to a patient of Asian descent?
   a. AST
   b. BUN
   c. Creatinine
   d. HLA-B*1502

29. The nurse instructs patients who have just received a prescription for carbamazepine (Tegretol) to avoid consuming grapefruit juice for which time period?
   a. Four hours after taking the medication
   b. No more than twice a week when taking the medication
   c. Not at all when taking the medication
   d. Two hours before taking the medication

*30. It would be of greatest priority for the patient to report which adverse effect of valproic acid?
   a. Abdominal pain
   b. Belching
   c. Hair loss
   d. Weight gain

31. A woman who is of childbearing age must take valproic acid to control seizures. Which statement, if made by the patient, suggests a need for further teaching?
   a. "Folic acid supplements are a good idea in case I accidentally get pregnant."
   b. " I should stop taking the drug if I find out that I am pregnant."
   c. "I need to inform all of my health care providers that I am taking valproic acid."
   d. "To be safe, I need to use two reliable forms of birth control."

32. Which would be the best goal for a child who is prescribed ethosuximide for absence seizures?
   a. Control of seizures allows for normal participation in activities
   b. No adverse effects from drug
   c. Plasma levels within therapeutic range
   d. Suppression of neurons in the thalamus

33. A patient is admitted with phenobarbital overdose. Which prescribed action would be of greatest priority?
   a. Assess respiratory status.
   b. Initiate IV fluids.
   c. Obtain drug level.
   d. Perform seizure precautions.

34. A patient with a history of hypertension and complex partial seizures has been prescribed oxcarbazepine (Trileptal) 100 mg twice a day and hydrochlorothiazide (Microzide). It is important for the nurse to assess for which condition that suggests possible hyponatremia? (Select all that apply.)
   a. Dry mucous membranes and flushed skin
   b. Hyperactive bowel sounds and tall tented T waves on electrocardiogram (ECG)
   c. Muscle spasms and weakness
   d. Headache and nausea

35. If a patient who is receiving lamotrigine (Lamictal) develops a rash, what should the nurse do?
   a. Assess vital signs.
   b. Continue nursing care.
   c. Immediately consult with the prescriber.
   d. Review laboratory test results.

*36. Pregabalin (Lyrica) can cause angioedema. What should the nurse teach the patient to do if he or she notes symptoms of angioedema?
   a. Get to a safe place to prevent injury during the seizure.
   b. Elevate the extremities.
   c. Seek emergency medical care.
   d. Take the drug with food.

37. What is true about levetiracetam (Keppra)?
   a. It can cause muscle weakness.
   b. It can decrease the effectiveness of warfarin (Coumadin).
   c. Its mechanism of action is blockade of sodium channels.
   d. It should be administered with food to decrease gastrointestinal adverse effects.

38. A ketogenic diet is especially dangerous when a patient with epilepsy is prescribed which drug?
   a. Levetiracetam
   b. Pregabalin
   c. Tiagabine
   d. Topiramate

39. Which laboratory test result would be of most concern to the nurse when a patient is prescribed topiramate (Topamax)?
   a. Creatinine 1.5 mg/dL
   b. HCO_3 20 mEq/L
   c. Hct 32%
   d. WBC 4600/mm³

40. Which symptom suggests a critical adverse effect when a patient is prescribed topiramate (Topamax) in addition to carbamazepine (Tegretol) for tonic-clonic seizures?
    a. Ataxia
    b. Difficulty concentrating
    c. Sudden eye pain
    d. Weight loss

41. What is the most appropriate action if the nurse notes that tiagabine (Gabitril) is ordered but no other AEDs are prescribed?
    a. Administer the medication.
    b. Administer the medication and ask the patient why he or she taking the medication.
    c. Withhold the medication.
    d. Withhold the medication and consult the prescriber.

42. The nurse would consult the prescriber before administering zonisamide (Zonegran) if the nurse notes that the patient had a known anaphylactic reaction to which drug?
    a. Acarbose (Precose)
    b. Insulin aspart (NovoLog)
    c. Glipizide (Glucotrol)
    d. Metformin (Glucophage)

DOSE CALCULATION QUESTIONS

43. The 5-year-old patient who weighs 35 lb is newly prescribed phenytoin 20 mg every 12 hours. The suggested initial dose is 2.5 mg/kg/day in divided doses. Is this a safe and effective dose for this child?

44. Phenytoin mg is available as a suspension of 125 mg/mL. How much drug should be administered if the prescribed dose is 20 mg twice a day?

CASE STUDY

A 26-year-old patient who is 8 months pregnant is admitted to the neurologic intensive care unit with the diagnosis of head injury. An automobile accident has left the patient unconscious. On admission, an intravenous (IV) line of D$_5$½ NS at 50 mL/hr is started. Within the first 24 hours on the unit, the patient has several tonic-clonic seizures. Standing orders on the unit allow the nurse to administer diazepam (Valium) 5 mg IV push. The prescriber is notified of the seizure and orders an IV loading dose of phenytoin (Dilantin) 800 mg followed by 100 mg every 6 hours, a phenytoin level the next day, and IV cimetidine 300 mg twice a day.

1. What nursing precautions are needed when administering phenytoin and cimetidine intravenously?

2. Phenytoin is available for IV infusion in a concentration of 50 mg/mL. How long should the nurse take when administering the 800-mg loading dose?

3. What symptoms should the nurse be alert for because of the possible interaction of phenytoin and cimetidine?

4. The next day, the phenytoin level is 14 mcg/mL. Why is it critical for the nurse to closely monitor plasma drug levels of phenytoin?

5. One week later, the patient goes into labor. Based on initiation of phenytoin near the end of the pregnancy, what fetal effects are most likely to occur?

6. What precautions might be taken to protect the fetus during drug therapy, during delivery, and after delivery?

7. Two weeks later, the patient is stabilized and has been transferred to the neurologic progressive unit. On admission the nurse notes a fine maculopapular rash on the patient's trunk. What should the nurse do and why?

8. Phenytoin (Dilantin) is discontinued. Carbamazepine (Tegretol) is substituted as the patient's antiseizure drug. The patient is concerned about taking seizure medication because she wants to have more children. She has been advised about possible adverse effects to the fetus. In addition to referring concerns to the prescriber, what information could the nurse provide about seizures, AEDs, and pregnancy?

25

Drugs for Muscle Spasm and Spasticity

STUDY QUESTIONS

True or False

For each of the following statements, enter T for true or F for false.

1. ____ Most drugs used to treat spasticity do not relieve acute muscle spasm.
2. ____ Muscle relaxant drugs shorten time of rehabilitation from traumatic injuries that cause muscle spasm.
3. ____ The therapeutic effects of muscle relaxants are similar to the effect of taking aspirin.
4. ____ Diazepam (Valium) is the most effective muscle relaxant.
5. ____ Most centrally acting muscle relaxants are not effective in treating spasticity associated with cerebral palsy.
6. ____ The nurse should assess all patients who are prescribed a centrally acting muscle relaxant for feelings associated with depression.
7. ____ Dark brown or black urine should be reported to the prescriber of methocarbamol (Robaxin).
8. ____ It is important for the nurse to review the BUN lab results when a patient is prescribed tizanidine, metaxalone, or dantrolene.
9. ____ Blocking the neurotransmitter GABA reduces spasticity.
10. ____ Baclofen decreases spasticity.

CRITICAL THINKING, PRIORITIZATION, AND DELEGATION QUESTIONS

✳11. The nurse knows that the priority nursing interventions and teaching for a patient receiving a centrally acting muscle relaxant are related to
    a. elimination.
    b. emotional support.
    c. nutrition.
    d. safety.

12. Which assessment finding does not suggest a possible significant adverse effect when a patient is prescribed metaxalone (Skelaxin)?
    a. Nausea and vomiting
    b. Right upper quadrant pain
    c. Sensitivity to light
    d. Tea-colored urine

13. The nurse should teach a patient who is prescribed a centrally acting muscle relaxant to avoid which drug?
    a. Diphenhydramine (e.g., Benadryl)
    b. Ibuprofen (e.g., Motrin)
    c. Multiple vitamins with iron
    d. Polyethelene glycol (e.g., MiraLax)

14. A resident is writing orders for hospitalized patients. The nurse would consult the prescriber if baclofen (Lioresal) was prescribed to relieve muscle spasms for a patient with which condition?
    a. Cerebral palsy
    b. Cerebrovascular accident
    c. Multiple sclerosis
    d. Spinal cord injury

DOSE CALCULATION QUESTIONS

15. Diazepam (Valium) 2 mg orally every 8 hours is prescribed for muscle spasms. The drug is available as 5 mg/mL. How much should the nurse administer at each dose?

16. Dantrolene 250 mg by rapid IV infusion is prescribed. The recommended dose to treat malignant hyperthermia is initially 2 mg/kg. The patient weighs 185 lb. Is this a safe dose?

CASE STUDIES

Case Study 1

A 19-year-old man is admitted to the neurologic intensive care unit after a motorcycle accident. He is paraplegic with severe lower extremity muscle spasms. He is receiving intrathecal baclofen. A pump is being used to infuse the drug because abrupt discontinuation can cause rhabdomyolysis and multiple organ system failure.

1. What is rhabdomyolysis, what organ is particularly sensitive to its effects, and what assessment findings would suggest that this is occurring?

2. The patient is transferred to a rehabilitation unit. Baclofen 20 mg is prescribed 4 times a day. What assessments should be included in the nurse's plan of care for this patient relating to drug therapy?

3. Developmentally, this patient is at risk for nonadherence to therapy. Why should the patient be discouraged from abrupt discontinuation of baclofen?

4. Dantrolene (Dantrium) would be more convenient for this patient because it only needs to be taken once a day. Why is it not a good choice for this patient?

Case Study 2

A patient with multiple sclerosis is admitted with pneumonia. She is receiving cyclobenzaprine (Flexeril) to relieve muscle spasms.

5. What are common anticholinergic adverse effects associated with this drug and nursing interventions relating to these effects?

6. What nonpharmacologic interventions and teaching could the nurse provide to help relieve the patient's discomfort and prevent complications?

Case Study 3

A patient returns to the postanesthesia care unit after general anesthesia. The vital signs have increased from normal to a temperature of 103.6° F, pulse 116 beats/min, respirations 22 breaths/min, and BP 145/99 mm Hg. The patient is developing muscular rigidity.

7. Why are antipyretics not appropriate to treat this fever?

8. The patient is prescribed dantrolene (Dantrium) 150 mg IV push. Why is it important to position the patient on his or her side with the side rails up?

26
Local Anesthetics

STUDY QUESTIONS

True or False

For each of the following statements, enter T *for true or* F *for false.*

Using a vasoconstrictor, such as epinephrine, with a local anesthetic

1. ____ allows for the use of less anesthetic.
2. ____ causes local vasoconstriction.
3. ____ can cause adverse effects from systemic absorption of the vasoconstrictor.
4. ____ causes local vasodilation.
5. ____ delays onset of anesthesia.
6. ____ delays systemic absorption.
7. ____ improves blood flow to the affected area.
8. ____ increases the risk of toxicity.
9. ____ reduces blood flow to the affected area.
10. ____ reduces the risk of toxicity.
11. ____ requires the use of a larger dose of anesthetic.

CRITICAL THINKING, PRIORITIZATION, AND DELEGATION QUESTIONS

▶12. The nurse is assisting the emergency department provider with anesthetizing and suturing multiple wounds on the extremities of a patient who was attacked by a dog. Which of these new developments would be of most concern to the nurse?
   a. Numbness and tingling around the mouth
   b. Rash
   c. Respirations 24/min
   d. Restlessness

▶13. A pregnant patient received an epidural anesthetic 10 minutes before delivering at 39 weeks of gestation. The neonate is brought to the nursery from the delivery room. Which finding would be a concern to the nursery nurse?
   a. Apical pulse 160 beats/min
   b. Positive Babinski's sign
   c. Respirations 22/min
   d. Temperature 36.8° C (98.2° F)

✳14. A patient is admitted to a surgical floor at 10 AM (1000) after a total abdominal hysterectomy performed with spinal anesthetic. During the assessment at 2 PM (1400), the nurse notes that the patient has not voided. The patient denies a need to void. What is the priority action by the nurse at this time?
   a. To administer bethanechol 5 mg subcutaneously ordered as needed for urinary retention
   b. To tell the patient that she needs to go to the bathroom to attempt to void
   c. To sit the patient upright on a bedpan to attempt to void
   d. To perform a bladder scan

15. Topical local anesthetic should be applied in what way? (Select all that apply.)
   a. Followed by heat to increase absorption
   b. Using the lowest effective dose
   c. Gently to areas of skin that are abraded
   d. As a thick film over the entire affected area
   e. Only to the affected area

✳16. Which symptoms, if occurring after a patient has received a local anesthetic with epinephrine, is a priority to report to the prescriber?
   a. Pulse 120 beats/min
   b. BP 100/60 mm Hg
   c. Respirations 24/min
   d. Temperature 38° C (100.4° F)

17. It is most important for the nurse to notify the physician of allergy concerns if the patient has a known allergy to chloroprocaine (Nesacaine) and is to receive which medication?
   a. Bupivacaine
   b. Lidocaine
   c. Mepivacaine
   d. Tetracaine

18. Cocaine differs from other ester-type local anesthetics in which way?
   a. It can be particularly dangerous if given to a patient with heart failure.
   b. It causes intense vasoconstriction.
   c. It is known to cause physical dependence.
   d. It produces CNS excitement, then depression.

19. A patient received intravenous regional anesthetic containing lidocaine without epinephrine when she had ankle surgery. It is a priority to assess for bradycardia, hypotension, and respiratory depression from the lidocaine at which time?
    a. Immediately after injection of the lidocaine
    b. When the surgeon makes the incision
    c. When the patient is in the postanesthesia care unit
    d. When the patient is in her hospital room on the medical-surgical unit

CASE STUDIES

Case Study 1

An 8-year-old child, accompanied by her parents, comes to the emergency department with a scalp laceration sustained when she fell off of her bicycle. The plan includes administration of lidocaine with epinephrine to close the wound with 6-8 interrupted sutures. The child is tearful but cooperative.

1. What are the nursing responsibilities for this procedure?

Case Study 2

A patient received lidocaine for the removal of an ingrown toenail. Seeping blood made it difficult to visualize the work area. Epinephrine is a vasoconstrictor that is often combined with lidocaine to delay systemic absorption of the lidocaine. As a vasoconstrictor, it would have decreased the blood seepage.

2. Why was it not used in this situation?

3. The patient has had this procedure before and is concerned about pain. She verbalizes a desire to use ice immediately to prevent pain. What precautions should the nurse provide regarding the use of cold?

4. The patient asks if she can use over-the-counter topical lidocaine anesthetic on her toe when sensation returns to relieve discomfort. What teaching should the nurse provide?

27

General Anesthetics

STUDY QUESTIONS

Matching

Match the anesthetic drug to the adverse effect.

1. ___ High risk of bacterial infection
2. ___ Hypotension can occur from vasodilation
3. ___ Can induce seizures
4. ___ Delirium and psychotic symptoms can occur postoperatively or days or weeks after surgery
5. ___ Can produce heat and fire in administration apparatus
6. ___ May prolong QT interval
7. ___ Tachycardia and hypertension can occur if blood levels drop suddenly

a. Desflurane
b. Enflurane
c. Droperidol
d. Isoflurane
e. Ketamine
f. Propofol
g. Sevoflurane

CRITICAL THINKING, PRIORITIZATION, AND DELEGATION QUESTIONS

8. General anesthesia involves the absence of
   a. sensibility to pain.
   b. consciousness and sensibility to pain.
   c. consciousness and sensibility to pain and temperature.
   d. consciousness and sensibility to pain, temperature, and taste.

9. The primary goal of using multiple agents to achieve anesthesia is to do what?
   a. Decrease the pain after the procedure
   b. Make the patient unable to feel pain during the procedure
   c. Permit full anesthesia with fewer adverse effects
   d. Prevent the patient from remembering the experience

10. Nitrous oxide has an extremely high minimum alveolar concentration (MAC). Because of this, which statement is true?
    a. The drug can be administered at low doses and achieve adequate anesthesia.
    b. Surgical anesthesia cannot be obtained with nitrous oxide alone.
    c. The drug can achieve adequate, safe anesthesia if a high enough dose is administered slowly.
    d. The drug will make the patient unresponsive to painful stimuli.

11. The nurse is caring for a patient in the postanesthesia care unit (PACU). What is the highest priority assessment by the nurse?
    a. Breathing
    b. Level of consciousness
    c. Pain
    d. Urinary output

12. The nurse should assess all postoperative patients who have received inhaled anesthesia for what condition?
    a. Diarrhea
    b. Excessive salivation
    c. Urinary urgency
    d. Wheezing

▶ 13. The nurse is completing the preoperative checklist for a same-day surgery patient who has been called to the operating room (OR). The patient makes a comment to the nurse that he hopes they "really knock me out" because he needs a lot of a drug to get a good effect. On further discussion, the patient reveals that he has been using oxycodone (OxyContin) illegally for 2 years and that his last dose was 6 hours ago. What should the nurse do?
    a. Call the OR and cancel the surgery.
    b. Note the medication on the patient's chart and send the patient to the OR.
    c. Notify anesthesiologist and the surgeon of the finding.
    d. Nothing, the medication should be out of the patient's system at this time.

▶ 14. A male patient who has received midazolam (Versed), a periprocedure benzodiazepine, has just been admitted to the postcolonoscopy recovery area. He informs the nurse that he needs to urinate. The nurse should initially do what?
    a. Assist the patient to the bathroom, staying with the patient at all times.
    b. Provide the patient a urinal and ask him to try to use it while still in bed.
    c. Provide the patient with a urinal and assist him with standing.
    d. Insert a Foley catheter.

▶ 15. What is the assessment finding that would warrant the nurse withholding morphine from a postoperative patient?
    a. Blood pressure 160/92 mm Hg
    b. Pain 9 on a scale of 1 to 10
    c. Respirations 8/min
    d. Temperature 38.2° C

✳ 16. A 14-month-old patient received isoflurane and succinylcholine during surgery. Which immediate postoperative assessment findings would be a priority concern?
    a. Blood pressure 86/54 mm Hg
    b. Pulse 68 beats/min
    c. Respirations 30/min
    d. Temperature 103.6° F (39.8° C)

✳ 17. The emergency department has sent a patient to the OR for emergency surgery including general anesthetic with isoflurane. The family has just arrived, and the nurse has learned that the patient has been taking the calcium channel blocker amlodipine (Norvasc). This information needs to be communicated to the OR and PACU. Because of the similarity in effects of isoflurane and amlodipine, what is the priority assessment?
    a. Blood pressure for hypotension
    b. Pulse for bradycardia
    c. Respirations for hypopnea or apnea
    d. Temperature for malignant hyperthermia

18. Why is nitrous oxide widely used in surgery?
    a. Balanced anesthesia can be achieved with nitrous oxide alone.
    b. It has significant analgesic effects without significant cardiac or respiratory depression.
    c. It can produce a state of unconsciousness at very low doses.
    d. Postoperative nausea and vomiting are uncommon.

19. What is the purpose of administering methohexital in the OR?
    a. Decrease respiratory secretions
    b. Prevent muscle contraction
    c. Prevent sensation of pain
    d. Produce unconsciousness

20. A cataract surgery patient receives midazolam and fentanyl. The nurse would expect these medications to produce which effects? (Select all that apply.)
    a. Absence of anxiety
    b. Analgesia
    c. Flaccid paralysis
    d. Sedation
    e. Unconsciousness

21. What is required when propofol is being used?
    a. Sterile technique
    b. Storage in a freezer and thawing 15 minutes before use
    c. Use of a 25-26 gauge IV catheter for administration
    d. Usage within 30 minutes of preparation

22. What is the priority assessment when a patient has received propofol?
    a. Blood pressure
    b. Breathing
    c. Heart rate
    d. Intake and output

CASE STUDIES

Case Study 1

A 65-year-old man with a history of lung cancer has been admitted the evening before surgery and is scheduled for a thoracotomy at 8 AM under balanced general anesthetic. He is 5 feet 6 inches tall and weighs 210 lb. The patient has a productive cough and admits to tobacco use for the last 40 years, smoking one pack of cigarettes per day. He has hypertension and takes hydrochlorothiazide, which has been effective in keeping his blood pressure under control.

1. Describe the ideal anesthetic for this patient.

2. What would be priority concerns of the PACU nurse for this patient relating to general anesthetic?

3. What actions should the PACU nurse employ relating to this concern?

Case Study 2

The nurse is admitting a patient with a history of type 2 diabetes mellitus and hypertension to the same-day surgery unit. The patient is scheduled for an inguinal herniorrhaphy.

4. What type of agents would be included if this patient is to receive balanced anesthesia?

5. What data are important for the nurse to collect relating to scheduled general anesthesia?

6. The patient is in the PACU and has just awakened, but is very drowsy. Describe nursing interventions relating to the effects of inhalation anesthetic that are needed when a patient first awakens.

7. The postoperative patient reports having awakened during surgery and being in pain, but being unable to tell the surgeon. What should the nurse do?

28

Opioid (Narcotic) Analgesics, Opioid Antagonists, and Nonopioid Centrally Acting Analgesics

STUDY QUESTIONS

True or False

For each of the following statements, enter T *for true or* F *for false.*

1. ____ An opiate is a drug that contains compounds found in opium, while an opioid may be a laboratory-created compound.
2. ____ The term *narcotic* refers only to synthetic compounds that relieve pain.
3. ____ Enkephalins, endorphins, and dynorphins are body substances with opioid properties.
4. ____ The respiratory depression, physical dependence, and euphoria that occur with opioid analgesics are related to activation of mu opioid receptors.
5. ____ Buprenorphine (Buprenex) has less constipation and sedative effects than morphine.
6. ____ An agonist-antagonist blocks pain when taken alone but improves the pain-relieving effect of another opioid if in the blood at the same time.
7. ____ The dose of oral morphine is higher than the intravenous (IV) dose because hepatic first pass metabolizes some of the drug before it reaches the central nervous system.

CRITICAL THINKING, PRIORITIZATION, AND DELEGATION QUESTIONS

8. Four patients return to the nursing unit from the postanesthesia care unit (PACU) at 1600. Which of these patients would be most likely to experience respiratory depression during the 0700-1530 shift the next day?
   a. 45-year-old female patient, postop open cholecystectomy, who is reluctant to cough and deep-breathe and who had the last dose of 2 mg of morphine IV at 1430
   b. 84-year-old female patient who had an open reduction and internal fixation of a right hip fracture who has had no morphine in PACU but received a subcutaneous dose of 5 mg of morphine at 1930
   c. 5-year-old male patient who is postop appendectomy and received 0.1 mg/kg of morphine IV at 2045
   d. 63-year-old male patient post–total knee arthroplasty who received 5 mg of morphine epidural at 1125 during surgery

9. The nurse is ambulating a postoperative patient in the hall who is receiving an opioid analgesic for pain. The patient complains of severe nausea. What is the priority nursing action at this time?
   a. Administer the prescribed antiemetic.
   b. Assist the patient to sit down.
   c. Get an emesis basin.
   d. Walk the patient back to his room.

▶ 10. A patient who has received morphine becomes slightly disoriented. If this adverse effect is due to the morphine, which intervention by the nurse might aid in reversing it?
   a. Assist the patient to ambulate.
   b. Instruct the patient to change positions slowly.
   c. Instruct the patient to take slow, deep breaths.
   d. Keep the room well-lit.

＊11. A neonate is born to a known heroin addict. The infant is exhibiting symptoms of opioid withdrawal. Which of these nursing issues is of the highest priority as the nurse cares for the neonate in the nursery?
a. Altered nutrition
b. Disturbed sleep
c. Fluid deficit
d. Parenting

12. A cancer patient who is receiving oxycodone (OxyContin) for pain relief develops a rash after being prescribed an antibiotic. The prescriber discontinues the antibiotic and prescribes diphenhydramine (Benadryl). The nurse would include in the plan of care assessment and interventions for which possible effects of the combination of oxycodone and diphenhydramine?
a. Delirium
b. Fever
c. Hypotension
d. Urinary retention

＊13. A patient who has overdosed on oxycodone (OxyContin), an opiate, is brought into the ED unresponsive with severely depressed respirations. The patient receives IV naloxone HCl (Narcan), a narcotic antagonist, with an improvement in level of consciousness and respiratory rate and effort within minutes. The nurse is scheduled to go to lunch in 15 minutes. What is the nursing priority that guides information that must be communicated before the nurse leaves for lunch?
a. Prevention of abstinence syndrome
b. The short half-life of naloxone
c. The short half-life of oxycodone
d. History of substance abuse

14. A fentanyl (Duragesic) patch has been prescribed for a patient after multiple musculoskeletal injuries. The most important reason why the nurse should teach the patient not to apply heat in the area of the patch is because it might
a. inactivate the drug.
b. loosen the patch from the skin.
c. prolong the drug's effect.
d. cause respiratory depression.

15. The nurse should assess for respiratory depression for 24 hours after a patient has discontinued use of which medication?
a. Intrathecal morphine
b. Intramuscular meperidine (Demerol)
c. Oral methadone (Dolophine)
d. Transmucosal fentanyl (Actiq)

16. What would be most likely to cause a life-threatening reaction?
a. The patient chews the pellets in a morphine/naltrexone capsule.
b. The patient crushes and snorts the pellets in a morphine/naltrexone capsule.
c. The patient consumes a shot and a beer while taking morphine/naltrexone as prescribed.
d. The patient does not take the prescribed morphine/naltrexone.

17. What is a reason to withhold a newly prescribed fentanyl transdermal system patch?
a. The patient has not taken any opioids in the past 30 days.
b. The patient is also prescribed a short-acting opioid for breakthrough pain.
c. The patient rates pain as 5/10.
d. The patient weighs more than 200 lb.

＊18. The nurse answers a call to the ED from a woman who is prescribed fentanyl lozenge on a stick (Actiq). She states that she found her 2-year-old grandson with the medication in his mouth. She took it away from him, and he is standing next to her crying. Which action would be of greatest priority?
a. Call 911.
b. Assess how much drug was consumed.
c. Contact the poison hotline.
d. Rinse out the child's mouth.

19. Which is the appropriate method of administering fentanyl buccal film (Onsolis)?
a. Apply the patch to dry skin that is not hairy to ensure adhesion.
b. Place the drug between the cheek and the lower gum and actively suck on it.
c. Place the drug on the floor of the mouth directly under the tongue, and allow it to dissolve completely. Do not chew, suck, or swallow the drug.
d. Press the pink side of the film against a moist area of inside of the cheek for 5 seconds, and then leave it there.

20. An aphasic patient, who has been receiving meperidine 75 mg every 3-4 hours for pain for the past 36 hours, has suddenly become restless and irritable. The last dose of meperidine was 4 hours ago. Why is it important for the nurse to withhold the meperidine, do a complete assessment on the patient, and contact the prescriber with the findings?
    a. Respiratory depression is imminent.
    b. The patient is becoming physiologically dependent on the meperidine.
    c. Tolerance to the meperidine has developed.
    d. Toxicity from a metabolite may be occurring.

21. Which ordered diagnostic test would be a priority to review when a patient is prescribed methadone?
    a. ALT
    b. ECG
    c. eGFR
    d. Potassium

▶22. A cancer patient has been taking increasing doses of oxycodone (OxyContin) for pain relief. Which teaching can prevent the adverse effect that is most likely to persist with long-term use of this drug?
    a. Consume adequate fluids and fiber.
    b. Change positions slowly.
    c. Do not operate dangerous machinery.
    d. Take deep breaths every hour.

23. A cancer patient has received instructions regarding administration of oxycodone (OxyContin). Which of these statements made by the patient would indicate that the patient needs further teaching?
    a. "I need to inform my doctor if I experience episodes of pain between doses."
    b. "If I have difficulty swallowing the pill, I should crush it and take it with a small amount of applesauce."
    c. "I should tell all of my health care providers that I am taking this drug regularly."
    d. "I should not take this drug if I am allergic to Percocet, but it is OK if I am only allergic to acetaminophen (Tylenol)."

▶24. What is a potential cause of a patient experiencing agitation, rhinorrhea, and yawning after administration of pentazocine, nalbuphine, butorphanol, or buprenorphine?
    a. The patient has an opioid agonist in her system.
    b. The patient is allergic to the drug.
    c. The patient is experiencing a common adverse effect of the drug.
    d. The patient is unable to excrete the drug.

✳25. A patient is admitted to the ED after a traumatic injury and is in severe pain from compound fractures. Which chronic condition would be of greatest concern when administering an opioid?
    a. Asthma
    b. Diabetes
    c. Head injury
    d. Hypertension

26. The nurse would consult the prescriber if the nurse identified that a patient had a history of which chronic condition and was prescribed tramadol (Ultram) for pain relief?
    a. Heart failure (HF)
    b. Chronic obstructive pulmonary disease (COPD)
    c. Dementia
    d. Seizure disorder

▶27. A cancer patient is prescribed clonidine (Duraclon) for burning pain. What should be reported to the prescriber before administering the drug? (Select all that apply.)
    a. Blood pressure 86/60 mm Hg
    b. Creatinine 1.1 mg/dL
    c. INR 2.8
    d. Pulse 88 beats/min
    e. Temperature 99.8° F

✳28. What is the most common nursing concern when a patient is receiving intrathecal ziconotide (Prialt)?
    a. Breathing
    b. Circulation
    c. Elimination
    d. Safety

DOSE CALCULATION QUESTIONS

29. A patient is prescribed 3 mg of morphine by intravenous route every 3 hours as needed for postoperative pain. Available are vials containing 5 mg/mL. How many mL of morphine will the nurse administer at each dose? The drug handbook recommends that morphine be diluted in 5 mL of sterile water and administered slowly over 5 minutes. The 10-mL syringe is marked in 0.2-mL increments. How many seconds should elapse between each push of 0.2 mL of the diluted morphine?

30. Naloxone 10 mcg/kg is prescribed to treat respiratory depression for a 7-lb neonate. The drug is available as 0.4 mg/mL. What is the amount of naloxone that should be administered?

CASE STUDIES

Case Study 1

The nurse is providing preoperative teaching to a 35-year-old female patient who has been admitted for an abdominal hysterectomy. Patient-controlled analgesia (PCA) is anticipated as the mechanism of postoperative pain relief.

1. What preoperative teaching should the nurse provide this patient to enhance pain relief and prevent adverse effects, including respiratory depression?

2. Postoperatively, the patient is ordered morphine IV via PCA pump for her postoperative pain. The pump is set to deliver 1 mg of morphine per injection and up to a maximum of 5 mg/hr. What are the advantages and disadvantages of PCA?

3. The patient appears to be sleeping. Her skin is pale, and her respiratory rate is 8/min and shallow. What should the nurse do at this time in order of priority?

4. What measures, other than drug therapy, can the nurse employ to reduce this patient's pain?

Case Study 2

A patient continues to require morphine long after the usual time frame for opioids after the type of surgery that was performed. She tells the nurse that she has no tolerance for pain, but the prescriber has decided that she must stop the morphine. The nurse is concerned that the patient may have been dependent on drugs before coming to the hospital and that withdrawing the morphine may lead to abstinence syndrome.

5. How should the nurse address these concerns?

6. What are the symptoms of abstinence syndrome that the nurse should include in patient assessment?

7. Is it possible that the patient could be having uncontrolled pain, not be a substance abuser, and not have any other medical problems?

8. How does physical dependence on opioid analgesics differ from abuse and addiction?

9. Describe a situation where physical dependence on opioid analgesics is rarely a complication.

29

Pain Management in Patients with Cancer

STUDY QUESTIONS

Matching

Match the types of pain to their origin.

1. ____ Injury to bone, joint, muscle
2. ____ Peripheral nerve injury
3. ____ Injury to organs
4. ____ Tissue injury pain

    a. Neuropathic
    b. Nociceptive
    c. Somatic
    d. Visceral

CRITICAL THINKING, PRIORITIZATION, AND DELEGATION QUESTIONS

5. What is the most reliable indicator of the need for pain relief in the oncology patient?
   a. Changes in vital signs that can occur with pain
   b. Extensiveness of the cancer involvement
   c. Patient's expressions and reluctance to move
   d. Patient's report of a need for pain relief

✳ 6. When developing a plan of care for pain management for the cancer patient, achievement of _____ is the priority outcome.
   a. a rating of pain less than 3 on a scale of 0 to 10
   b. comfort that allows the patient to complete all activities of daily living
   c. pain relief that is acceptable to the patient
   d. total pain relief

7. A cancer patient whose history includes type 2 diabetes mellitus informs the nurse that she is experiencing constant burning pain in her feet. Based on the type of foot pain commonly experienced by diabetics, the nurse would consult the prescriber regarding possibly ordering which drug?
   a. An analgesic, such as acetaminophen (Tylenol)
   b. An antiseizure adjunct drug, such as gabapentin (Neurontin)
   c. A nonsteroidal anti-inflammatory drug (NSAID), such as naproxen (Aleve)
   d. An opioid-agonist analgesic, such as morphine

✳ 8. Which of these laboratory test results would be a priority to report to the prescriber when a cancer patient treated with chemotherapy is taking a pain reliever that contains ibuprofen?
   a. ALT 40 international units/L
   b. BUN 22 mg/dL
   c. Platelet count 60,000/mm^3
   d. WBC 5500/mm^3

9. A postoperative cancer patient was receiving morphine sulfate IV 10 mg every 4 hours for pain. The prescriber has discontinued the IV morphine and ordered morphine sulfate 20-mg tablet every 4 hours. How does the oral dose compare with the IV dose?
   a. The oral dose cannot be compared with the IV dose.
   b. These are equianalgesic doses.
   c. The oral dose produces less analgesia than the IV dose.
   d. The oral dose produces more analgesia than the IV dose.

▶10. The nurse knows that respiratory depression is most likely to occur with which pain regimen?
   a. A loading dose of 10 mg of morphine before starting PCA
   b. Increased long-term IV dose of morphine from 5 mg to 7 mg
   c. Patient-controlled analgesia (PCA) morphine at 1 mg of morphine per injection up to a maximum of 5 mg/hr
   d. 60 mg of IV morphine every hour to a patient who has been receiving steadily increasing doses of morphine

11. A patient has been taking oral opioids for moderate pain associated with prostate cancer that has metastasized to the spine. Surgery is performed, and the patient is experiencing moderate to severe postoperative pain. Which analgesic is most appropriate in this case?
   a. Buprenorphine IV
   b. Fentanyl transdermal patch
   c. Intermittent IM dosing of meperidine
   d. Morphine sulfate via PCA pump

∗12. What is of most concern to the nurse when a patient is prescribed an NSAID analgesic on a regular basis?
   a. Lack of adequate pain relief
   b. Heartburn
   c. Rigid abdomen
   d. Swollen ankles

13. Celecoxib 200 mg twice a day is prescribed for a patient with cancer that has metastasized to the bone. Which adverse effect is more likely to occur with celecoxib than with other NSAIDs?
   a. BP elevation
   b. Cerebrovascular accident
   c. GI bleed
   d. Physical dependence

∗14. Which laboratory test result would be of greatest priority to report to the prescriber of an NSAID drug to a cancer patient?
   a. BUN 23 mg/dL
   b. FBG 233 mg/dL
   c. Platelets 40,000/mm^3
   d. WBC 4700/mm^3

∗15. What is of greatest priority when naloxone is administered to combat respiratory depression associated with opioid use for cancer patients?
   a. Hydration
   b. Level of consciousness
   c. Presence of gag reflex
   d. Return of pain

16. The nurse is preparing to administer metoclopramide (Reglan) to a cancer patient who is experiencing nausea associated with opioid use. How should the nurse respond when the patient asks how this drug works?
   a. "The drug counteracts gastric slowing caused by opioid use."
   b. "The drug decreases the release of histamine."
   c. "The drug relaxes smooth muscle."
   d. "The drug works on the nausea center in the brain."

∗17. What is the priority concern when a patient combines prescribed opioids with alcohol?
   a. Nausea and vomiting
   b. Orthostatic hypotension
   c. Physical dependence
   d. Respiratory depression

DOSE CALCULATION QUESTION

18. Hydromorphone (Dilaudid) 10 mg is prescribed via IV push. The drug book recommends administering at a rate of 2-5 mg/min. The drug is available as 10 mg/mL. The nurse prepares to administer the drug using a syringe marked in hundredths. If the nurse administers 0.02 mL every 5 seconds, will the rate be safe?

CASE STUDY

A cancer patient is being discharged on oxycodone and acetaminophen (Percocet).

1. What teaching should the nurse provide regarding the opioid and nonopioid components of this drug?

The patient's pain is not relieved by two Percocet (oxycodone 10 mg and acetaminophen 325 mg) tablets taken every 4 hours. The prescriber has discontinued the Percocet and ordered oxycodone CR (OxyContin) 40 mg twice a day, oxycodone IR 5 mg every 6 hours as needed, and acetaminophen 650 mg every 6 hours. The patient is overwhelmed by the multiple medications and asks why he cannot just take three Percocet tablets every 4 hours.

2. How should the nurse respond?

3. What interventions can the nurse offer to help the patient understand his analgesic regimen?

4. What teaching should the nurse provide regarding the adverse effect of constipation?

5. What teaching can the nurse provide to enable the patient to assist the prescriber with decisions regarding analgesic prescription?

30
Drugs for Headache

STUDY QUESTIONS

Matching

Match the drugs for prevention of migraines to the reasons to withhold the drug and contact the prescriber regarding the drug.

1. ___ Abdominal pain and amylase 500 international units/L
2. ___ Apical pulse 48 beats/min
3. ___ pH 7.32; HCO_3 19 mEq/L; pco_2 35 mm Hg
4. ___ Positive Homans' sign and swelling in left calf
5. ___ Postvoid bladder scan 600 mL
6. ___ Potassium 5.6 mEq/L
7. ___ Systolic BP drops 30 mm Hg when changing from sitting to standing

a. Amitriptyline (tricyclic antidepressant)
b. Candesartan (ARB)
c. Divalproex (antiseizure)
d. Estrogen (hormone)
e. Propranolol (beta blocker)
f. Topiramate (antiseizure)
g. Verapamil (CCB)

CRITICAL THINKING, PRIORITIZATION, AND DELEGATION QUESTIONS

8. A nurse knows the following about migraine headaches. (Select all that apply.)
   a. They cannot be treated effectively after the pain starts.
   b. They involve inflammation of intracranial blood vessels.
   c. They involve vasoconstriction of intracranial blood vessels.
   d. Their therapy includes regular schedule for eating, sleep, and exercise.
   e. Their therapy should start at the earliest sign of attack.

9. What is the primary reason why abortive medication for migraine headaches should not be used more than 1 or 2 days a week?
   a. Abuse potential
   b. Development of chest pain
   c. Development of tolerance so medication is not effective
   d. Medication-overuse headache

10. Which over-the-counter medication has not demonstrated effectiveness in relieving mild to moderate migraine headache pain?
    a. Aspirin
    b. Acetaminophen
    c. Acetaminophen, aspirin, and caffeine
    d. Ibuprofen

11. Which nursing concern would be of greatest priority when a patient is prescribed meperidine (Demerol) for migraine headaches?
    a. Abuse potential
    b. Potential for respiratory distress
    c. Constipation
    d. Relief of headache

✳12. Which assessment finding would be of greatest priority to report to the prescriber if the nurse was preparing to administer ergotamine to a patient who is experiencing the start of a migraine headache?
    a. ALT 30 international units/L
    b. Blood pressure 90/58 mm Hg
    c. Capillary refill of 12 seconds
    d. Flashes of light in visual fields

13. The rationale for administering both ergotamine and metoclopramide (Reglan) to a patient to abort a migraine headache includes that the metoclopramide
    a. decreases nausea and vomiting.
    b. minimizes sensitivity to light.
    c. prevents adverse effects of weakness and myalgia from ergotamine.
    d. provides additional vasoconstriction to relieve cranial vessel vasodilation.

14. The nurse would consult the prescriber before administering ergotamine or triptan drugs for migraine headache to a patient with which condition(s)? (Select all that apply.)
    a. Cardiovascular disease
    b. Diabetes mellitus
    c. Hypertension
    d. Infection
    e. Peptic ulcer disease

15. What is true about triptan therapy for migraine headaches?
    a. Administering an oral dose of the drug after subcutaneous administration will prevent recurrence of the headache.
    b. Combination with ergotamine provides more relief than triptan alone.
    c. Peripheral vasoconstriction is the primary cause of adverse effects.
    d. Therapy relieves headache, nausea, and sensitivity to sound and light.

*16. The nurse has administered sumatriptan (Imitrex)
► subcutaneously for migraine headache relief at 2100 (9 PM) to a 35-year-old smoker. One hour after administration, the patient complains of heavy arms and chest pressure. What is the priority action at this point?
    a. Activate the medical emergency team.
    b. Assess vital signs and evaluate the chest pain.
    c. Continue care; this is a normal adverse effect.
    d. Notify the prescriber.

17. A patient does not inform her primary care provider (PCP) that she is prescribed duloxetine (Cymbalta) by her rheumatologist. The PCP prescribes a triptan for migraines. What symptoms of serotonin syndrome are possible with this combination?
    a. Confusion and incoordination
    b. Extremities becoming cold, pale, and numb
    c. Hypotension and fainting
    d. Nausea and vomiting

18. The nurse would plan for which potential nursing problem when administering haloperidol (Haldol) for migraine headache?
    a. Altered tissue perfusion
    b. Fluid volume deficit
    c. Safety
    d. Skin integrity

*19. A patient is prescribed propranolol for migraine prevention. Which assessment finding would be a priority to report to the prescriber?
    a. BP 130/80 mm Hg
    b. Expiratory wheezing
    c. Hunger and thirst
    d. Pulse 98 beats/min

20. What would be a contraindication for estrogen use to prevent menstrual migraines?
    a. Asthma
    b. Dysuria
    c. Menorrhagia
    d. Thrombophlebitis

21. A patient is receiving lithium carbonate for prevention of cluster headaches. This drug has a narrow therapeutic index. Which drug level would fall into the safe and effective range?
    a. 0.1 mEq/L
    b. 0.2 mEq/L
    c. 0.5 mEq/L
    d. 0.8 mEq/L

DOSE CALCULATION QUESTIONS

22. Dihydroergotamine mesylate (D.H.E. 45) is available in solution (1 mg/mL). Prescribed is 1000 micrograms IM. How much drug should the nurse administer?

23. Naratriptan (Amerge) 5 mg is prescribed. Available are 2.5-mg tablets. How many should the nurse administer?

CASE STUDY

A 49-year-old patient is seen in the emergency department (ED) with a chief complaint of severe, frequent headaches that begin mid-morning and grow progressively worse throughout the day. She admits to occasional nausea and vomiting. Advil has been minimally successful in treating the headaches. Her headaches are pulsatile and usually unilateral. All of the patient's laboratory findings are within normal limits. Sumatriptan (Imitrex) 6 mg subcutaneously is prescribed to be administered now, along with a prescription for Imitrex STAT dose Pen 6 mg to be taken as directed.

1. Describe what the nurse should include in teaching this patient about administering the self-injecting pen.

2. The patient attempts to fill the prescription at the hospital outpatient pharmacy, but her insurance does not cover sumatriptan. Dihydroergotamine is prescribed in place of the sumatriptan. What teaching needs to be provided by the ED nurse regarding the administration of dihydroergotamine?

4. The patient tells the nurse that a friend takes ergotamine. Her friend "got hooked" on ergotamine and had to go to the hospital to "get off of it." What would the nurse include when comparing ergotamine and dihydroergotamine?

3. What teaching regarding preventing toxicity from dihydroergotamine should be provided to this patient?

5. The patient is instructed to seek follow-up with her PCP. The PCP discusses the use of prophylactic drugs to prevent the migraine headaches. What drugs might be considered?

31
Antipsychotic Agents and Their Use in Schizophrenia

STUDY QUESTIONS

True or False

For each of the following statements, enter T *for true or* F *for false.*

1. ___ High-potency antipsychotic drugs are more likely to be effective than low-potency drugs.
2. ___ High-potency antipsychotic drugs produce desired effects at lower doses than low-potency drugs.
3. ___ High-potency antipsychotic drugs treat both positive and negative symptoms more than low-potency drugs.
4. ___ Second-generation antipsychotic (SGA) drugs are often thought to be more effective.
5. ___ SGA drugs cost less than first-generation antipsychotics (FGAs).
6. ___ SGA drugs can affect thinking.
7. ___ SGA drugs only cause minor adverse effects.
8. ___ Antipsychotic drugs can cure schizophrenia if taken as prescribed.

CRITICAL THINKING, PRIORITIZATION, AND DELEGATION QUESTIONS

9. A patient who is receiving chemotherapy for breast cancer is prescribed chlorpromazine (Thorazine). There is no mention of other medical or psychiatric disorders in the patient's history. What is the most likely reason why this patient is receiving the drug?
   a. History of delusions
   b. History of hallucinations
   c. History of nausea
   d. History of tics

10. Which extrapyramidal adverse effect of antipsychotic drugs would the nurse expect to occur only after an extended period of drug therapy?
   a. Repetitive, slow, twisting movements of the tongue and face
   b. Severe spasms of the mouth, face, neck, or back
   c. Slow movement, tremor, and rigidity
   d. Uncontrollable need to be in motion

✳11. What is the greatest priority when a patient is experiencing acute laryngeal dystonia?
    a. Airway clearance
    b. Anxiety treatment
    c. Pain therapy
    d. Ensuring patient safety

✳12. Which of these findings, in a patient who has been receiving a neuroleptic antipsychotic, is of highest priority and should be reported to the prescriber immediately?
    a. Agitation
    b. Difficulty speaking
    c. Involuntary movements of the tongue
    d. Sudden, whole-body muscle contractions

✳13. What would be the priority action to reduce a patient's body temperature of 104° F (40° C) caused by neuroleptic malignant syndrome?
    a. Administering acetaminophen (Tylenol) prescribed every 4-6 hours as needed
    b. Administering dantrolene (Dantrium) immediately as prescribed
    c. Increasing fluid intake to 1500 mL/day
    d. Tepid bath

▶14. The nurse is assessing the orthostatic blood pressure and pulse of a patient who is prescribed a neuroleptic antipsychotic drug. Which assessment finding would be reason to withhold the drug and consult the prescriber?
    a. BP lying 110/66 mm Hg and pulse 76 beats/min; 2 minutes later BP standing 108/70 mm Hg and pulse 80 beats/min
    b. BP lying 120/84 mm Hg and pulse 70 beats/min; 2 minutes later BP standing 110/76 mm Hg; pulse 72 beats/min
    c. BP lying 116/70 mm Hg and pulse 72 beats/min; 2 minutes later BP standing 110/68 mm Hg and pulse 122 beats/min
    d. BP lying 146/90 mm Hg and pulse 73 beats/min; 2 minutes later BP standing 138/88 mm Hg; pulse 78 beats/min

15. A 68-year-old patient who is prescribed an FGA is diagnosed with benign prostatic hyperplasia. Which assessment would be of greatest priority related to the drug and this condition?
    a. Abdominal pain
    b. Blood pressure
    c. Dizziness
    d. Intake and output

16. Which symptom would be of greatest concern when administering an FGA that causes QT prolongation?
    a. Elevated fasting blood glucose
    b. Fatigue
    c. Sudden fainting
    d. Thirst

17. Which statements suggest that a family member needs additional teaching regarding administration of an oral liquid FGA? (Select all that apply.)
    a. "I must chill the drug for an hour after diluting in juice so it tastes better."
    b. "I need to dilute the drug in enough juice to make it taste OK but not too much so I am sure that he takes all of it."
    c. "I need to rinse my skin with water if I spill the drug."
    d. "I should keep the drug in the bottle that it comes in and put it in a dark cabinet."
    e. "I should let him take the drug himself so that he is not suspicious that I am poisoning him."

18. Which symptom of an adverse effect, if identified in a patient who is receiving thioridazine (Mellaril) or haloperidol (Haldol), should the nurse report to the prescriber immediately?
    a. Fainting not associated with sudden position changes
    b. Milk secretion from a male patient
    c. Stool hard and difficult to expel
    d. Sunburn

19. What is another name for second-generation antipsychotics (SGAs)?
    a. Atypical antipsychotics
    b. High-potency antipsychotics
    c. Low-potency antipsychotics
    d. Typical antipsychotics

20. It is important for the nurse to teach patients who are prescribed any neuroleptic antipsychotic drug to avoid taking which over-the-counter medication?
    a. Acetaminophen (Tylenol)
    b. Acetylsalicylic acid (aspirin)
    c. Diphenhydramine (Benadryl)
    d. Pseudoephedrine (Sudafed)

21. A patient is prescribed haloperidol decanoate (Haldol) 2 mg IM every 4 weeks. What site is no longer recommended for intramuscular (IM) injection?
    a. Deltoid
    b. Dorsogluteal
    c. Vastus lateralis
    d. Ventrogluteal

＊22. Which laboratory test result would be of greatest priority to report to the prescriber of haloperidol (Haldol)?
a. BUN 18 mg/dL
b. FBS 286 mg/dL
c. Potassium 3.2 mg/dL
d. Triglycerides 97 mg/dL

23. It is important for the nurse to assess for excessive hunger, thirst, and urination if a patient is prescribed which drug(s)? (Select all that apply.)
a. Chlorpromazine (Thorazine)
b. Clozapine (Clozaril)
c. Haloperidol (Haldol)
d. Olanzapine (Zyprexa)

＊24. It would be a priority to report which assessment
▶   finding in a patient who is receiving clozapine (Clozaril)?
a. Blood pressure drop of 10 mm Hg systolic when changing from lying to standing position
b. Residual of 150 mL of urine after voiding
c. Temperature 104° F (40° C)
d. Weight gain of 2 lb in 1 month

▶25. What laboratory tests are important for the nurse to monitor when caring for a patient who is prescribed risperidone (Risperdal)? (Select all that apply.)
a. ALT
b. Cholesterol
c. Creatinine
d. Hemoglobin A1c
e. INR

DOSE CALCULATION QUESTIONS

26. Chlorpromazine 100 mg IM three times a day is ordered. The drug will be administered in the ventrogluteal muscle. The drug is available as 25 mg/mL. How many mL should be injected at a dose?

27. Intravenous benztropine (Cogentin) 1 mg is prescribed STAT for acute dystonia associated with a FGA. Benztropine is available as 1 mg/mL and can be administered undiluted over at least 1 minute. The nurse decides to be cautious and administer the drug over 2 minutes. How much drug should the nurse administer every 10 seconds?

CASE STUDY

An 82-year-old patient who resides in a nursing facility is admitted to the hospital with pneumonia. She becomes agitated and is not oriented to place. The on-call hospitalist is consulted.

1. Why is it important to inform the hospitalist about the presence or absence of a history of dementia?

Haloperidol 0.5 mg every 8 hours is prescribed as needed when nonpharmacologic measures cannot control agitation. Two hours after administering the drug orally, the nurse notes that the patient is moaning. Her eyes are rolled upward, and her back is arched.

2. What action should the nurse take first?

3. What other assessment data are important for the nurse to collect and communicate to the prescriber?

32
Antidepressants

STUDY QUESTIONS

Completion

1. The most common symptom of depression in addition to depressed mood is _____ _____ or _____ in usual activities and pastimes.

2. Due to the risk of suicide, close observation is important during the first few months of antidepressant therapy and _____ _____.

3. Maximum response to antidepressant drugs occurs in _____ to _____ weeks.

4. Relapse is more likely if a patient discontinues pharmacotherapy sooner than _____ to _____ months after symptoms resolve.

5. Tricyclic antidepressants (TCAs) are reserved for patients who have not responded to first-line drugs because they have _____ _____ _____.

6. Selective serotonin reuptake inhibitors (SSRIs) should be administered in the morning because they are _____ and can cause _____.

7. Overdose of TCAs can cause death because of effects on the _____.

8. When taken at doses and times as prescribed, _____ antidepressants can still cause hypertensive crisis and death.

9. Patients who are prescribed amitriptyline hydrochloride (Elavil) for depression should consult the prescriber or pharmacist before taking any over-the-counter _____ or _____ _____.

10. When a drug has the possible adverse effect of bruxism, the nurse should assess the patient for _____, _____ _____ and _____ _____.

11. Patients who are prescribed MAO inhibitors should not eat foods containing _____.

CRITICAL THINKING, PRIORITIZATION, AND DELEGATION QUESTIONS

✳12. When assessing a patient who is receiving an antidepressant, which question would be of greatest priority for the nurse to ask?
   a. "Are you concerned about weight gain when you take medications?"
   b. "Are you having thoughts about doing anything that could harm you?"
   c. "Do you experience dizziness when you stand up?"
   d. "Have you had any difficulty voiding?"

13. Patient compliance with antidepressant drug therapy is most likely to be increased if the nurse explains the
   a. possible drug interactions.
   b. reason for limiting the number of units of the drug supplied with each prescription.
   c. seriousness of the adverse effects.
   d. expected timing of the therapeutic response.

✳14. When a patient who is receiving an antidepressant verbalizes suicidal ideation, what is the priority nursing action?
   a. Administer the antidepressant.
   b. Ask the patient why he or she feels this way.
   c. Notify the prescriber.
   d. Provide a safe environment.

15. Which antihypertensive drugs could increase the risk of hyponatremia if prescribed in addition to fluoxetine (Prozac)?
   a. Candesartan
   b. Enalapril
   c. Hydrochlorothiazide
   d. Spironolactone

＊16. Which laboratory test result, if identified in a patient who is receiving fluoxetine and warfarin, would be a priority to report to the prescriber?
   a. AST 30 international units/L
   b. Creatinine 0.8 mg/dL
   c. INR 4.5
   d. Platelets 250,000/mm^3

17. The nurse should consult the prescriber regarding which order?
   a. Take fluoxetine (Prozac) 20 mg by mouth once a day at bedtime.
   b. Take mirtazapine (Remeron) 15 mg by mouth once a day at bedtime.
   c. Take fluoxetine (Sarafem) 20 mg by mouth days 14-28 of menstrual cycle.
   d. Discontinue fluoxetine (Prozac) today and start enteric-coated fluoxetine (Prozac Weekly) 90 mg by mouth once a week in 7 days.

18. The nurse would be especially vigilant to assess the patient for unexplained bleeding when a patient is prescribed fluoxetine and
   a. an antihistamine.
   b. lithium.
   c. low-dose aspirin therapy.
   d. a thiazide diuretic.

19. The nursery nurse sees that a neonate, whose mother has been taking venlafaxine (Effexor XR) for major depression throughout pregnancy, is tremulous and very irritable. Which assessment finding, noted when the neonate is crying, would be of most concern to the nurse?
   a. Difficulty calming
   b. Flexed extremities
   c. Pulse 186 beats/min
   d. Respirations 20/min

＊20. The nurse is reviewing laboratory test results for a patient whose drug regimen includes desvenlafaxine (Pristiq). Which result would be of greatest priority to report to the prescriber?
   a. eGFR 75 mL/min
   b. hCG 900 milli-international units/mL
   c. Osteoarthritic changes in the spine
   d. Sodium 135 mEq/L

21. Which of these conditions, if identified in the history of a patient prescribed duloxetine (Cymbalta), would be of concern to the nurse?
   a. Back pain
   b. Cirrhosis
   c. Diabetic neuropathy
   d. Stress urinary incontinence

22. A patient complains to the nurse that he has been experiencing erectile dysfunction since he was prescribed paroxetine (Paxil). What would be the nurse's best response?
   a. Encourage the patient to share this concern with the prescriber.
   b. Instruct the patient to not take the antidepressant on weekends.
   c. Suggest that the patient ask the prescriber to change his prescription to bupropion (Wellbutrin).
   d. Withhold the drug until the issue is resolved.

＊23. What is the priority assessment when a patient is switched from a TCA antidepressant to an MAO inhibitor?
   a. Blood glucose
   b. Blood pressure
   c. Skin color
   d. Skin hydration

24. What is a property of TCAs and SSRIs? (Select all that apply.)
   a. Effect on neurotransmitters occurs rapidly.
   b. Effect on neurotransmitters occurs slowly.
   c. Serious adverse effects can occur if combined with MAO inhibitor antidepressants.
   d. Therapeutic effects occur rapidly.
   e. Therapeutic effects occur slowly.

25. Which change, when assessing the BP of a patient who is prescribed a TCA, suggests significant orthostatic BP change and risk of fainting?
   a. BP 136/76 and P 74 sitting; BP 112/60 and P 98 standing
   b. BP 172/96 and P 84 sitting; BP 166/90 and P 78 standing
   c. BP 114/76 and P 74 sitting; BP 102/60 and P 78 standing
   d. BP 120/82 and P 84 sitting; BP 108/76 and P 80 standing

26. Which data would be of greatest concern when a patient is prescribed clomipramine (Anafranil)?
   a. Patient reports experiencing "yawngasm."
   b. Patient reports frequent palpitations and a racing heart.
   c. Patient reports that he burns easily when in the sun.
   d. Patient reports use of polyethylene glycol (MiraLAX) weekly due to constipation.

✳27. The nurse has received a start of shift report on patients who have recently been prescribed antidepressant medications and are experiencing the following adverse effects. Which patient is of highest priority for the nurse to assess?
   a. Amitriptyline—sleepiness and constipation
   b. Fluoxetine—nausea and diarrhea
   c. Tranylcypromine (Parnate)—headache and vomiting
   d. Venlafaxine—anorexia and sweating

28. Which foods can cause a hypertensive crisis when a patient is prescribed an MAOI? (Select all that apply.)
   a. Apples, pears
   b. Baked goods that contain yeast
   c. Bologna, pepperoni, salami
   d. Milk, yogurt, cottage cheese, cream cheese
   e. Soy sauce

29. Which instruction should be included when teaching a patient who is prescribed an MAOI about orthostatic BP?
   a. Avoid certain foods to prevent orthostatic hypotension.
   b. Change positions from lying to sitting and standing slowly.
   c. Drink at least two servings of caffeinated beverages each day to decrease the risk of orthostatic hypotension.
   d. Stop taking the drug if you experience dizziness when standing from a sitting position.

30. The nurse assesses for shivering and fever when a patient who is prescribed an MAOI is receiving which drug for postoperative pain?
   a. Butorphanol (Stadol)
   b. Hydrocodone/acetaminophen (Vicodin)
   c. Hydromorphone (Dilaudid)
   d. Meperidine (Demerol)

✳31. It would be of greatest priority to report which new condition to the prescriber of bupropion (Wellbutrin)?
   a. Anemia
   b. Diabetes mellitus
   c. Epilepsy
   d. Glaucoma

✳32. Which laboratory result would be of greatest concern to the nurse when a patient is receiving nefazodone?
   a. AST 356 international units/L
   b. BUN 22 mg/dL
   c. Na 146 mEq/L
   d. WBC 11,000/mm³

33. It is most important for the nurse to teach a patient who has been prescribed trazodone (Oleptro) to do what?
   a. Drink at least 2500 mL of fluid each day.
   b. Increase fluid and fiber in diet to prevent constipation.
   c. Report any symptoms of a urinary tract infection.
   d. Seek medical care if erection does not subside after four hours.

34. What should be included in teaching the patient who reveals that he or she self-medicates with St. John's wort?
   a. Inform all health care providers that she is using this drug.
   b. Research has proven the product is as effective as antidepressant drugs for mild depression.
   c. The substance has not been proven to be effective.
   d. The substance is completely safe because it is natural and not a drug.

DOSE CALCULATION QUESTIONS

35. Paroxetine (Paxil) CR 50 mg is prescribed once a day. Available are 25-mg and 62.5-mg CR tablets. What should the nurse administer?

36. Venlafaxine (Effexor XR) ER 150 mg is prescribed. The hospital pharmacy stocks 75-mg ER capsules. How many capsules should the nurse administer?

CASE STUDIES

Case Study 1

A 28-year-old patient, who is a high school science teacher with two children, comes to the community mental health center at her family's urging because of lack of interest in usual activities, difficulty concentrating, excessive sleepiness, and feeling "down" every day for the past 3 months. Desipramine (Norpramin) 50 mg at bedtime is prescribed.

1. Developmentally, what are the advantages of this particular TCA for this patient?

2. The patient is hopeful that the medication will help. She asks "If the drugs work, why do I have to meet with the doctor every week?" What is the basis of the response to this question?

3. What symptoms should the patient, family members, and/or caregivers be told to report?

4. The patient asks why the drug is supposed to be taken at bedtime. How should the nurse respond?

5. What teaching should the nurse provide regarding these common adverse effects of TCAs? (1) sedation; (2) orthostatic hypotension; (3) anticholinergic effects

6. The patient is concerned about cost because the prescriber has prescribed only 1 week's supply at a time. What would be the rationale for such a small prescription amount?

7. The patient is admitted for an inguinal herniorrhaphy. When providing history information, the patient states that she has been taking desipramine (Norpramin) 200 mg at bedtime for 3 months. She tells the nurse that some nights she forgets to take the medication, but does not feel bad the next day. She states that she thinks she must not need the medication any more. How should the nurse respond?

Case Study 2

An adolescent patient who has been irritable, refusing to go to school, or eat meals for several months is admitted to an adolescent psychiatric unit. Cognitive behavioral therapy is started and the psychiatrist prescribes fluoxetine (Prozac).

8. What precautions teaching would the nurse provide because of the risk of serotonin syndrome?

The patient's insurance allows only 10 days of inpatient hospitalization, and the patient is to be discharged to the care of his parents. All antidepressants have a boxed warning for suicide risk, especially in children and adolescents.

9. The nurse would caution the patient's parents that suicide risk is greatest at what point in antidepressant therapy?

10. What actions should be taken because of this risk?

11. What rationale would support the use of antidepressants in this case?

33

Drugs for Bipolar Disorder

STUDY QUESTIONS

True or False

For each of the following statements, enter T *for true or* F *for false.*

1. ___ All patients with bipolar disorder (BPD) alternate between mania and depression, but length of episodes vary.
2. ___ BPD is a chronic condition.
3. ___ BPD requires treatment for the rest of the patient's life.
4. ___ Manic episodes are always distressing to the patient with BPD.
5. ___ The cause of BPD is an unstable personality.
6. ___ The pathophysiology of BPD involves atrophy of brain regions involved with emotion.
7. ___ The drug divalproex sodium (valproate) can promote neuronal growth and survival in the subgenual prefrontal cortex.
8. ___ Antipsychotic drugs should not be used in BPD unless the patient has symptoms of psychosis.

CRITICAL THINKING, PRIORITIZATION, AND DELEGATION QUESTIONS

✳ 9. A patient is admitted with an acute mixed episode of BPD. The patient is started on divalproex sodium (valproate) and bupropion. What is the priority nursing concern?
   a. Electrolyte imbalances
   b. Hydration
   c. Safety
   d. Toxicity

▶10. When administering lithium carbonate, which would be the most appropriate nursing outcome?
   a. Does not verbalize flight of ideas
   b. Exhibits pressured speech
   c. Sits long enough to watch a television program
   d. Sleeps 8 hours per night

▶11. A nurse is reviewing laboratory tests of a patient receiving lithium carbonate for an acute episode of BPD. Which result should the nurse report to the prescriber immediately?
   a. ALT 30 international units/L
   b. Creatinine 2.7 mg/dL
   c. Sodium 132 mEq/L
   d. Potassium 4 mEq/L

▶12. The nurse is caring for an acutely ill patient who is prescribed lithium carbonate for BPD. Which treatment(s) could increase lithium levels and cause toxicity? (Select all that apply.)
   a. Colonic cleansing preparation for colonoscopy
   b. Frequent dressing change on a diabetic wound
   c. Hemodialysis
   d. Repeated hypoglycemic episodes with diaphoresis
   e. Respiratory tract suctioning

✳13. It would be a priority to consult the prescriber of lithium carbonate about monitoring lithium levels if the BPD patient is diagnosed with hypertension and prescribed what drug?
   a. Amlodipine
   b. Atenolol
   c. Hydrochlorothiazide
   d. Valsartan

▶14. When administering divalproex sodium, which observation(s) would be a reason to withhold the drug and contact the prescriber? (Select all that apply.)
   a. Constant midepigastric pain radiating to the back
   b. Nausea, vomiting, and very dark-colored urine
   c. Pale conjunctiva
   d. Petechial rash
   e. Warm or hot skin and fruity breath

＊15. A patient with BPD is prescribed carbamazepine 200 mg twice a day. Trough levels drawn 30 minutes before the next prescribed dose are 6 mcg/mL. What is the priority nursing action at this time?
a. Administer the drug as prescribed.
b. Assess for seizure activity.
c. Consult the prescriber.
d. Elevate the side rails of the bed for safety.

►16. The CBC on a patient who is scheduled to receive the first dose of carbamazepine includes hemoglobin 14.5 g/dL, platelets 170,000/mm^3, reticulocyte count 2%, and WBC 6600/mm^3. What should the nurse do?
a. Administer the drug as ordered.
b. Hold the medication and assess the patient.
c. Hold the medication and consult the prescriber.
d. Hold the medication and consult the prescriber STAT.

＊17. A patient with BPD is taking lamotrigine (Lamictal) and the nurse notes a rash along with vesicles in the patient's oral cavity. What is the priority nursing action at this time?
a. Administer the drug as ordered.
b. Hold the medication.
c. Hold the medication and consult the prescriber during rounds.
d. Hold the medication and consult the prescriber immediately.

DOSE CALCULATION QUESTIONS

18. Lithium carbonate 0.6 g three times a day is prescribed. How many capsules should be administered if 300-mg capsules are available?

19. Divalproex sodium is available as a syrup containing 250 mg/5 mL. How many mL should be administered if the prescribed dose is 375 mg three times a day?

CASE STUDY

A 35-year-old patient who has a history of BPD has stopped taking her prescribed divalproex sodium (valproate/Depakote). She is brought to the hospital because she has become increasingly hyperexcitable over the past 5 days. She has talked on the phone almost continuously because she says she is trying to start a business. She has called friends and relatives all over the country at all hours of the night to tell them her news. She went on a spending spree to buy new clothes and equipment for her business venture and accumulated almost $10,000 worth of bills before she was caught for writing bad checks. Her husband was called when she tried to purchase a car, and the bank reported that she had insufficient funds to cover the check. She was brought to the hospital in an acute manic state. On admission she moves about restlessly, waving her arms in a threatening manner while loudly berating her husband and the hospital staff. She demands to be released from "this jail" and curses the nurse who interviews her.

1. Why might this patient have stopped taking her medication?

2. Lithium carbonate 300 mg is prescribed 4 times a day. Why must lithium be taken in divided daily doses?

3. The patient complains that she cannot play cards or write a letter. What should the nurse do?

4. The nurse has explained to the patient and family the importance of monitoring plasma lithium levels every 2-3 days until therapeutic levels have been reached and maintained and every 1-3 months once maintenance level dose has been established. What should the nurse teach about other times that the patient should consult the prescriber about the need for additional monitoring?

5. What measures can the nurse teach the patient to prevent fluctuations in lithium levels?

6. What is the therapeutic range of plasma lithium for maintenance therapy, and at what point are lithium levels critical?

7. Adherence to drug therapy is often an obstacle to managing BPD. How can the nurse increase the likelihood of this patient taking her medication and participating in therapy as prescribed?

8. What teaching does the nurse need to provide to the patient and family relating to prescribed and over-the-counter drugs that relate to the patient's medical history?

9. What nonpharmacologic measures can the nurse teach the patient and family that may help modulate mood?

34
Sedative-Hypnotic Drugs

STUDY QUESTIONS

Matching

Match the effect of benzodiazepines with the affected area of the brain.

1. ____ Cerebral cortex and hippocampus
2. ____ Cortical areas
3. ____ Limbic system
4. ____ Supraspinal motor areas

    a. Anterograde amnesia and confusion
    b. Muscle relaxation
    c. Promote sleep
    d. Reduce anxiety

True or False

For each of the following statements, enter T for true or F for false.

Benzodiazepine-like drugs

5. ____ can intensify the effects of alcohol.
6. ____ are metabolized into an inactive compound.
7. ____ produce moderate muscle relaxation.
8. ____ are used to prevent seizures.
9. ____ prolong periods of uninterrupted sleep.
10. ____ promote falling asleep.
11. ____ have a rapid onset.

12. ____ reduce REM sleep.
13. ____ require reduced doses for people with liver impairment.
14. ____ can cause significant rebound insomnia if suddenly discontinued.

CRITICAL THINKING, PRIORITIZATION, AND DELEGATION QUESTIONS

15. What does the lipid-solubility of benzodiazepines do? (Select all that apply.)
    a. Causes induction of hepatic metabolizing enzymes
    b. Decreases the risk that the drug will cause congenital defects
    c. Extends plasma half-life
    d. Increases absorption
    e. Improves distribution to the CNS

▶ 16. What does the nurse know about most benzodiazepines?
    a. They are absorbed from the GI tract very slowly.
    b. They intensify the effects of GABA.
    c. Their metabolites are not pharmacologically active.
    d. They are short-acting.

▶ 17. A patient asks for a sleeping pill at 2200. She states that she can fall asleep but awakens during the night and has difficulty getting back to sleep. The medication administration record (MAR) lists triazolam (Halcion) 0.125 mg at hour of sleep (hs) as needed. What should the nurse do?
a. Administer the triazolam.
b. Administer the triazolam and communicate the need to assess for effectiveness during shift report.
c. Contact the prescriber and discuss the need for a slower-onset hypnotic.
d. Hold the triazolam because it is not effective in this situation.

✳ 18. The nurse in the emergency department administers progressive doses of flumazenil (Romazicon) to a patient who has overdosed on a benzodiazepine and alcohol. What is a nursing priority in this situation?
a. Ensuring adequate fluids
b. Monitoring breathing
c. Reducing anxiety
d. Monitoring renal function

✳ 19. What is the nursing priority when administering a long-acting benzodiazepine as prescribed?
a. Gastric distress
b. Potential for abuse
c. Respiratory depression
d. Safety

20. When caring in the morning for a patient who has received zolpidem (Ambien) for sleep the night before, the nurse would monitor for symptoms of which common adverse effect?
a. Dizziness
b. Hypertension
c. Sweating
d. Tremors

21. A patient falls asleep without difficulty but frequently awakens during the night. The nurse would consult the prescriber if which drug was prescribed for sleep? (Select all that apply.)
a. Eszopiclone (Lunesta)
b. Ramelteon (Rozerem)
c. Temazepam (Restoril)
d. Zaleplon (Sonata)
e. Zolpidem (Ambien CR)

22. Tolerance to barbiturates does not produce cross-tolerance to which substance?
a. Alcohol
b. Benzodiazepines
c. General anesthetics
d. Opiates

23. A child with a severe head injury is in a barbiturate-induced coma. The child's parents ask the nurse why he is being kept unconscious. They want the drug to be stopped so they can see if he will respond. The best explanation is that this therapy
a. decreases the brain's need for oxygen and glucose.
b. produces amnesia so the child will not remember the accident.
c. relaxes skeletal muscle so the patient is not uncomfortable.
d. stabilizes the patient's blood pressure and pulse.

24. The nurse should assess for which symptoms in a patient with a suspected barbiturate overdose?
a. Apnea and hyperthermia
b. Respiratory depression and constricted pupils
c. Hypertension and hypothermia
d. Hypotension and dilated pupils

✳ 25. A nursing priority for a patient during immediate care after overdose on a barbiturate is to monitor what?
a. Bowel sounds
b. Deep tendon reflexes
c. Peripheral pulses
d. Oxygen saturation

26. Patients with depression sometimes experience insomnia. The nurse recognizes that in addition to being a symptom of the disorder, insomnia is an adverse effect of some antidepressants. Which antidepressants are effective in treating depression-associated insomnia? (Select all that apply.)
a. Bupropion (Wellbutrin)
b. Doxepin (Silenor)
c. Fluoxetine (Prozac)
d. Fluvoxamine (Luvox)
e. Trazodone (Desyrel)

27. The lowest prescribed dose of doxepin for depression is approximately how many times greater than the highest dose of doxepin (Silenor) prescribed for insomnia?
a. 2
b. 3
c. 12
d. 20

28. An older adult patient occasionally uses diphen-hydramine (Sominex) for insomnia. What should the nurse include in patient education to prevent a very common adverse effect?
    a. Increase fiber in the diet.
    b. Limit fluid intake.
    c. Eat a low-fat diet.
    d. Take the medication with food.

29. The nurse is caring for a hospitalized patient who states that he has difficulty falling asleep when away from home. Which intervention should the nurse employ first?
    a. Assess for a possible reason for insomnia.
    b. Discuss the benefits of melatonin for insomnia.
    c. Medicate with prescribed as-needed zolpidem (Ambien).
    d. Offer a backrub.

30. Which statement(s) are true regarding use of melatonin for insomnia? (Select all that apply.)
    a. Research suggests melatonin is effective but may cause difficulty awakening.
    b. Melatonin is a dietary supplement and is not closely regulated.
    c. Melatonin relieved insomnia in a blinded study of insomniacs.
    d. Studies have shown that melatonin is effective in preventing jet lag.
    e. There is no guarantee that the product contains the amount of melatonin as listed on the label.

DOSE CALCULATION QUESTIONS

31. Zolpidem 10 mg as needed at hs is prescribed. Available are 5-mg immediate-release tablets. How many tablets would be administered at one dose?

32. Flumazenil (Romazicon) 0.2 mg is ordered for a patient with a benzodiazepine overdose, followed by a second dose of 0.3 mg 30 seconds later by intravenous push. The drug is available in 0.1 mg/mL. How much drug should the nurse administer for each dose?

CASE STUDIES

Case Study 1

An 18-year-old college student comes to the outpatient department of a local mental health center. She expresses worries about upcoming exams and states that she cannot sleep, cannot concentrate on her studies, has felt her heart pound, is dizzy, and has trouble catching her breath. These symptoms are unusual for her and began several weeks ago.

1. What additional data should the nurse collect about the patient's symptoms?

2. Why is it imperative that patients on benzodiazepines be cautioned against combining them with alcohol?

3. What information should be included in the nurse's health teaching plan for this patient?

Case Study 2

A patient who has been receiving benzodiazepine therapy for a long time has been notified that her insurance will no longer cover the medication.

4. What are possible effects of sudden discontinuation of the drug?

5. What can the nurse do to help this patient if she can no longer afford a drug to treat insomnia?

35

Management of Anxiety Disorders

STUDY QUESTIONS

True or False

For each of the following statements, enter T for true or F for false.

1. ____ Social anxiety, generalized anxiety, obsessive-compulsive, panic, and posttraumatic stress disorders are all primary anxiety disorders.
2. ____ Benzodiazepines are approved for use for three major anxiety disorders—generalized anxiety disorder, obsessive-compulsive disorder, and phobias.
3. ____ Cognitive behavioral therapy combined with drug therapy is effective for panic disorder.
4. ____ Depression often coexists with anxiety disorders.
5. ____ Generalized anxiety disorder (GAD) is an acute condition.
6. ____ Onset of relief from anxiety with lorazepam (Ativan) and buspirone (BuSpar) is rapid.
7. ____ Principal adverse effects of buspirone (BuSpar) include sedation and psychomotor slowing.
8. ____ Selective serotonin reuptake inhibitors (SSRIs) are effective against anxiety even when depression is not present.
9. ____ Supportive, cognitive behavioral, and/or relaxation therapy is usually all that is needed in mild to moderate anxiety disorders.
10. ____ Symptoms of situational anxiety may be intense, but they are temporary.

Completion

Fill in the blank with the disorder being described.

11. Anxiety when patient thinks he or she cannot leave a room or situation: _____

12. Chronic uncontrollable worrying: _____ _____ _____

13. Intense irrational fear of embarrassment:

_____ _____ _____

14. Persistent uncontrollable thinking and repetitive actions: _____ _____ _____

15. Reexperiencing, avoidance, and/or emotional, numbing, and hyperarousal: _____ _____ _____ _____

16. Sudden anxiety attacks that may include fear of dying or going crazy: _____ _____

CRITICAL THINKING, PRIORITIZATION, AND DELEGATION QUESTIONS

＊17. A nurse is admitting a patient who is scheduled for outpatient surgery. The patient was instructed to take her levothyroxine with a sip of water in the morning before coming to the hospital. The patient reveals that she was extremely anxious, so she also took a lorazepam, but only with the same sip of water "about 1 hour ago." Which nursing action would be the greatest priority?
    a. Assessing for abuse of benzodiazepines
    b. Determining if the patient signed the needed consents before coming to the hospital
    c. Ensuring that the patient understands the preoperative teaching
    d. Notifying anesthesia of the medications taken this morning

18. The nurse is preparing to administer buspirone (BuSpar) to a patient who has been taking the drug for 2 months. What do nursing considerations include?
    a. Importance of administering on an empty stomach
    b. Safety precautions because sedation is common
    c. Teaching to avoid drinking grapefruit juice
    d. Teaching to not discontinue this drug suddenly

19. A patient has been taking paroxetine (Paxil) for anxiety for 3 months. The nurse expects that the drug has been most effective in reducing which symptoms? (Select all that apply.)
    a. "Butterflies" in the stomach
    b. Palpitations
    c. Poor concentration
    d. Tension headache
    e. Worrying

*20. A patient with a history of GAD has been admitted with exacerbated COPD. It is of greatest priority to consult with the prescriber regarding continuation of which drug, if the patient has been taking the drug at home?
    a. Alprazolam
    b. Buspirone
    c. Duloxetine
    d. Paroxetine

21. The nurse is caring for a patient who has been diagnosed with panic disorder. Teaching should include which information?
    a. Avoid strenuous exercise because it increases anxiety.
    b. Drug therapy helps the patient be more comfortable with situations and places he or she has been avoiding.
    c. It is important to maintain adequate, regular sleep habits.
    d. Symptoms usually only last 1-2 hours.

22. It would be a priority for the nurse to report that a patient with panic attacks and depression has admitted to attempting suicide in the past if the patient were currently prescribed which drug?
    a. Clomipramine
    b. Clonazepam
    c. Fluoxetine
    d. Imipramine

*23. The priority outcome when teaching a patient about phenelzine prescribed for panic disorder with depression is that the patient will state the
    a. actions needed to prevent constipation.
    b. importance of avoiding aged cheese, meats, and fish.
    c. importance of exercise.
    d. possible adverse sexual effects.

24. The nurse notes that a patient becomes very upset when the nurse rearranges any object in the room. The nurse would expect to find which diagnosis in the patient's history?
    a. Obsessive-compulsive disorder
    b. Panic disorder
    c. Social anxiety disorder
    d. Situational anxiety

▶25. When the nurse administers sertraline (Zoloft) to a patient for social anxiety disorder, which outcome would indicate that therapy has achieved the desired effect?
    a. Patient goes on errands without experiencing palpitations, chest pain, dizziness, or fear of losing control.
    b. Patient presents teaching to nursing students.
    c. Patient rides in elevators without experiencing an anxiety attack.
    d. Patient touches people without fear of contamination.

26. Experiencing which event is most likely to precipitate posttraumatic stress disorder (PTSD)?
    a. Earthquake
    b. Flood
    c. Rape
    d. Tornado

DOSE CALCULATION QUESTIONS

27. Buspirone (BuSpar) 7.5 mg PO twice a day is ordered. Available are 5-mg tablets. How many tablets should the nurse administer per dose?

28. What is the safe dose range of lorazepam (Ativan) intravenous push for a 121-lb adult patient when the recommended dose is 0.02-0.06 mg/kg?

CASE STUDY

A 58-year-old woman with a history of 70 pack-years of tobacco use is admitted with exacerbated chronic obstructive pulmonary disease (COPD). The patient is very demanding. During care, the patient states that she constantly worries about things that might go wrong. She has not been sleeping and has difficulty completing daily tasks because of weakness and fatigue.

1. What should the nurse do first?

2. The nurse tries nonpharmacologic interventions to relieve the patient's anxiety without success. The prescriber orders alprazolam (Xanax) 0.5 mg 3 times a day. What should the nurse include in her teaching about this benzodiazepine drug?

3. The patient's daughter comes to visit and expresses concern about her mother receiving a benzodiazepine drug. She states that her mother has a history of alcohol abuse but has not had a drink for several years. How should the nurse respond to this information?

4. A consult is ordered, and the patient is diagnosed with GAD and history of alcohol abuse. Routine alprazolam (Xanax) is discontinued, and buspirone (BuSpar) 7.5 mg twice a day is ordered. Why is this drug a good choice for this patient?

5. The patient complains that the drug is not working like the Xanax. She asks if she can take an extra dose of buspirone (BuSpar). How should the nurse respond?

6. The patient is referred for cognitive behavioral therapy to augment drug therapy. What are the principles of this therapy?

36

Central Nervous System Stimulants and Attention-Deficit/Hyperactivity Disorder

STUDY QUESTIONS

Matching

Match the drug with its description.

1. ____ Amphetamine
2. ____ Dexmethylphenidate
3. ____ Lisdexamfetamine
4. ____ Methamphetamine
5. ____ Methylphenidate
6. ____ Methylxanthine
7. ____ Theophylline

a. Found in coffee, tea, soda, and energy drinks
b. The drug is not effective if injected or inhaled
c. A 50:50 mixture of dextroamphetamine and levamphetamine
d. Has stimulant effects but is used for bronchodilation
e. Approved for obesity, although not preferred treatment for the condition
f. The dosage is one-half the dosage of methylphenidate
g. Structurally dissimilar from the amphetamines but the pharmacologic actions are essentially the same

True or False

Indicate whether these statements relating to atomoxetine (Strattera) are true or false.

8. ___ It is approved for use for attention-deficit/hyperactivity disorder (ADHD) in adults.

9. ___ It has a moderate potential for abuse.

10. ___ It has a risk of liver injury.

11. ___ It takes 2-3 weeks before therapeutic effects develop.

12. ___ Patients doing well on stimulant drugs should be switched to Strattera because it is safer and more effective.

13. ___ Patients with an atypical form of the CYP2D6 metabolizing enzyme of cytochrome P450 need higher doses of the drug to be effective.

14. ___ Sexual dysfunction and urinary retention are possible adverse effects in adults.

CRITICAL THINKING, PRIORITIZATION, AND DELEGATION QUESTIONS

15. Central nervous system (CNS) stimulants are appropriately used for which conditions? (Select all that apply.)
    a. ADHD
    b. CNS depressant poisoning
    c. Depression
    d. Narcolepsy
    e. Diabetes

▶16. The elementary school nurse cares for a 5-year-old child who receives a CNS stimulant drug for ADHD. The child comes into the office complaining of not feeling well. Which assessment finding would be a concern?
    a. BP 120/84 mm Hg
    b. Heart rate 100 beats/min
    c. Respirations 25/min
    d. Weight gain of 2 lb since last year

17. A patient asks the nurse why her physician will not prescribe amphetamines to help her lose weight. She claims that her mother took them and lost weight. The nurse's response should be based on what knowledge about amphetamines?
    a. They are ineffective for weight loss.
    b. They can cause hypotension and bradycardia.
    c. They can cause physical and psychological dependence.
    d. They can unmask latent bipolar disorder.

▶18. A patient with a history of narcolepsy, treated with Dexedrine Spansules, is first day postoperative after a right knee replacement. He has become agitated and is refusing all treatments, including pain medications. He accuses the staff of trying to hurt him. What should the nurse do?
    a. Consult the attending physician.
    b. Administer doxapram.
    c. Continue nursing care; the symptoms will abate within hours.
    d. Restrain the patient so that he does not injure the surgical site.

19. A child who has been prescribed Metadate CD for ADHD is having difficulty swallowing the medication. What is a logical nursing action?
    a. Crush the medication and mix it in a small amount of applesauce.
    b. Notify the prescriber because the medication must be taken whole.
    c. Open the capsule and sprinkle the beads in a small amount of soft food, telling the child to be careful not to chew the beads.
    d. Open the capsule and dissolve the contents in liquid.

20. A fifth-grade student with ADHD has been prescribed Daytrana transdermal methylphenidate patch. He normally awakens at 7:30 AM, attends school from 8:30 AM until 2:45 PM, and does his homework as soon as he gets home from school. He goes to bed at 9:00 PM. The nurse will teach the parents that which is the best time to apply the patch?
    a. 5:30 AM
    b. 8:00 AM
    c. 4:00 PM
    d. 9:00 PM

21. The nurse teaches a parent to apply Daytrana transdermal methylphenidate patch to unbroken skin on which part of the child's body?
    a. Arm
    b. Back
    c. Buttock
    d. Hip

22. A nurse's aide is experiencing a headache aura. Caffeine often helps prevent a full-blown migraine. She asks the nurse which item has the most caffeine. What is the best response by the nurse?
    a. Cola, 12 oz
    b. Iced tea, 12 oz
    c. Chocolate bar, 1.5 oz
    d. Orange soda, 12 oz

23. Research suggests that caffeine consumption during human pregnancy is associated with
    a. birth defects.
    b. low birth weight.
    c. first trimester spontaneous abortion.
    d. preterm birth.

24. Modafinil (Provigil) has been prescribed for a 22-year-old woman who works rotating shifts. When teaching about this drug, the nurse should include which instruction?
    a. Not taking with food because absorption of the drug will decrease
    b. Orthostatic blood pressure precautions
    c. Taking immediately after waking because the drug can cause insomnia
    d. Using a second form of birth control if oral contraceptives are used

✶25. When a child is prescribed guanfacine or clonidine for ADHD, it is a priority to teach parents to report to the prescriber if the child experiences what?
    a. Difficulty completing homework
    b. Dizziness with position changes
    c. Weight gain of greater than 2 lb in 1 year
    d. Pulse less than 70 beats/min

DOSE CALCULATION QUESTIONS

26. The recommended initial dose of caffeine citrate (Cafcit) for neonatal apnea is 20 mg/kg IV administered over 30 minutes. Caffeine citrate (Cafcit) 60 mg has been prescribed for a neonate who weighs 6 lb 10 oz. Is the dose safe?

27. Caffeine citrate (Cafcit) comes in a concentration of 20 mg/mL. What is the infusion rate in drops per minute if 60 mg is to be administered over 30 minutes and the drip factor is 60 drops/mL?

CASE STUDIES

Case Study 1

The school nurse cares for a seventh-grade child who recently was diagnosed with ADHD, combined type. The parents rejected the diagnosis previously because they do not like the idea of their child using medication. The child is prescribed methylphenidate (Ritalin) 10 mg 3 times a day. The parents speak with the nurse when they deliver the medication and medication administration forms to the school. They verbalize concern that they will be "drugging" their son and ask why behavioral therapy would not be sufficient.

1. Based on current research, how will the nurse explain the rationale for drug therapy?

2. The nurse has been administering the second dose at 11:00 AM. The nurse is planning for the individual education plan (IEP) meeting with teachers, a counselor, and parents. She notes that the child has not been gaining weight. The child admits that he is not very hungry. In the meeting, the nurse learns that the parents give the child methylphenidate at 6:30 AM. The child eats his breakfast at school. The last dose is administered at 5:00 PM with dinner. What changes can be made to help improve the appetite of this child?

3. Most teachers at the IEP meeting share that the child's behavior has improved since starting medication. However, his organization and study skills are still very weak. Based on the expected therapeutic response to methylphenidate, what information can the nurse provide?

4. The fourth-period (10:15-11:00 AM) teacher states that the child is very sleepy in his class. What could be happening to cause this sleepiness?

5. Several weeks later, the child's parents come to see the nurse, stating that the pediatrician has recommended that their son be switched to Metadate CD 20 mg once a day. The parents are concerned because "This is a newer drug, and they don't know enough about it." How should the nurse respond?

6. The child does well at school on Metadate CD but has difficulty once home getting his homework done and socially at after-school activities. The prescriber puts the child on Concerta. How does the nurse explain the difference between Concerta and Metadate CD?

7. What teaching should be provided about administration of Concerta?

Case Study 2

A 25-year-old woman is seeking medical help for amphetamine dependence. She was prescribed amphetamines for weight loss several years ago and lost 100 lb. She is now 5 feet 6 inches tall and weighs 130 lb. She continued taking amphetamines after she reached her goal weight and now wants to stop taking the drug, but she says she cannot do it alone. When she stops taking the amphetamines, she experiences withdrawal symptoms and becomes frightened, so she continues to use the drug.

8. What signs and symptoms would you expect the patient to exhibit when she is using amphetamines?

9. It is important to decrease the amphetamine slowly since the patient has previously experienced withdrawal symptoms. What withdrawal symptoms should the nurse be alert for when a patient is withdrawing from amphetamine use, and what nursing interventions can help the patient cope with these symptoms?

37

Drug Abuse I: Basic Considerations

STUDY QUESTIONS

Completion

1. _____ is when a particular dose elicits a less intense response.

2. When a person is _____ _____ on a drug, withdrawal syndrome will develop if the drug is stopped.

3. _____ _____ is the intense subjective need for a drug.

4. When a person experiences _____ _____, symptoms are often opposite of the normal effects of the drug.

5. Higher doses of a drug are needed in _____ because the person has abused another drug, usually in the same class.

6. _____ is when one drug can prevent withdrawal from another drug.

7. _____ is the neurotransmitter involved in the reward circuit of the brain.

8. Drug addiction is a(n) _____, _____ illness.

CRITICAL THINKING, PRIORITIZATION, AND DELEGATION QUESTIONS

9. Which statements are true regarding addictive behavior? (Select all that apply.)
   a. It involves physical, psychological, or social harm.
   b. It involves reinforcement of pleasure or reduction in intensity of an unpleasant experience.
   c. It involves activation of the brain's endorphin reward circuit.
   d. It is a treatable disease.
   e. It is present if the patient is physically dependent on a psychoactive substance.

10. Psychological factors associated with tendencies toward drug abuse would make it important for the nurse to provide drug abuse prevention education to children who have been diagnosed with which condition? (Select all that apply.)
    a. Attention-deficit/hyperactivity disorder (ADHD)
    b. Anxiety
    c. Cerebral palsy
    d. Depression
    e. Developmental delay

11. An example of addiction is when an individual experiences withdrawal symptoms if he or she stops taking which substance?
    a. Amphetamines used to reduce symptoms of ADHD
    b. OxyContin used for cancer pain
    c. Phenobarbital used to prevent seizures
    d. Tobacco used to reduce stress

12. Drugs that the nurse can administer and that have the highest potential for abuse and dependence are classified by the Controlled Substances Act as which schedule?
    a. Schedule I
    b. Schedule II
    c. Schedule III
    d. Schedule IV
    e. Schedule V

13. A patient has been prescribed hydrocodone 5 mg and acetaminophen 500 mg (Vicodin), a schedule IV drug. What do federal regulations state regarding refills of this drug?
    a. It cannot be refilled.
    b. It may be refilled two times within 3 months.
    c. It may be refilled five times within 6 months.
    d. It may be refilled as many times as the prescriber specifies within 12 months.

14. When there are different laws on the state and federal levels regarding prescribing controlled substances, which law takes precedence?
    a. The most restrictive law
    b. The least restrictive law
    c. The federal law
    d. The state law

CASE STUDY

The nurse is working on a drug and alcohol detoxification unit. Describe how the nurse's expertise can be applied to address the following issues of drug abuse.

1. Diagnosis and treatment of toxicity

2. Diagnosis and treatment of secondary medical complications

3. Facilitating withdrawal

4. Educating and counseling drug abusers in hope of maintaining long-term abstinence

38

Drug Abuse II: Alcohol

STUDY QUESTIONS

True or False

For each of the following statements, enter T *for true or* F *for false.*

1. ___ Pattern of drinking alcohol is more important than type of alcohol when evaluating cardiovascular effects.
2. ___ Moderate alcohol consumption may decrease the risk of type 1 diabetes mellitus (T1DM).
3. ___ Alcohol consumption speeds the development of osteoporosis.
4. ___ A person with COPD should never drink alcohol because even 1-2 drinks can slow respirations.
5. ___ It is common for alcoholics to take antacids on a regular basis.
6. ___ Chronic alcohol drinkers develop hepatitis more often than cirrhosis.
7. ___ Diuresis that occurs with alcohol consumption occurs because of increased release of antidiuretic hormone (ADH).
8. ___ Alcohol enhances sexual desire and performance.
9. ___ Moderate alcohol intake is a risk factor for several common cancers.
10. ___ Valid research suggests drinking a maximum of 1-2 drinks a week is safe during pregnancy.
11. ___ Alcohol is an effective treatment for insomnia.
12. ___ Drinking one alcoholic beverage with a meal can promote gastric functioning.

Matching

Match the substance with the effect when combined with alcohol.

13. ___ High alcohol intake counteracts effects.
14. ___ Increases risk of injury to GI mucosa.
15. ___ Increases risk of liver damage.
16. ___ Intensifies CNS depression.
17. ___ Produces nausea and vomiting; can produce death.

   a. Acetaminophen
   b. Antihypertensives
   c. Benzodiazepines
   d. Disulfiram
   e. Nonsteroidal anti-inflammatory drug (NSAID)

CRITICAL THINKING, PRIORITIZATION, AND DELEGATION QUESTIONS

18. The nurse is caring for a patient with a history of chronic alcohol abuse. The patient is prescribed thiamin to prevent Wernicke's encephalopathy. The nurse should assess for which symptoms of this disorder? (Select all that apply.)
   a. Abnormal ocular movements
   b. Confabulation
   c. Confusion
   d. Inability to convert short-term memory to long-term memory
   e. Nystagmus

19. Research on older adults suggests that consumption of one alcoholic drink per day has been associated with what?
   a. Atrophy of the cerebrum
   b. Lower levels of high-density lipoproteins (HDLs)
   c. Improving the quality of sleep
   d. Preservation of cognitive functioning

20. Research suggests that alcohol consumption has positive effects in which situations?
   a. A woman who eats nutritious foods, exercises regularly, and has a drink in the evening 1-2 times a week
   b. A man who has a drink with dinner 3-4 times a week
   c. A person who drinks 5-6 drinks 1-2 times a month
   d. A person who drinks 1-2 drinks to prevent hypothermia when outside in the cold

▶21. A patient who has been a heavy drinker for 30 years is admitted with constant, severe midepigastric pain radiating to the flank. It would be a priority for the nurse to report which laboratory test result to the prescriber?
a. Amylase 500 international units/L
b. BNP 33 pg/mL
c. Bilirubin 1 mg/dL
d. Protein 6.5 g/dL

22. For the average person with normal liver functioning, alcohol levels in the blood will begin to increase if a person consumes which drink in 1 hour? (Select all that apply.)
a. One Long Island iced tea
b. One 1.5-oz shot of whiskey
c. One 8-oz glass of wine
d. One 24-oz glass of beer
e. One 8-oz wine cooler

23. Chronic alcohol consumption does not produce tolerance to which condition?
a. Activation of the reward circuit
b. Decreased alertness
c. Diminished reflexes
d. Respiratory depression

24. Which benzodiazepine regimen has been shown to protect against seizures and breakthrough symptoms of alcohol withdrawal while promoting speedier withdrawal?
a. Administered as needed in response to symptoms
b. Administered as needed in response to symptoms in combination with another drug to reduce withdrawal symptoms
c. Administered around the clock on a fixed schedule
d. Administered around the clock in declining doses on a fixed schedule

25. Which symptoms suggest the most serious effect when a patient is admitted after taking disulfiram (Antabuse) and then drinking several bottles of beer?
a. Dizziness and palpitations
b. Flushing and sweating
c. Nausea and vomiting
d. Thirst and headache

26. Disulfiram (Antabuse) reactions can occur if a patient is exposed to alcohol and takes which antimicrobial medication?
a. Azithromycin (Zithromax)
b. Gentamicin (Garamycin)
c. Metronidazole (Flagyl)
d. Cefazolin (Ancef)

27. A patient is admitted with a fractured hip and scheduled for surgery. Why is it important to inform the surgeon of the patient's history of alcohol abuse and use of naltrexone (ReVia) to assist with abstinence?
a. There are specific analgesic drugs that the patient should not receive.
b. The patient is at risk for addiction to opioids used for postoperative pain.
c. The patient should not receive any opioid analgesics for postoperative pain.
d. Usual doses of opioid analgesics for postoperative pain may be ineffective.

28. Why does naltrexone for IM injection need to be administered only once a month?
a. It has a long half-life.
b. It is lipid-soluble.
c. It is slowly absorbed from the muscle.
d. This prevents adverse effects.

＊29. Which teaching would be of greatest priority when a patient is prescribed acamprosate (Campral)?
a. The importance of seeking help if thoughts of self-harm occur
b. That the full effects do not occur for about a week
c. That the patient must increase fluid and fiber in the diet if diarrhea occurs
d. The importance of including psychosocial support in therapy

30. Dietary counseling for a patient with alcohol abuse should include adequate servings of what type of food to prevent thiamin deficiency?
a. Citrus fruits
b. Green, leafy vegetables
c. Low-fat milk
d. Pork products

DOSE CALCULATION QUESTIONS

31. Disulfiram (Antabuse) 125 mg orally at bedtime is prescribed for a patient motivated to abstain from alcohol. Available are 250-mg tablets. The nurse will teach the patient to self-administer how many tablets per dose?

32. Diazepam (Valium) 10 mg intravenous push is prescribed for a patient in alcohol withdrawal. Available is 5 mg/mL to be administered over 3 minutes. To make it easier to inject the drug over this period of time, the nurse decides to dilute the drug to a total of 3 mL. How much diluent should the nurse add to the drug solution in the syringe to achieve a total of 3 mL?

CASE STUDIES

Case Study 1

The nurse is caring for a 45-year-old man with a history of alcohol abuse and cirrhosis of the liver who is newly admitted with gastrointestinal bleeding from ulcers.

1. What would be appropriate nursing diagnoses and related assessments for this patient?

2. The patient's blood alcohol level is 0.320%. Chlordiazepoxide (Librium) was ordered at 100 mg IM STAT followed by high doses via the oral route with the dose decreasing every 3 days. What is the rationale for this treatment regimen?

3. What would be an appropriate nursing outcome for this patient relating to the reason for administering chlordiazepoxide (Librium)?

4. The patient has been admitted once before for detoxification. He was discharged at that time on a maintenance dose of chlordiazepoxide (Librium). Based on the believed effects of alcohol on the CNS, why would this patient revert back to alcohol abuse?

5. After detoxification the patient states he is motivated to quit. He asks for disulfiram (Antabuse) to help him refrain from drinking. What teaching should the nurse provide to the patient and family about this drug?

Case Study 2

Senior-level student nurses have just finished clinical hours in a local hospital emergency department (ED) and are having a postconference. They are discussing a 21-year-old male patient who was brought in during their shift and was resuscitated in the ED after acute overdose of alcohol. A fellow college student accompanying the patient reported that he had drunk four shots in 15 minutes while playing a drinking game. The students had not eaten anything for more than 3 hours before starting the game.

6. The nursing students identify which priority nursing problem for this patient at this time?
    a. Airway clearance
    b. Anxiety
    c. Knowledge deficit
    d. Sensory perceptual alterations

7. The parents of the patient arrived at the ED. The patient's father asked how this could happen. He states that he has had more than five drinks in an evening and has been fine. What factors should the nurse identify as having contributed to the patient's extreme intoxication?

8. Why would discussion about alcohol's effects on the heart, liver, stomach, and kidneys not be likely to motivate this patient to abstain from alcohol?

9. Developmentally, discussion of what adverse effects of alcohol might motivate this young man to drink responsibly?

39

Drug Abuse III: Nicotine and Smoking

STUDY QUESTIONS

True or False

For each of the following statements, enter T for true or F for false.

1. ____ Tobacco is a product that, when used exactly as directed, kills adults and children.
2. ____ Medical costs from smoking are greater than nonmedical costs such as lost time at work and disability.
3. ____ The prevalence of smoking in the USA in the 21st century is approximately 30%.
4. ____ Tobacco smoke contains nicotine, carbon monoxide, hydrogen cyanide, ammonia, nitrosamines, and tar.
5. ____ Nicotine in cigar smoke is absorbed primarily from the mouth.
6. ____ It takes approximately 5 minutes for the nicotine from inhaled smoke to reach the brain of a fetus.
7. ____ Nicotine elevates BP and heart rate in new and chronic smokers.
8. ____ Nicotine slows gastric motility, which is why new smokers often vomit.
9. ____ The effects of nicotine on the pleasure system are mild compared to the effects of cocaine and amphetamines.
10. ____ Nicotine replacement is safer than tobacco smoke during pregnancy.
11. ____ Research suggests that gradual reduction in tobacco use prolongs withdrawal symptoms.
12. ____ Nicotine is the active ingredient in some insecticides.
13. ____ The risk of COPD and death from myocardial infarction equals that of those who have never smoked 20 years after quitting.
14. ____ Health care providers can predict which smoking cessation product will be best for a particular patient.
15. ____ Counseling increases the chance that smoking cessation drugs will be effective.
16. ____ E-cigarettes are effective devices to promote smoking cessation.
17. ____ The most troubling side effects of Varenicline [Chantix, Champix] are mood changes, erratic behavior, and suicidality.

CRITICAL THINKING, PRIORITIZATION, AND DELEGATION QUESTIONS

18. A 9-month-old child is admitted to the emergency department after eating a cigarette. Which assessment finding would be of most concern to the nurse?
    a. Apical pulse 145 beats/min
    b. Blood pressure 66/48 mm Hg
    c. Respirations 15/min
    d. Temperature 37° C

19. Which nicotine product produces the most similar effect on the pleasure system as tobacco use?
    a. Chewing gum
    b. Lozenges
    c. Nasal spray
    d. Transdermal patch

20. Which statement, if made by a patient who is planning to use nicotine gum for smoking cessation, suggests the need for more teaching?
    a. "Chewing releases the nicotine."
    b. "I might burp more often when using the gum."
    c. "I should chew soon after eating to avoid upset stomach."
    d. "I should chew the gum slowly."

21. When using a transdermal patch, what should the person attempting smoking cessation be instructed to do?
    a. Change the patch daily following brand instructions.
    b. Change the site of application once a week.
    c. Report mild redness and itching at the patch site if present when the patch is removed.
    d. Shave the area before applying the patch.

22. The nurse is teaching a patient how to use a nicotine nasal spray. The nurse teaches the patient to do what? (Select all that apply.)
    a. Administer 2 sprays per dose.
    b. Administer up to 5 doses per hour.
    c. Administer up to 60 doses per day.
    d. Direct the spray away from the nasal septum.
    e. Use the hand that is opposite the nostril.

23. The nurse will withhold which smoking cessation drug and contact the prescriber if the patient exhibits seizure activity?
    a. Bupropion (Zyban, Wellbutrin)
    b. Nicotine patch (Nicotrol, Nicoderm CQ)
    c. Nicotine lozenge (Commit)
    d. Nortriptyline (Aventyl, Pamelor)

＊24. Which is the greatest teaching priority for a patient who has been prescribed varenicline (Chantix)?
    a. How to manage dry-mouth symptoms
    b. To increase fiber in diet to reduce the risk of constipation
    c. That the drug will decrease the pleasurable effect of nicotine from tobacco use
    d. To report thoughts of self-harm

25. Why should e-cigarettes not be used for smoking cessation? (Select all that apply.)
    a. The doses of nicotine vary.
    b. Products of known safety are available.
    c. Their vapor contains contaminants.
    d. They are not regulated by the FDA.
    e. They are proven to be ineffective.

DOSE CALCULATION QUESTIONS

26. Bupropion (Zyban) 450 mg SR is prescribed. Bupropion (Zyban) 150 mg SR is available. How many tablets should the nurse administer?

27. Varenicline (Chantix) 500 mcg is prescribed for the first 3 days of smoking cessation therapy. Available are 0.5-mg tablets. How many tablets should the patient self-administer?

40
Drug Abuse IV: Major Drugs of Abuse Other Than Alcohol and Nicotine

STUDY QUESTIONS

True or False

For each of the following statements, enter T *for true or* F *for false.*

1. ____ Nurses should teach hospitalized patients who are prescribed opioids for pain relief to not take the drug unless the pain is unbearable, to prevent the risk of addiction to the opioid.

2. ____ Nurses are at greater risk for opioid abuse than teachers, engineers, or architects.

3. ____ Heroin is the most commonly abused opioid among street users.

4. ____ A person who tries heroin for the first time is at greater risk for respiratory depression than a person who has used the heroin for years.

5. ____ Research suggests that new OxyContin OP tablets are less likely to be abused than the older OC formulation.

6. ____ Meperidine causes less miosis than most other abused opioids.

7. ____ Opioid drug abusers must be hospitalized during withdrawal because opioid withdrawal syndrome can be life-threatening.

8. ____ A patient who is stable after receiving a dose of naloxone (Narcan) for a life-threatening overdose of heroin is still at risk for fatal respiratory depression.

9. ____ Buprenorphine is only available through certified opioid treatment programs.

10. ____ Naltrexone is a drug that blocks the desired effects of opioids that can be administered as a depot injection once a month.

11. ____ Methadone therapy should not be offered to a patient who admits that he or she is not interested in detoxification at this time.

12. ____ Sudden withdrawal of opioids is more likely to cause severe symptoms and possible death than sudden withdrawal of barbiturates.

13. ____ A person who has required increased doses of barbiturates will also need higher doses of morphine in order to achieve adequate pain relief after surgery.

14. ____ During surgery, a person who has developed tolerance to barbiturates might be awake and experiencing pain despite anesthesia but be unable to speak or move due to muscle paralysis.

15. ____ Naloxone can reverse the physical effects of opioids, barbiturates, cocaine, and methamphetamines.

16. ____ Research suggests that psychological dependence on methamphetamines is greater than physical dependence.

17. ____ Marijuana has several approved medical uses.

18. ____ Marijuana increases the incidence of psychotic episodes in people diagnosed *or* not diagnosed with schizophrenia.

19. ____ Chronic use of LSD produces tolerance and physical dependence.

20. ____ LSD can cause permanent visual disturbances.

21. ____ Deaths associated with LSD are primarily related to the effect on the heart.

22. ____ Dissociative drugs were developed for use in surgery.

23. ____ Phencyclidine (PCP) can prevent muscle contraction and cause hypothermia.

24. ____ There is no known effective treatment for PCP overdose.

CRITICAL THINKING, PRIORITIZATION, AND DELEGATION QUESTIONS

✳25. What is the priority concern when caring for an opioid addict who is experiencing withdrawal syndrome?
   a. Central nervous system (CNS) depression
   b. Preventing respiratory arrest
   c. Relapse to opioid use
   d. Timing of doses of nalmefene (Revex)

✳26. A patient who has a history of heroin abuse is brought into the emergency department (ED) unresponsive with pinpoint pupils. The nurse assesses that the patient has stopped breathing. In addition to supporting respirations, the patient is prescribed intravenous (IV) naloxone HCl (Narcan). The nurse notes an improvement in level of consciousness, respiratory rate, and effort within minutes of administration of naloxone. What is the priority action by the nurse 30-40 minutes after administration of the drug?
   a. Assessing the patient for withdrawal symptoms
   b. Identifying the abused opioid
   c. Monitoring of pulse and blood pressure
   d. Reassessing for respiratory depression

▶27. Which would be the most accurate indicator to the nurse that the dose of methadone prescribed to minimize withdrawal syndrome is inadequate?
   a. The patient has difficulty arising in the morning.
   b. The patient is experiencing daily vomiting and diarrhea.
   c. The patient is exhibiting fatigue throughout the day.
   d. The patient states that the dose is inadequate.

▶28. Which statement, if made by a patient who has been prescribed clonidine to assist with withdrawal from addiction to oxycodone (OxyContin), would indicate a need for further teaching?
   a. "I'm glad that I won't feel like I need the drug."
   b. "I need to be careful not to jump up out of bed too quickly."
   c. "I should have less muscle pain if I take this drug."
   d. "The medication should help prevent vomiting and diarrhea."

29. A patient has been prescribed sublingual buprenorphine-naloxone (Suboxone) for long-term management of heroin addiction. What would occur if the patient crushed, dissolved, and injected the drug IV?
   a. An overdose
   b. Heroin-induced euphoria
   c. Respiratory depression
   d. Withdrawal symptoms

30. What has been associated with maintenance therapy with methadone?
   a. Early death
   b. Inability to form relationships with other people
   c. Lack of productivity at work
   d. No significant impairment in health

✳31. A patient with a suspected barbiturate overdose is brought into the ED unresponsive with pinpoint pupils. What is the nursing intervention of greatest priority?
   a. Administering phenobarbital
   b. Maintaining respirations
   c. Preventing withdrawal symptoms
   d. Starting an intravenous line

▶32. When responding to acute overdose of cocaine, which outcome would best indicate that therapy has been successful?
   a. Blood pressure 110/70-145/90 mm Hg
   b. No adventitious lung sounds
   c. Sensory perceptions normal
   d. Temperature 98° F to 99° F

▶33. The nurse is caring for a patient whose assessment findings include T 99.4° F, BP 178/102 mm Hg, P 110 beats/min, respirations 25/min, rhinorrhea, and coryza. The patient admits to a history of amphetamine abuse. Which drug should not be administered to this patient?
   a. Chlorpheniramine (Chlor-Trimeton)
   b. Diphenhydramine (Benadryl)
   c. Guaifenesin (Humibid)
   d. Pseudoephedrine (Sudafed)

34. A patient has been admitted with adverse effects of taking MDMA (ecstasy). Which assessment finding would warrant consulting the physician regarding possible administration of dantrolene?
   a. Extreme anxiety and confusion
   b. Hallucinations and delusions
   c. Spasmodic jerking and elevated temperature
   d. Suicidal thoughts and behavior

35. Which condition would increase the risk of serious adverse effects if the patient used ecstasy?
   a. Anxiety
   b. Attention deficit/hyperactivity disorder
   c. Anorexia
   d. Obsessive-compulsive disorder

36. Which are potential effects of high doses of dextromethorphan found in cough medications? (Select all that apply.)
   a. Disorientation
   b. Euphoria
   c. Hallucinations
   d. Paranoia
   e. Sedation

▶37. Which nursing concern is appropriate when a patient has taken excessive amounts of amyl nitrate?
   a. Confusion
   b. Constipation
   c. Fluid volume deficit
   d. Safety

38. Which vital sign finding suggests that a 14-year-old patient may have inhaled (huffed) nail polish remover?
   a. BP 135/82 mm Hg
   b. P 48 beats/min
   c. R 16/min
   d. T 102.2° F (39° C)

DOSE CALCULATION QUESTIONS

39. A patient with known opioid addiction is prescribed buprenorphine/naloxone, 4 mg/1 mg sublingual. Available are buprenorphine/naloxone 2 mg/0.5 mg sublingual tablets. How many tablets should be administered?

40. Dantrolene (Dantrium) 1 mg/kg is prescribed for an 80-kg patient experiencing malignant hyperthermia associated with MDMA use. The drug is available as 20 mg/mL. The drug is prescribed to be administered by IV push over 2 minutes. How many mL should the nurse administer?

CASE STUDY

At an outpatient substance abuse support group, a new member shares her story of drug abuse. She began drinking in high school and by tenth grade was getting drunk several times a week. She married an alcoholic and drank with him for many years. She then began taking diazepam (Valium) with her alcohol. She says she had hangovers in the mornings, so she would have a beer or two and some amphetamines to "get myself together." She would also take a few aspirins for the headache and go to work feeling sick. As a rule, she would leave work at 5:00 PM, stop by the liquor store, and then go home to watch TV, drink, and take a few diazepam to calm down. After a few years of this, she began to buy crack cocaine. She was unable to do her job because she was either high or was in need of a fix, so she was fired. She stayed home and drank and found she was having difficulty buying drugs. She would get into violent arguments with her husband. He physically abused her, and she finally left him and sought help at a women's shelter. She tried to stop using drugs many times over the years, but could only stop for a few days before she began to feel ill. She started stealing to support her habit. After being arrested for stealing, she was required to enter a treatment program.

1. How has tolerance and physical dependence contributed to this person's drug abuse?

2. What assessments should the nurse perform to assess for drug withdrawal?

3. What interventions might the nurse employ to decrease the adverse effects of withdrawal?

41
Diuretics

STUDY QUESTIONS

Matching

Match the terms and descriptors.

1. ____ Most significant regulator of urine composition
2. ____ Moves passively following osmotic gradient
3. ____ Filtered then reabsorbed by active transport
4. ____ Nonselective process that does not regulate urine composition
5. ____ Uses pumps selective for organic acids and organic bases for active transport

    a. Filtration
    b. Reabsorption
    c. Active tubular secretion
    d. Solutes
    e. Water

True or False

For each of the following statements, enter T for true or F for false.

This food is a good source of potassium when a patient is receiving a potassium-excreting diuretic.

6. ____ Bananas
7. ____ Beans
8. ____ Cheese
9. ____ Red meat
10. ____ Oranges
11. ____ Pork
12. ____ Raisins
13. ____ Spinach
14. ____ Yogurt

Completion

15. The kidney produces approximately _____ mL of filtrate each day.

16. The normal amount of urine excreted in 24 hours is _____ mL.

17. Most diuretics work by blocking _____ and _____ reabsorption.

18. Diuretics that produce the most significant diuresis affect reabsorption in the

    _____ _____
    of the _____
    _____ of the
    _____ _____
    _____ .

19. Diuretics can affect blood levels of

    _____, _____,
    _____, _____,
    _____, _____,
    _____, _____,
    _____, _____,
    and _____ .

CRITICAL THINKING, PRIORITIZATION, AND DELEGATION QUESTIONS

20. Antidiuretic hormone affects kidney reabsorption of which substance?
    a. Glucose
    b. Potassium
    c. Sodium
    d. Water

▶ 21. A liter of water weighs approximately 1 kg. A patient with heart failure (HF) who weighs 176 lb has been prescribed a high-ceiling diuretic with the goal of loss of 1000 mL of additional urine output in the next 24 hours. The next morning, if this goal is met, the nurse would expect the patient's weight to be what?
    a. 170 lb
    b. 172 lb
    c. 174 lb
    d. 175 lb

22. A patient in chronic renal failure has been retaining fluid despite dialysis. Which diuretic would the nurse expect to administer?
    a. Bumetanide
    b. Hydrochlorothiazide (Oretic, HydroDIURIL)
    c. Metolazone (Zaroxolyn)
    d. Spironolactone (Aldactone)

23. Which food is a good source of potassium when a patient is prescribed a potassium-wasting diuretic? (Select all that apply.)
    a. Baked potato
    b. Cantaloupe
    c. Pork
    d. Raisins
    e. Spinach

▶ 24. A patient with left-sided HF has been prescribed a high-ceiling diuretic. Which assessment most accurately reflects a therapeutic effect of this drug?
    a. Drop in systolic blood pressure of 10 mm Hg
    b. Normal heart sounds
    c. Clear lung sounds
    d. Pulse 80 and regular

▶ 25. A patient who has been diagnosed with HF and type 2 diabetes mellitus (T2DM) has been prescribed furosemide (Lasix) 20 mg by mouth once a day. Based on the effect of furosemide on the patient's T2DM, it is important for the nurse to assess this patient for which symptoms?
    a. Irritability, paresthesias, and muscle weakness
    b. Diaphoresis, shakiness, and tachycardia
    c. Increased thirst; confusion; and dry, hot skin
    d. Nausea, vomiting, and diarrhea

✱ 26. The nurse takes orthostatic BP readings before administering diuretics to a group of patients. It would be a priority to teach orthostatic BP precautions to a patient with which orthostatic blood pressure readings?
    a. 150/90 mm Hg lying; 125/70 mm Hg sitting
    b. 140/82 mm Hg lying; 125/72 mm Hg sitting
    c. 130/90 mm Hg lying; 118/78 mm Hg sitting
    d. 116/70 mm Hg lying; 110/68 mm Hg sitting

27. Which laboratory test results should the nurse monitor when a patient is prescribed a high-ceiling diuretic? (Select all that apply.)
    a. Electrolytes
    b. Glucose
    c. LDL/HDL
    d. Uric acid
    e. WBC

✱ 28. A patient has been prescribed furosemide (Lasix). Which symptom is a priority for the nurse to monitor that suggests possible excessive loss of potassium?
    a. Hunger and fatigue
    b. 4+ deep tendon reflexes
    c. Muscle weakness and cramping
    d. Tall, tented T waves on ECG

29. Which over-the-counter medication can counteract the effects of diuretics?
    a. Acetaminophen
    b. Ibuprofen
    c. Iron
    d. Multiple vitamins

30. What is the recommended diuretic for initial therapy of essential hypertension?
    a. High-ceiling diuretic
    b. Osmotic
    c. Potassium-sparing diuretic
    d. Thiazide

31. Which symptoms suggest ototoxicity when a patient has been prescribed a high-ceiling diuretic?
    a. Photophobia
    b. Telangiectasia
    c. Tinnitus
    d. Xeroderma

▶ 32. The nurse is reviewing the lab values for a patient who has been prescribed lithium carbonate for bipolar disorder and furosemide for heart failure (HF). Which result would be a reason for concern?
    a. Chloride 100 mEq/L
    b. Magnesium 1.8 mEq/L
    c. Potassium 4.1 mEq/L
    d. Sodium 128 mEq/L

33. Which new symptom suggests hypomagnesemia when a patient is prescribed a thiazide or high-ceiling diuretic?
    a. Confusion
    b. Muscle weakness and tremor
    c. Systolic BP drop of 20 mm Hg
    d. Swollen and painful big toe

34. A patient who is prescribed valsartan (Diovan) does not mention that she is taking Yasmin, an oral contraceptive that contains the potassium-saving ingredient drospirenone. She is admitted to the ED with chest pain. Which ECG finding suggests that the combination of drugs is causing hyperkalemia?
    a. Prolonged ST interval
    b. Tall, tented T waves
    c. Depressed ST segments
    d. Extra P waves

▶35. Which laboratory result should be reported to the prescriber if a diabetic patient is prescribed hydrochlorothiazide 50 mg once a day and metformin/glyburide (Glucovance) 500 mg/2.5 mg twice a day?
    a. FBS 90 mg/dL
    b. A1c 8.2%
    c. Potassium 4 mEq/L
    d. Sodium 136 mg/dL

✳36. A 20-year-old patient has been prescribed spironolactone (Aldactone) for primary polycystic ovary syndrome (POS). Developmentally, what would be a priority nursing diagnosis?
    a. Activity intolerance related to loss of sodium
    b. Altered body image related to hirsutism and deepening of the voice
    c. Decisional conflict related to treatment options
    d. Fluid volume excess related to excessive salt intake

37. The nurse is preparing to administer mannitol (Osmitrol) to a patient. The nurse notes crystals in a clear solution. What should the nurse do first?
    a. Administer the solution.
    b. Discard the solution.
    c. Use an inline filter.
    d. Warm the solution to dissolve the crystals.

38. Because of the risk of hyperkalemia, the nurse consults the prescriber and monitors potassium levels if a patient is prescribed spironolactone and a drug with which suffix? (Select all that apply.)
    a. -floxacin
    b. -olol
    c. -pril
    d. -sartan
    e. -statin

✳39. It is a priority for the nurse to question a patient about which home feature when a patient has been prescribed a diuretic?
    a. Central air
    b. Forced air furnace
    c. Water softener
    d. Well or city water

DOSE CALCULATION QUESTIONS

40. Furosemide (Lasix) 40 mg orally once a day is prescribed. Available is furosemide (Lasix) 80-mg tablets. How many tablets will the nurse administer?

41. The drug handbook states that 40 mg of furosemide (Lasix) can be administered undiluted over 1-2 minutes; do not exceed 4 mg/min in patients with renal impairment. The nurse is unsure of the patient's renal status and plans to administer the drug over 10 minutes (4 mg/min). The furosemide (Lasix) vial states 40 mg/4 mL. The 5-mL syringe is marked with a line every 0.2 mL. The nurse will administer 0.2 mL (one line) of furosemide (Lasix) over what time period?

CASE STUDY

An 80-year-old nonsmoking woman has been taking spironolactone (Aldactone) 100 mg/day for about 6 years to control her moderate hypertension and mild HF. She comes to the emergency department with bilateral crackles (rales) in the lower and middle lobes and a blood pressure of 190/120 mm Hg. She is short of breath, very anxious, tachycardic (HR 134 beats/min), and diaphoretic. Her family assures you that she has been taking her medication. The family tells you she has been getting worse over the past 2 weeks since having friends bring her favorite lunch of hot dogs and potato chips every day. Pulmonary edema is diagnosed. Orders include STAT intravenous push furosemide (Lasix) 40 mg and morphine sulfate 2 mg, 3 L of oxygen via nasal cannula, electrolytes, and complete blood count, and an indwelling Foley catheter.

1. How will furosemide (Lasix) help relieve this patient's symptoms?

2. What information must the nurse know about furosemide (Lasix) administration before administering the drug via intravenous push?

3. Why was the Foley catheter ordered?

4. It has been 45 minutes since the patient received her furosemide (Lasix). Her Foley catheter is in place. She says that she is very thirsty. What assessments should be made at this point?

5. Lab results, drawn before she received any medication, have returned. Her sodium is 140 (normal: 135-145 mEq/L), chloride is 110 (normal: 98-106 mEq/L), and potassium is 3.5 (normal: 3.5-5 mEq/L). Knowing that she received her furosemide (Lasix) after these lab values were drawn, what should be included in the nurse's plan of action?

6. The patient improves significantly within the first 6 hours. Her blood pressure is 138/90 mm Hg, pulse 102, respirations 20, and rales are heard only in her bases bilaterally. She asks you how this could have happened since she had been taking her medicine as prescribed. What should the nurse discuss with the patient as possible reasons for her condition?

7. What nursing assessments would be made on at least a daily basis while she is in the hospital?

8. The patient continues to improve and is being discharged home on furosemide (Lasix) 20 mg twice a day and spironolactone (Aldactone) 50 mg daily. What teaching should be provided regarding dietary patterns, activity, and signs and symptoms of further problems?

9. What information should the nurse provide to prevent problems with drug interactions?

10. The patient will need to be started on digoxin. What must the nurse remember now that the patient is on digoxin and furosemide (Lasix)? What laboratory values need to be monitored?

42

Agents Affecting the Volume and Ion Content of Body Fluids

STUDY QUESTIONS

Completion

1. Cirrhosis of the liver can cause _____ _____.

2. Diuretics and chronic kidney disease can cause _____ _____.

3. Extensive burns can cause _____ _____.

4. Vomiting and diarrhea can cause _____ _____.

5. Total osmolality of plasma is equal to approximately _____ _____ _____ _____.

6. NaCl plus KCl to increase excretion of bicarbonate is used to treat _____ _____.

7. _____ _____ treatment includes rebreathing CO_2.

8. Sodium bicarbonate is used to treat _____ _____.

Matching

Match the conditions with the appropriate descriptor.

9. ___ Metabolic acidosis
10. ___ Respiratory acidosis
11. ___ Metabolic alkalosis
12. ___ Respiratory alkalosis

    a. Can occur with salicylate toxicity.
    b. Lung changes from smoking are a risk for this condition.
    c. May be associated with prolonged gastric suctioning.
    d. Seen in uncontrolled diabetes mellitus.

CRITICAL THINKING, PRIORITIZATION, AND DELEGATION QUESTIONS

✴13. When infusing an intravenous (IV) solution in cases of isotonic contraction, it is a priority for the nurse to do what?
    a. Assess for crackles in the lung fields.
    b. Calculate the infusion rate in drops per minute and hang by gravity.
    c. Infuse the fluid quickly.
    d. Infuse 0.45% sodium chloride.

14. Why are intravenous solutions of 5% dextrose ($C_6H_{12}O_6$) in water technically isotonic in the bag but hypotonic in the body?
    a. The body uses the dextrose for energy.
    b. The kidneys rapidly excrete the dextrose.
    c. Dextrose is a nonabsorbable sugar.
    d. The dextrose is metabolized in the blood to H_2O and CO_2.

▶15. A 15-year-old patient with bulimia who abuses laxatives is admitted to the hospital after experiencing extreme leg weakness. Potassium chloride 40 mEq by mouth twice a day has been prescribed. The nurse reviews the most recent laboratory tests before administering the drug. Results include Na 137 mEq/L, K 3.5 mEq/L, and Cl 100 mEq/L. What should the nurse do?
    a. Page the prescriber STAT.
    b. Administer the medication.
    c. Hold the medication and contact the prescriber.
    d. Administer the medication and contact the prescriber.

▶16. The nurse is administering furosemide (Lasix) and sustained-release potassium chloride (K-Dur) to a patient with HF. The nurse notes that the patient is chewing the potassium chloride. The patient states that she cannot swallow the large pill. What should the nurse do?
   a. Crush the pill and mix it with applesauce or pudding.
   b. Instruct the patient to drink at least 8 ounces of water after chewing the potassium pill.
   c. Contact the prescriber.
   d. Page the prescriber STAT.

17. Which assessment finding would be a priority to report to the prescriber when a patient is taking KCl tablets?
   a. Black stool
   b. Constipation
   c. Muscle weakness
   d. Nausea

✳18. Which laboratory result would be a priority to report to the prescriber when a patient is receiving intravenous fluids containing potassium?
   a. Blood urea nitrogen (BUN) 28 mg/dL
   b. Creatinine 4.2 mg/dL
   c. Potassium 3.5 mEq/L
   d. Serum glucose 220 mg/dL

19. A diabetic patient is admitted with hyperosmolar hyperglycemic syndrome (HHS). His serum glucose level is 750 mg/dL and his blood pH is 7.41. Intravenous regular insulin in normal saline (0.9% NaCl) is prescribed to lower the patient's blood sugar. When administering the IV insulin, the nurse needs to assess the patient for which symptoms of a possible electrolyte disorder that can be caused by this treatment?
   a. Skeletal muscle weakness and absent bowel sounds (hypokalemia)
   b. Disorientation, psychosis, and seizures (hypomagnesemia)
   c. Muscle weakness, hypotension, and sedation (hypermagnesemia)
   d. Confusion, anxiety, heavy legs, and tall T waves on ECG (hyperkalemia)

20. Which medication used to treat hypertension can increase the risk of hyperkalemia if prescribed with potassium or with each other? (Select all that apply.)
   a. Amlodipine (Norvasc)
   b. Atenolol (Tenormin)
   c. Furosemide (Lasix)
   d. Ramipril (Altace)
   e. Spironolactone (Aldactone)

✳21. Which action is of greatest priority when a patient is diagnosed with hyperkalemia?
   a. Administer sodium polystyrene sulfonate.
   b. Initiate cardiac monitoring.
   c. Question the patient about medical history.
   d. Teach foods that should be avoided because of high potassium content.

22. Which condition might prevent oral magnesium supplementation from being effective?
   a. The patient has impaired renal functioning.
   b. The patient is a diabetic.
   c. The patient has hypertension.
   d. The patient experiences diarrhea.

✳23. The nurse reviews laboratory test results that include a magnesium level of 1 mEq/L on a newly admitted patient. It is of greatest priority for the nurse to inform the prescriber of this result if the patient has a history of which disorder?
   a. Asthma
   b. AV heart block
   c. Gastroesophageal reflux disease (GERD)
   d. Rheumatoid arthritis

24. Because of the risk of neuromuscular blockade when administering magnesium, the nurse must know how to obtain which IV medication?
   a. Calcium gluconate
   b. Potassium chloride
   c. Sodium chloride
   d. Sodium polystyrene sulfonate

DOSE CALCULATION QUESTIONS

A 165-lb patient is admitted to the burn unit with burns over 36% of her total body surface area (TBSA). Because of evaporative and intracellular fluid loss, burns over 15% of TBSA require more rapid fluid replacement than other cases of hypertonic contraction. This facility uses the Parkland (Baxter) formula for fluid replacement. Crystalloid replacement is lactated Ringer's solution 4 mL/kg × %TBSA/24 hr.

25. What is the total amount of lactated Ringer's solution that needs to be infused in the first 24 hours?

26. Half of the fluid is to be administered during the first 8 hours. What rate in mL/hour should the nurse program into the IV pump?

CASE STUDIES

Case Study 1

A patient is admitted with prolonged diarrhea. An IV solution of 0.45% sodium chloride with 40 mEq of potassium chloride is prescribed at 150 mL/hr.

1. What laboratory tests does the nurse need to monitor when administering potassium supplements?

2. What assessments does the nurse need to perform to ensure safe infusion of the potassium solution?

3. What measures should the nurse take to ensure accurate infusion of the prescribed dose of fluid and electrolytes?

4. What assessments should the nurse perform to assess for possible fluid overload?

Case Study 2

A postoperative patient has been NPO for 4 days with a nasogastric tube set to low intermittent suction. The patient develops muscle cramping and disorientation. Serum Mg is 1.0 mEq/L. The prescriber orders an IV solution of 10% magnesium sulfate to infuse at 100 mL/hr.

5. What should the nurse do before initiating this IV therapy?

6. The prescriber changes the infusion rate to 90 mL/hr. What critical assessment should the nurse perform while administering magnesium?

7. What assessment findings would warrant the nurse stopping the infusion and consulting the prescriber?

43

Review of Hemodynamics

STUDY QUESTIONS

True or False

For each of the following statements, enter T *for true or* F *for false.*

1. ___ Arteries readily stretch in response to pressure changes.
2. ___ Arterioles determine blood flow to tissue.
3. ___ Cardiac output is determined by the rate of the heart contraction times the amount of blood ejected from the heart with each beat.
4. ___ Conditions that decrease chest expansion with breathing decrease blood return to the heart.
5. ___ Conditions that cause an inability of skeletal muscle to contract (or severe weakness) can cause peripheral edema.
6. ___ Normal adult blood volume is 8 L.
7. ___ Stimulation of the vagal nerve, such as bearing down to defecate, speeds the heart rate.
8. ___ The average amount of blood ejected from the heart at each beat is slightly over 2 ounces.
9. ___ The heart of a normal adult pumps the entire blood volume in approximately 1 minute.

10. ___ The majority of the blood in the body is in the arteries and the heart.
11. ___ Vasodilation increases resistance to blood flow.

Matching

Match the terms and descriptors.

12. ___ Afterload
13. ___ Aldosterone (renin-angiotensin-aldosterone system)
14. ___ Baroreceptors
15. ___ Beta$_2$-adrenergic receptors
16. ___ Cardiac output
17. ___ C-natriuretic peptide
18. ___ Preload
19. ___ Muscarinic receptors
20. ___ Natriuretic peptides ANP and BNP
21. ___ Sinoatrial node
22. ___ Stroke volume
23. ___ Systemic filling pressure

a. Amount of blood pumped out of the heart in 1 minute
b. Constricts vessels and increases kidney water retention
c. Force that returns blood to the heart
d. Force with which the ventricles of the heart contract
e. The amount of stretch in the ventricle before it contracts
f. Pressure in the aorta that the heart must overcome to eject blood out of the heart
g. Pressure sensors in the aortic arch and carotid sinus
h. Primarily promotes vasodilation
i. Shift fluid from vascular to extravascular compartment, increase diuresis, dilate arterioles and veins
j. Where stimulation of heartbeat originates
k. Stimulation of these receptors decreases heart rate
l. Stimulation of these receptors increases heart rate

CRITICAL THINKING, PRIORITIZATION, AND DELEGATION QUESTIONS

24. Individuals who have plaque lining their arteries experience an increase in vessel resistance. The nurse should assess for which reaction that is the body's attempt to compensate?
a. Peripheral edema
b. Rise in blood pressure (BP)
c. Shifting of point of maximal impulse (PMI)
d. Slowing of heart rate

25. Drugs that can be used to lower BP decrease venous resistance by doing what? (Select all that apply.)
a. Dilating veins
b. Reducing right atrial pressure
c. Reducing volume of blood
d. Stimulating auxiliary muscle pumps

26. A patient with early heart failure (HF) has an average heart rate of 90 beats/min and a stroke volume of 55 mL. What is true about this patient's per-minute cardiac output?
a. It is extremely low.
b. It is low.
c. It is high.
d. It is within normal limits

▶27. The nurse is researching a drug. The handbook states that it decreases afterload. Before the nurse administers this medication to a patient, which assessment would be most critical?
a. BP for hypotension
b. Pulse for tachycardia
c. Respirations for tachypnea
d. Temperature for fever

✳28. The nurse is assessing a patient who is receiving medication for acute HF. Which assessment would be a priority to report to the prescriber?
a. Cough with frothy sputum
b. Expiratory wheezes of bronchi and bronchioles
c. Pulse 100 beats/min
d. Respirations 25/min

▶29. The nurse is reassessing a patient 1 hour after administering a vasodilator to treat hypertension. Assessment findings include BP 116/70 mm Hg (down from 145/88 mm Hg), pulse 88 (up from 80 beats/min), and respirations 22 (up from 20). What should the nurse do? (Select all that apply.)
a. Continue collecting additional assessment data.
b. Document the findings.
c. Explain orthostatic BP precautions.
d. Page the prescriber STAT.
e. Raise all four bed side rails for safety.
f. Reassess the vital signs within 1 hour.

►30. A patient is receiving a vasodilator that has a high incidence of orthostatic hypotension. Before administering the medication and after the patient has rested supine for 10 minutes, the nurse assesses the BP and pulse. Results are BP 145/80 mm Hg, P 68 beats/min. The nurse assists the patient to stand, ensuring safety, and after 1 minute reassesses the BP and pulse. Which reading would be of most concern to the nurse?

a. BP 110/70 mm Hg, pulse 92 beats/min
b. BP 126/70 mm Hg, pulse 78 beats/min
c. BP 134/70 mm Hg, pulse 72 beats/min
d. BP 140/82 mm Hg, pulse 70 beats/min

CASE STUDIES

Case Study 1

A patient newly diagnosed with coronary artery disease (CAD) has been prescribed a nitroglycerin patch 12 hours on and 12 hours off. The nurse is explaining the medication to the patient. Nitroglycerin is a drug that causes extensive venous vasodilation. The drug handbook states that the therapeutic effect is to decrease the workload of the heart. The patient wants to know how this helps her heart.

1. How should the nurse explain this effect?

2. The patient verbalizes understanding of nitroglycerin, but states that she is afraid to take off the patch because she might have a heart attack. What is the rationale for not using nitroglycerin patches continuously?

a. Absorption is decreased if patches are left on too long.
b. Skin irritation occurs if patches are left on too long.
c. Tolerance to the drug's effect develops if patches are left on too long.
d. Toxicity develops if patches are left on too long.

Case Study 2

The student nurse is caring for a patient with HF. The heart is enlarged and weak, and its muscle fibers are stretched beyond the point of effective recoil. The student nurse must do a teaching project.

3. Describe how the student nurse could use a balloon to demonstrate the pathophysiology of HF to the patient.

44

Drugs Acting on the Renin-Angiotensin-Aldosterone System

STUDY QUESTIONS

Matching

1. ____ Catalyzes the conversion of angiotensin I (inactive) into angiotensin II (highly active).
2. ____ Drug that dilates blood vessels by decreasing level of angiotensin II formation from angiotensin I, increasing renal excretion of sodium and water, slightly decreasing heart remodeling, and causing dry cough by increasing bradykinin levels.
3. ____ Drug that acts on renin to inhibit the conversion of angiotensinogen into angiotensin I suppressing the renin-angiotensin-aldosterone system (RAAS).
4. ____ Drug that blocks the action of angiotensin II causing dilation of blood vessels and potassium-sparing diuresis, but does not cause cough or prevent myocardial remodeling.
5. ____ Drug that produces selective blockade of aldosterone receptors causing potassium-sparing diuresis and significant prevention of myocardial remodeling.

6. ___ Hormone that causes retention of sodium and water and retention of potassium and hydrogen by the kidneys to maintain adequate filtering pressure in the glomerulus.

7. ___ Secreted by kidney, regulates angiotensin II formation.

8. ___ System where renin is released from kidneys, resulting in aldosterone release from adrenals.

9. ___ Vasoconstricts and stimulates aldosterone release.

a. Aldosterone
b. Aldosterone receptor antagonist
c. Angiotensin II
d. Angiotensin-converting enzyme (kinase II)
e. Angiotensin-converting enzyme (ACE) inhibitor
f. Angiotensin II receptor blocker (ARB)
g. Direct renin inhibitor (DRI)
h. RAAS
i. Renin

CRITICAL THINKING, PRIORITIZATION, AND DELEGATION QUESTIONS

10. The nurse recognizes that the generic names of ARB drugs end in which suffix?
a. -mycin
b. -olol
c. -pril
d. -sartan

11. The nurse recognizes that the generic names of ACE inhibitor drugs end in which suffix?
a. -mycin
b. -olol
c. -pril
d. -sartan

12. A nurse understands how drugs that block the effects of angiotensin II can be beneficial for heart failure patients. What information would not be correct about ARBs?
a. The drug improves cardiac function primarily by decreasing electrical conduction through cardiac tissue.
b. The drug can help heart function by increasing excretion of sodium and water by the kidneys.
c. The drug can decrease the formation of pathologic changes in cardiac structure.
d. The drug can help heart function by preventing pathologic changes to the structure and function of blood vessels.

13. What would not stimulate renin release by the kidneys?
a. Dehydration
b. Hemorrhage
c. Hypernatremia
d. Stimulation of beta$_1$-adrenergic receptors

14. Which adverse effect, reflecting accumulation of bradykinin, may a patient may experience from taking an ACE inhibitor?
a. Dehydration
b. Dry cough
c. Hyperkalemia
d. Hyponatremia

▶15. When the nurse is scheduled to administer lisinopril to a patient, which laboratory values should be reviewed? (Select all that apply.)
a. Creatinine
b. Fasting blood sugar
c. Sodium
d. Potassium
e. Uric acid

✻16. It would be a priority to teach orthostatic BP precautions to a patient before the first dose of an ACE inhibitor if laboratory tests include which result?
a. ALT 35 IU/L
b. BUN 24 mg/dL
c. Potassium 4.1 mEq/L
d. Sodium 132 mg/dL

17. The nurse receives laboratory test results, including AST 22 international units/L, ALT 33 international units/L, BUN 32 mg/dL, and creatinine 2.2 mg/dL, for a patient who is scheduled to receive an ACE inhibitor drug. Which ACE inhibitor could be administered without concern of toxicity?
a. Captopril
b. Enalapril
c. Fosinopril
d. Lisinopril

✻18. A patient who is prescribed an ACE inhibitor complains of tongue swelling and is experiencing obvious dyspnea. What is the priority action by the nurse?
a. Administer prescribed PRN epinephrine
b. Assess BP
c. Assess lung sounds
d. Consult the prescriber

▶19. Which of these ECG findings would suggest hyperkalemia in a patient who is prescribed an ACE inhibitor and who was using a salt substitute?
a. Flat T waves
b. Prolonged QT interval
c. Shortened QT interval
d. Tall, peaked T waves

20. A patient who has been taking an ACE inhibitor for hypertension is concerned because she has just discovered that she is 7 weeks pregnant. The nurse knows that research suggests that if the patient stops taking the ACE inhibitor now, the risk for adverse effects on the fetus is
a. unknown.
b. low.
c. medium.
d. high.

✳21. When a patient is prescribed an ACE inhibitor, it is a priority to teach the patient not to take which OTC drug without consulting the prescriber?
a. Antacids
b. Cough suppressant
c. Laxative
d. NSAID

22. ARB drugs are similar to ACE inhibitors except that they are also associated with a decreased potential for which adverse effect?
a. Cancer
b. Cough
c. Fetal harm
d. Renal failure

23. What is an advantage of the direct renin inhibitor aliskiren (Tekturna) over ARBs?
a. Reduced incidence of cough
b. Fewer gastrointestinal (GI) adverse effects
c. No drug interactions
d. Unclear advantage

24. Spironolactone (Aldactone) is less selective than eplerenone (Inspra). The nurse knows that this means what about spironolactone?
a. It causes more adverse effects.
b. It has fewer drug interactions.
c. It is less effective.
d. It produces therapeutic effects more rapidly.

25. The nurse assesses a hypertensive, diabetic patient who is prescribed eplerenone (Inspra) for adverse effects, which may be related to electrolyte imbalance. These symptoms include
a. flushed, dry skin.
b. diarrhea.
c. irritability.
d. weak hand grasps.

✳26. When taking a history from a patient who is prescribed an ACE inhibitor, ARB, or eplerenone (Inspra), which question would be most important for the nurse to ask?
a. "Are you bothered by a frequent nonproductive cough?"
b. "Do you eat 4-5 servings of fruits and vegetables each day?"
c. "Have you ever been diagnosed with iron-deficiency anemia?"
d. "What do you use to season your food?"

▶27. A patient who has been prescribed quinapril (Accupril) for hypertension has not had the expected reduction in blood pressure. Regular use of which over-the-counter medications may be contributing to lack of therapeutic effect of the ACE inhibitor?
a. Acetaminophen
b. Calcium carbonate
c. Ibuprofen
d. Milk of magnesia

DOSE CALCULATION QUESTIONS

28. Aliskiren (Tekturna) is available as 150-mg tablets. How many tablets are administered for a 300-mg dose?

29. Enalapril (Vasotec) 1.25 mg is prescribed IV push over 5 minutes. It is available in solution of 1.25 mg/mL. The nurse can take longer, but not shorter, than the prescribed infusion time. The nurse should push 0.1 mL every how many seconds?

CASE STUDY

A 68-year-old man was admitted to the medical unit with complaints of a 10-lb weight gain over the past week, swollen ankles, and increasing shortness of breath. Although furosemide (Lasix) was partially effective, the prescriber chooses to add an ACE inhibitor. The patient is prescribed captopril (Capoten) 2.5 mg by mouth three times a day. His blood pressure is currently 140/74 mm Hg. Significant history includes an anterior myocardial infarction 12 months ago and renal artery stenosis involving the right kidney.

1. What question should the nurse ask when consulting the prescriber about this new medication order?

2. What teaching should the nurse provide about the timing of the doses of captopril (Capoten)?

3. What assessments and actions should the nurse perform when administering the first dose of captopril (Capoten)?

4. What teaching should the nurse provide to the patient and family about reasons to contact the prescriber?

5. The patient's spouse has a friend who used to take captopril (Capoten), but the friend's prescriber discontinued the ACE inhibitor and prescribed the newer drug valsartan (Diovan). The patient's spouse would like the patient to be prescribed valsartan because it is "newer and better." How should the nurse respond?

45
Calcium Channel Blockers

STUDY QUESTIONS

Completion

1. Calcium channel blockers (CCBs) lower blood pressure by _____.

2. CCBs differ from nitrates in that they do not cause vasodilation of _____.

3. Dihydropyridine CCBs primarily affect _____.

4. The three net effects of the CCBs verapamil and diltiazem on the heart are _____, _____, and _____ _____.

5. The suffix of the generic name of dihydropyridine CCBs is _____.

CRITICAL THINKING, PRIORITIZATION, AND DELEGATION QUESTIONS

✳ 6. In addition to assessing blood pressure, what is the priority assessment before administering diltiazem (Cardizem)?
   a. Ankle edema
   b. Apical pulse
   c. Peripheral pulses
   d. Respiratory rate

7. The lowering of blood pressure and improvement of arterial blood flow to the heart counteract the negative effects of reduced heart rate and reduced force of contraction caused by verapamil (Calan).
   a. True
   b. False

8. The nurse is caring for a patient who is scheduled to receive verapamil (Calan) and atenolol (Tenormin), a beta$_1$-adrenergic blocker, at 0900. It is important for the nurse to assess for what critical adverse effects based on the combination of these two drugs before administration? (Select all that apply.)
   a. Crackles or pulmonary edema
   b. Muscle pain
   c. Shortness of breath
   d. Urinary output of at least 45 mL/hr
   e. Weight gain of 3 lb in 24 hours

9. The drop in blood pressure (BP) produced by the CCB activates baroreceptors and stimulates the sympathetic nervous system. Which of these CCBs is most likely to have the adverse effect of reflex tachycardia?
   a. Diltiazem (Cardizem)
   b. Nifedipine (Procardia)
   c. Verapamil (Calan)

►10. The nurse is caring for a patient who is scheduled to receive verapamil (Calan SR) 180 mg and atenolol (Tenormin) 50 mg at 0900. The patient has had a gastric tube (G-tube) inserted, and drugs are to be administered via the tube. Which action should the nurse take before administering these two drugs?
   a. Change the time of the drug administration so that they are administered via the G-tube at least 2 hours apart.
   b. Consult the prescriber.
   c. Crush both tablets separately.
   d. Flush the G-tube with 5-15 mL of water between administering the drugs.

＊11. A patient is prescribed diltiazem (Cardizem). It would be a priority to withhold the drug and contact the prescriber if which assessment finding is present?
   a. BP 150/85 mm Hg
   b. Constipation
   c. Dizziness with position changes
   d. Pulse 50 beats/min

►12. Which dermatologic finding in an older adult would warrant consultation with the prescriber regarding administration of diltiazem (Cardizem)?
   a. Burrows and erythematous papules between the fingers
   b. Erythematous, oozing vesicles on the chin and inside of elbows
   c. Silvery, scaling plaques on the elbows
   d. White, cheesy plaque on the tongue

13. The nurse is administering the Verelan PM form of verapamil. The patient states she takes all of her medications in the morning when she awakens. The nurse's response should be based on what knowledge?
   a. Verelan PM produces maximal effects in the morning when most cardiac events occur.
   b. Verelan PM is given at night so it peaks during sleep to prevent orthostatic hypotension.
   c. Verelan PM should not be administered with any other medication.
   d. Verelan PM should be taken at night because it causes sedation.

14. A patient on a surgical unit has been prescribed intravenous (IV) diltiazem (Cardizem) for atrial fibrillation. What should the nurse do?
   a. Move the resuscitation cart into the patient's room.
   b. Arrange for the patient to be transferred to a unit where constant monitoring of BP and electrocardiogram is possible.
   c. Continuously monitor the patient's oxygen saturation and pulse during infusion.
   d. Have another nurse check the calculated drip rate before hanging the medication by gravity feed.

15. A patient taking both verapamil (Calan) and digoxin (Lanoxin) is at greater risk for digitalis toxicity. The nurse should assess and monitor the patient for early symptoms of digitalis toxicity, which include
   a. nausea and vomiting.
   b. slurred speech.
   c. tachycardia.
   d. photophobia.

▶16. The nurse is administering medications on a medical-surgical unit in a hospital. The medication administration record states that the patient should receive Cardizem LA 120 mg once a day. The patient's drug supply includes Cardizem SR. What should the nurse do?
   a. Administer the medication.
   b. Administer the medication and notify the prescriber of the change.
   c. Contact the pharmacy.
   d. Hold the medication and contact the prescriber.

17. Which drug might be prescribed to counteract the reflex tachycardia associated with administration of dihydropyridine CCB?
   a. Digoxin (Lanoxin)
   b. Enalapril (Vasotec)
   c. Furosemide (Lasix)
   d. Metoprolol (Lopressor)

18. A patient who has experienced palpitations (reflex tachycardia) while taking nifedipine (Procardia) 20 mg three times a day has had his prescription changed to nifedipine (Procardia XL) 60 mg once a day. The patient asks the nurse how taking the same medication once a day instead of three times a day will help prevent palpitations. What should the nurse's response include?
   a. Rapid-acting formulas of nifedipine are more potent than sustained-release formulas.
   b. Blood levels of rapid-acting formulas of nifedipine rise more rapidly than with sustained-release formulas.
   c. Sustained-release formulas of nifedipine cause a more gradual drop in BP.
   d. Sustained-release formulas of nifedipine suppress the automaticity of the heart like verapamil.

19. A patient has been prescribed extended-release nifedipine (Procardia). Teaching regarding administration should include which instruction?
   a. Administer 1 hour before or 2 hours after meals.
   b. Do not crush or chew tablet.
   c. Take with grapefruit juice to improve absorption.
   d. Take on an empty stomach.

✱20. It would be a priority to assess for cardiac effects and toxicity in a patient who is receiving nifedipine (Procardia) if laboratory test results include
   a. ALT 30 IU/L.
   b. BNP 100 picograms/mL.
   c. BUN 22 mg/dL.
   d. eGFR 32 mL/min.

DOSE CALCULATION QUESTIONS

21. Diltiazem is prescribed for IV infusion for a patient in atrial fibrillation. A dose of 5 mg/hr has been prescribed. The pharmacy has supplied the drug in a concentration of 0.45 mg/mL. How many mL/hr will the nurse program into the IV infusion pump?

22. The recommended initial dose of diltiazem (Cardizem) IV push is 0.25 mg/kg for adult patients. What is the recommended safe dose for a patient who weighs 178 lb?

CASE STUDY

A 75-year-old female patient who is a nonsmoker with a history of hypertension, esophageal cancer, and type 2 diabetes mellitus comes to the emergency department with fatigue and extreme shortness of breath. She is diagnosed with atrial fibrillation. The prescriber orders verapamil (Calan) 5 mg IV push.

1. The nurse is administering the verapamil (Calan) IV push. While administering the medication, the nurse notes a sudden reduction in heart rate and prolongation of the PR interval on the cardiac monitor. What should the nurse do?

2. Thirty minutes after injecting the IV verapamil, the patient requests assistance with getting up and using the toilet to void. What should the nurse do?

3. The patient is stabilized, and the prescriber has prescribed verapamil (Calan) 120 mg three times a day. The nurse is reviewing the patient's laboratory tests. Which laboratory value would require consultation with the prescriber regarding administration of verapamil? (Select all that apply and explain why.)
   a. Alanine aminotransferase (ALT) 250 units/L
   b. Blood urea nitrogen (BUN) 28 mg/dL
   c. Creatinine 3.2 mg/dL
   d. Fasting blood glucose (FBS) 250 mg/dL
   e. Hemoglobin (Hgb) 10 mg/dL
   f. International normalized ratio (INR) 1.8
   g. Potassium (K^+) 3.3 mEq/L
   h. Sodium (Na^+) 146 mg/dL

4. The nurse is reviewing the patient's prescribed medications. In addition to verapamil 80 mg three times a day, the patient is taking nateglinide (Starlix) 120 mg, a medication that increases production of insulin by the pancreas and lowers the blood sugar to treat the patient's diabetes mellitus. Both verapamil and nateglinide are metabolized by the CYP3A4 hepatic enzyme. Verapamil inhibits the action of this enzyme. Because of this interaction, the nurse knows the patient is at increased risk for hypoglycemia. What symptoms suggest that the patient's blood glucose has dropped below normal?

5. What teaching should the nurse provide that can prevent problems with common adverse effects of verapamil?

46
Vasodilators

STUDY QUESTIONS

True or False

For each of the following statements, enter T *for true or* F *for false.*

1. ____ Hydralazine (Apresoline) reduces the work of the heart by reducing afterload.
2. ____ Hydralazine (Apresoline) lowers blood pressure by causing vasodilation and diuresis.
3. ____ An adverse effect of minoxidil is impairment in tissue perfusion.
4. ____ The effects of an IV infusion of nitroprusside end within minutes of stopping the infusion.
5. ____ Nitroglycerin is used to treat angina because it dilates arterioles in the heart, allowing more oxygen to get to heart muscle cells.
6. ____ Orthostatic hypotension is more likely to occur when a patient is receiving a drug that dilates veins than one that dilates arterioles.
7. ____ Reflex tachycardia only occurs with drugs that dilate both arterioles and veins.
8. ____ Drugs with the suffix -lol are used to slow the heart when reflex tachycardia occurs.
9. ____ When a patient is receiving nitroprusside, the nurse would report a thiocyanate level greater than 0.1 mg/mL.

CRITICAL THINKING, PRIORITIZATION, AND DELEGATION QUESTIONS

✳10. Which would be a priority to report to the prescriber of hydralazine (Apresoline)?
   a. Ankle edema
   b. BP 150/80 mm Hg
   c. Pulse 120 beats/min
   d. 10 mm Hg drop in BP when sitting up from a reclining position

11. Which drug is commonly prescribed for patients with heart failure when prescribed hydralazine (Apresoline) because of the adverse effect of sodium retention?
   a. Atenolol
   b. Furosemide
   c. Isosorbide dinitrate
   d. Minoxidil

✳12. When caring for a patient who is prescribed minoxidil, it is most important for the nurse to assess for what?
   a. Abnormal hair growth
   b. Bradycardia
   c. Fluid volume deficit
   d. Shortness of breath

► 13. A patient with severe hypertension is prescribed minoxidil (Loniten). The nurse should contact the prescriber STAT if assessment findings include what?
   a. Distended neck veins, muffled heart sounds, and narrow pulse pressure
   b. Exertional dyspnea, 1+ ankle edema, and anxiety
   c. Headache, dizziness, and blurred vision
   d. Shift of point of maximal impulse (PMI) 2 cm to left and bruits over carotid arteries

14. The nurse is caring for a nonambulatory patient who is receiving hydralazine (Apresoline). When monitoring for adverse effects, the nurse would expect that edema would first appear where?
   a. Around the medial malleolus of the ankle
   b. Fingers
   c. Sacral area
   d. Dorsal aspect of the feet

✳15. Laboratory test results on a patient receiving hydralazine (Apresoline) include elevated antinuclear antibodies (ANA). When notifying the prescriber of these lab results, it is a priority to include which assessment finding?
   a. Fatigue
   b. Headache
   c. Respirations 22/min
   d. Temperature 101° F (38.3° C)

► 16. The nurse is administering nitroprusside (Nitropress) in a cardiac care unit. The prescriber also orders administration of oral antihypertensives. The patient's blood pressure is still elevated, but dropping slowly. The nurse should do what?
   a. Administer both medications.
   b. Hold both the nitroprusside and the oral antihypertensives until the prescriber can be consulted.
   c. Hold the nitroprusside and administer the oral antihypertensives until the prescriber can be consulted.
   d. Hold the oral antihypertensives and administer the nitroprusside until the prescriber can be consulted.

17. The nurse is preparing to administer intravenous (IV) nitroprusside sodium (Nipride). The patient has an IV of 5% dextrose with 20 mEq of potassium running at 75 mL/hr. What would be the best action by the nurse?
   a. Connect the nitroprusside sodium (Nipride) to the Y-port of the primary line above the intravenous pump and run both fluids simultaneously.
   b. Disconnect the primary intravenous line and administer the nitroprusside sodium (Nipride) then reconnect the primary line.
   c. Start a second intravenous site and administer the nitroprusside sodium (Nipride) using a separate intravenous pump.
   d. Stop the primary fluid infusion and connect the nitroprusside sodium (Nipride) to a port below the intravenous pump.

18. A patient who weighs 165 lb is receiving intravenous (IV) nitroprusside sodium (Nipride) 300 mcg/min. An important nursing assessment at this dose is for what?
   a. Adequate fluid intake and urinary output
   b. Anorexia, nausea, and vomiting
   c. Fever, flushing, and chills
   d. Palpitations, disorientation, and respiratory depression

19. The nurse is preparing to administer nitroprusside sodium (Nipride). The solution has just been prepared in the pharmacy, but has a faint brown discoloration. What should the nurse do?
   a. Administer the medication.
   b. Consult the prescriber before administering the solution.
   c. Discard the solution and get a new bag from the pharmacy.
   d. Warm the IV bag and reassess to see if the brown color clears.

DOSE CALCULATION QUESTIONS

20. Hydralazine (Apresoline) 40 mg intravenous bolus dose is prescribed. The drug comes in a concentration of 20 mg/mL. The dose is to be administered undiluted over 1 minute. How many tenths of a mL should be administered every 10 seconds?

21. What rate of infusion of nitroprusside would the nurse program into the IV pump if administering 3 mcg/kg/min to a patient who weighs 176 lb (80 kg) if the drug dilution is 50 mg in 250 mL of 5% dextrose in water?

CASE STUDY

A 78-year-old patient is seen in the emergency department in hypertensive crisis. She is 5 feet 2 inches tall and weighs 125 lb. Her BP is 230/130 mm Hg, and she is very edematous. She has a history of alcohol abuse. IV nitroprusside sodium (Nipride) at 0.3 mcg/kg/min is prescribed.

1. What assessments of the solution and precautions should the nurse take when administering this medication?

2. Knowing that nitroprusside sodium (Nipride) creates a rapid response (within 1 to 2 minutes), what and how often should the nurse assess to follow the results of the drugs and the patient's response?

3. The patient suddenly becomes diaphoretic and complains of nausea, palpitations, and headache. What should the nurse do?

4. The patient has improved significantly. The prescriber orders hydralazine, metoprolol, and hydrochlorothiazide on a long-term basis to control her blood pressure. Explain the rationale for this combination of medications.

5. The nurse checks the drug handbook, and the dose recommendation for adults for hydralazine is listed as 10-50 mg 4 times a day or 100 mg 3 times a day. What are possible reasons for the low dose being extended to every 8 hours?

47

Drugs for Hypertension

STUDY QUESTIONS

Matching

Match primary mechanism(s) of action with classes of antihypertensive drugs.

1. ___ Because of their ability to conserve potassium, these drugs can play an important role in an antihypertensive regimen.
2. ___ Promote dilation of arterioles and have direct suppressant effects on the heart, reducing reflex tachycardia.
3. ___ Promote dilation of arterioles; no significant dilation of veins; risk of orthostatic hypotension is low. Lowering of BP may be followed by reflex tachycardia, renin release, and fluid retention.

4. ___ Blood pressure reduction results from dilation of arterioles and veins; reduction of heart rate and contractility; and suppression of renin release.
5. ___ Lower BP by promoting renal excretion of sodium and water; produces diuresis through aldosterone receptor blockade.
6. ___ Act directly on renin to inhibit conversion of angiotensinogen into angiotensin I.
7. ___ Produce much greater diuresis than the thiazides; they lower BP by reducing blood volume and promoting vasodilation.
8. ___ Reduce BP by two mechanisms: reduction of blood volume and reduction of arterial resistance.

9. ___ Decrease heart rate and contractility; suppress reflex tachycardia caused by vasodilators; block receptors on juxtaglomerular cells of the kidney and reduce release of renin; long-term use reduces peripheral vascular resistance.

10. ___ Act within the brainstem to suppress sympathetic outflow to the heart and blood vessels.

11. ___ Depletes norepinephrine from postganglionic sympathetic nerve terminals reducing sympathetic stimulation of the heart and blood vessels; can cause deep emotional depression.

12. ___ Promote dilation of arterioles; can cause reflex tachycardia.

13. ___ Prevent stimulation of receptors on arterioles and veins, thereby preventing sympathetically mediated vasoconstriction; not recommended as first-line therapy for hypertension.

14. ___ Prevent angiotensin II–mediated vasoconstriction and release of aldosterone by blocking the actions of angiotensin II.

15. ___ Lower BP by preventing formation of angiotensin II, thereby preventing angiotensin II–mediated vasoconstriction and aldosterone-mediated volume expansion.

a. Adrenergic neuron blockers
b. Aldosterone antagonists
c. Alpha$_1$ (α_1) androgenic receptor blockers (alpha$_1$ blockers)
d. Alpha$_1$ (α_1)/beta androgenic receptor blockers (alpha$_1$/beta blockers)
e. Angiotensin-converting enzyme inhibitors (ACEI)
f. Angiotensin receptor blockers (ARBs)
g. Beta (β) androgenic receptor blockers (beta blockers)
h. Centrally acting alpha$_2$ agonists
i. Dihydropyridine calcium channel blockers (CCB)
j. Direct-acting vasodilators
k. Direct renin inhibitors
l. High-ceiling diuretics
m. Nondihydropyridine calcium channel blockers (CCB)
n. Potassium-sparing diuretics
o. Thiazide diuretics

CRITICAL THINKING, PRIORITIZATION, AND DELEGATION QUESTIONS

16. Hypertension in which case would be classified as primary hypertension?
    a. Diabetic in end-stage renal failure
    b. Hyperthyroid adult
    c. Postmenopausal African-American woman
    d. Young adult male with an adrenal tumor

17. When possible, the nurse should assess the patient's BP with the patient in which position?
    a. Lying flat in bed
    b. Lying in bed with the head elevated at least 45 degrees
    c. Sitting with feet dangling
    d. Sitting with feet on the floor

▶18. It is important for the nurse to discuss adverse effects of the antihypertensive drugs that are prescribed because the nurse knows what about the drugs' adverse effects?
    a. They affect adherence.
    b. They are life-threatening.
    c. They are necessary if the antihypertensive is at a dose that is effective.
    d. They reflect the cause of hypertension.

19. The teaching plan for a patient taking antihypertensive drugs should include which information? (Select all that apply.)
    a. Cigarette smoking and consuming more than two alcoholic drinks per day can reduce the effectiveness of antihypertensive drugs.
    b. Eating produce like fresh bell peppers, oranges, and tomatoes can help the patient lower his or her blood pressure.
    c. Certain foods, such as milk, have substantial amounts of sodium even though they do not have a salty taste.
    d. The patient's symptoms of hypertension are the best indicators of the need for antihypertensive drugs.

20. When administering an antihypertensive drug to a patient who has a history of hypertension and type 2 diabetes mellitus, what would be an appropriate outcome for therapy?
    a. BP 100/60 to 110/70 mm Hg
    b. BP 110/70 to 130/80 mm Hg
    c. BP 120/80 to 130/85 mm Hg
    d. BP 128/80 to 138/90 mm Hg

►21. Which laboratory results should be reported to the prescriber if a patient is receiving a thiazide or loop diuretic?
a. Blood urea nitrogen (BUN) 20 mg/dL
b. Hemoglobin A1c 5.5%
c. Potassium (K$^+$) 3.2 mEq/L
d. Uric acid 20 mg/dL

22. The nurse would teach a patient who is on which diuretic to avoid use of potassium-containing salt substitutes and excessive consumption of bananas and orange juice?
a. Ethacrynic acid (Edecrin)
b. Furosemide (Lasix)
c. Hydrochlorothiazide (HydroDIURIL)
d. Triamterene (Dyrenium)

23. Acebutolol (Sectral), penbutolol (Levatol), and pindolol are beta blockers that have intrinsic sympathomimetic activity. This decreases the incidence of what adverse effect?
a. Bradycardia at rest
b. Bronchoconstriction
c. Heart block
d. Hypoglycemia

24. Which nursing concern is of greatest priority when a patient starts therapy with an alpha$_1$ blocker?
a. Adequate exercise
b. Hydration
c. Safety
d. Urinary output

25. A patient would most likely experience reflex tachycardia if receiving which antihypertensive drug?
a. ACE inhibitors
b. Beta blockers
c. Direct-acting vasodilators
d. Nondihydropyridine calcium channel blockers

26. Which action is of greatest priority when caring for a patient who has just been prescribed a drug for hypertension?
a. Identifying obstacles to adherence to therapy
b. Teaching how the prescribed drug works
c. Teaching the patient how to assess his BP sitting and standing
d. Telling the patient his target BP

27. Which teaching would most likely prevent the most serious effect when a patient is prescribed clonidine for hypertension?
a. Change positions slowly.
b. Consult the prescriber before stopping the drug.
c. Exercise regularly.
d. Use sugar-free candy.

28. Which intervention is most likely to decrease adverse effects of hypertension in African-American adults?
a. Explaining measures to respond to adverse effects of antihypertensive drugs
b. Identifying adverse effects of antihypertensive drugs
c. Prescribing of the appropriate drug for hypertension
d. Promoting regular screening of BP

29. Which drug class is recommended as first-line treatment for an African-American patient with hypertension?
a. ACE inhibitor
b. Calcium channel blocker
c. Diuretic
d. Vasodilator

30. What is the recommended time goal for lowering BP when a patient is in acute congestive heart failure?
a. 30 minutes
b. 60 minutes
c. 90 minutes
d. 2 hours

31. A positive hCG would be of most concern if the patient is prescribed
a. captopril (Capoten).
b. hydrochlorothiazide (HydroDIURIL).
c. prazosin (Minipress).
d. propranolol (Inderal).

32. What is the best treatment for severe preeclampsia?
a. Delivery of the fetus
b. Labetalol (Normodyne)
c. Lisinopril (Zestril)
d. Methyldopa (Aldomet)

33. Which magnesium level is within the target range for a patient being treated for eclampsia?
a. 1 mEq/L
b. 2 mEq/L
c. 5 mEq/L
d. 8 mEq/L

34. It would be of greatest priority to monitor capillary blood sugar rather than rely on symptoms that suggest hypoglycemia if a patient is prescribed which class of antihypertensive drugs?
    a. ACE inhibitor
    b. Beta blocker
    c. High-ceiling (loop) diuretic
    d. Thiazide diuretic

CASE STUDY

A 48-year-old African-American man with a history of type 2 diabetes mellitus comes to the emergency department (ED) with a frontal headache and generalized complaints of "not feeling well." Upon examination, his BP is 210/120 mm Hg, his pulse is 98, and his respirations are 24 and labored.

1. What risk factors does this patient have for a cardiovascular event?

2. When is it important to lower this patient's BP within 1 hour rather than slowly as for most hypertensive patients?

3. The resident writes an order for intravenous nitroprusside 80 mcg/min. What precautions should the nurse take while administering this medication?

4. The patient is stabilized and discharged on hydrochlorothiazide and diltiazem (Cardizem). On the follow-up visit, the patient's BP is 160/90 mm Hg. The patient asks why the prescriber does not just give him a high enough dose to bring his BP down to normal. How should the nurse respond?

48

Drugs for Heart Failure

STUDY QUESTIONS

Matching

Match the patient symptoms of heart failure (HF) with the most appropriate nursing diagnosis.

1. ___ Faint peripheral pulses, decreased urine output
2. ___ Lack of exercise, high-fat diet
3. ___ Orthopnea, jugular venous distention (JVD)
4. ___ Palpitations, pallor
5. ___ Shortness of breath when walking to bathroom

    a. Activity intolerance
    b. Cardiac output, decreased
    c. Fluid volume excess
    d. Health maintenance, ineffective
    e. Perfusion, ineffective peripheral

Match the drug with its description.

6. ___ Improve LV ejection fraction, reduce HF symptoms, increase exercise tolerance, decrease hospitalization, enhance quality of life, and reduce mortality. However, they do not increase levels of kinins; therefore, they have no effect on cardiac remodeling.

7. ___ Produce profound diuresis; can promote fluid loss even when GFR is low.

8. ___ Increase myocardial contractile force, thereby increasing cardiac output. Alter the electrical activity of the heart, and favorably affect neurohormonal systems.

9. ___ Block production of angiotensin II, decrease release of aldosterone, and suppress degradation of kinins, thereby improving hemodynamics and favorably altering cardiac remodeling.

10. ___   Block aldosterone receptors in the heart and blood vessels.

11. ___   Produce moderate diuresis; used when edema is not too great. Are ineffective when GFR is low; cannot be used if cardiac output is greatly reduced.

12. ___   Can improve LV ejection fraction, increase exercise tolerance, slow progression of HF, reduce the need for hospitalization, and prolong survival.

13. ___   Synthetic catecholamine that causes selective activation of beta$_1$-adrenergic receptors; can increase myocardial contractility, and can thereby improve cardiac performance.

   a. Aldosterone receptor antagonist
   b. Angiotensin-converting enzyme (ACE) inhibitors
   c. Angiotensin receptor blockers (ARBs)
   d. Beta-adrenergic receptor blockers (beta-blockers)
   e. Cardiac glycosides
   f. High-ceiling (loop) diuretics
   g. Sympathomimetic drugs
   h. Thiazide diuretics

CRITICAL THINKING, PRIORITIZATION, AND DELEGATION QUESTIONS

14. Which statement, if made by a patient with HF, would indicate a need for further teaching?
   a. "If blood cannot get through my heart, the backup of fluid will make it hard for me to breathe."
   b. "My heart is stretching so much it is losing the ability to squeeze out the blood."
   c. "The changes in my heart started when I began to feel tired and short of breath."
   d. "When my heart beats too fast, it cannot fill properly."

15. Elevation of B-natriuretic peptide (BNP) suggests HF because BNP is released when the
   a. heart beats faster.
   b. heart's atria stretch.
   c. heart does not get enough oxygen.
   d. heart muscle thickens.

✳16. The nurse would be most concerned if a patient with HF exhibits which symptom? (Select all that apply.)
   a. Peripheral edema
   b. Urine output of 825 mL in 24 hours
   c. Distention of the jugular veins
   d. Weight gain

17. The nurse cannot hear the apical pulse of a patient with the diagnosis of HF when assessing at the fifth intercostal space at the midclavicular line. Which direction should the nurse move the stethoscope diaphragm/bell to be more likely to hear the pulse?
   a. Toward the clavicle
   b. Toward the left side
   c. Toward the sternum
   d. Toward the waist

✳18. A patient with HF is prescribed spironolactone (Aldactone) and enalapril (Vasotec). It would be a priority to consult the prescriber regarding evaluation of the patient's potassium levels if the patient exhibited
   a. confusion.
   b. constipation.
   c. weakness.
   d. shallow respirations.

✳19. What is a priority assessment when administering dopamine?
   a. Bowel sounds
   b. Capillary refill
   c. Temperature
   d. Urine output

▶20. A maintenance intravenous (IV) infusion of inamrinone is prescribed for a patient who has a current infusion of 5% dextrose and 0.45% NaCl running at 45 mL/hr. How should the nurse administer the inamrinone?
   a. After flushing the primary line
   b. Using a second IV site
   c. As a secondary infusion through the primary line
   d. Over 2-3 minutes via the primary line

21. Nitrates, including nitroglycerin and isosorbide, reduce the workload of the myocardium by
   a. decreasing the amount of blood returning to the heart.
   b. decreasing conduction of impulses through the heart.
   c. decreasing the volume of blood in the vascular system.
   d. increasing myocardial remodeling.

*22. The nurse is preparing to administer hydralazine (Apresoline) for HF. Because this drug has been associated with drug-induced lupus-like syndrome, it would be a priority to report what symptom to the prescriber? (Select all that apply.)
a. Facial rash
b. Heartburn
c. Joint pain
d. Fever

23. Before administering nitroglycerin to a newly admitted patient, it would be most important for the nurse to identify if the patient has recently self-medicated with a drug for what condition?
a. Erectile dysfunction
b. Fever
c. Itching
d. Pain

24. A possible explanation for why digoxin has not demonstrated an improvement in mortality is that the drug does not
a. decrease heart rate.
b. improve heart remodeling.
c. increase cardiac output.
d. increase urine production.

▶25. When a patient with HF is prescribed digoxin and furosemide, the nurse should carefully assess the patient for which symptoms of digoxin toxicity?
a. Anorexia and nausea
b. Anxiety and abdominal cramps
c. Bone pain and constipation
d. Muscle spasms and convulsions

▶26. What findings in a patient with HF would warrant that the nurse not administer digoxin and notify the prescriber?
a. Blood pressure 100/76 mm Hg
b. Digoxin 2.4 ng/mL
c. Heart rate 100 beats/min
d. Potassium 5.3 mEq/L

27. The nurse would consult the prescriber if a patient with HF who is experiencing pain is prescribed which drug?
a. Acetaminophen
b. Imipramine
c. Ibuprofen
d. Morphine

28. A fixed dose of hydralazine and isosorbide (BiDil) has been approved to treat HF in people of which self-reported race?
a. American Indian
b. Asian
c. Caucasian
d. Black

29. It is a priority to assess for digitalis toxicity if a patient is receiving digoxin (Lanoxin), the digoxin level is 1.3 ng/mL, and the patient has which other laboratory result?
a. BNP 1813 picograms/mL
b. INR 1.5
c. Potassium (K) 3.0 mEq/L
d. Sodium 150 mEq/L

DOSE CALCULATION QUESTIONS

30. Dobutamine HCl is prescribed at a rate of 2.5 mcg/kg/min. The patient weighs 165 lb (55 kg). The drug is available as 2 mg/mL of 5% dextrose. The IV pump is calibrated in mL/hr. What rate should the nurse program into the IV pump?

31. An IV bolus of 50 mg of inamrinone is prescribed for a patient who weighs 154 lb. Is the dose safe if the recommended dose is 0.75 mg/kg?

CASE STUDIES

Case Study 1

An 81-year-old male patient with chronic HF who resides in a long-term care facility has been treated with digoxin (Lanoxin) 0.125 mg, furosemide 80 mg, and potassium chloride (K-Dur) 20 mEq once a day by mouth for a long time. Recently, the prescriber added eplerenone (Inspra) 50 mg orally once a day to the medication regimen.

1. When consulting the prescriber about this patient, what questions might the nurse ask?

2. Why is it important for the nurse to monitor electrolyte and digoxin levels on this patient?

3. The long-term care nurse notes during the report from the night shift that the patient has become increasingly restless, "coughs all night," and seems very fatigued when the staff is providing care. His appetite has been poor, even for things he normally enjoys. Assessment findings include BP 90/70 mm Hg; alternating weak and strong pulse at a rate of 118 beats/min; S$_3$ ventricular gallop; rales throughout lung fields; and a 5-lb weight gain in the last week. What action should the nurse take at this time?

4. The patient is admitted to an acute care facility. Based on the knowledge of digoxin and its relationship to potassium, how could these blood levels have contributed to the patient's decompensation?

Case Study 2

A 64-year-old male patient is a direct admission to the nursing unit with the complaint of abdominal pain, nausea, and extreme weakness. The patient has a history of diabetes, chronic renal failure, and sleep apnea. Admission nursing assessment findings include temperature 99.3° F, BP 174/110 mm Hg, pulse 96 and irregular, PMI shifted to the left, JVD 4.5 cm above the angle of Louis, 3+ pitting edema in the lower extremities, and tenderness in the RUQ with abdominal palpation.

5. What nursing diagnosis is most appropriate for this patient?

6. The nurse obtains laboratory results from tests drawn on admission including BNP 1275 pg/mL; K$^+$ 5.4 mEq/L, creatinine 2.7 mg/dL, BUN 42 mg/dL. The nurse contacts the prescriber who orders a STAT electrocardiogram, which shows S-T changes. What action should the nurse take at this point?

7. The patient is transferred to the coronary care unit. Oxygen is administered along with furosemide (Lasix), nitroglycerin, and enalapril (Vasotec). What is the rationale for administration of these drugs?

8. The patient is stabilized and is transferred to the nursing unit. Prescribed drugs include carvedilol, enalapril, and furosemide. What laboratory values does the nurse need to monitor when a patient is receiving these drugs?

9. What teaching should the nurse provide to prepare this patient for discharge?

10. The patient lives in an apartment building with 12 stairs to climb to his apartment. After climbing the stairs, he needs to rest because he is short of breath. He can, however, perform most activities of daily living. According to the New York Heart Association (NYHA), what is this patient's HF classification?

49
Antidysrhythmic Drugs

STUDY QUESTIONS

Completion

1. *Arrhythmia* is not as accurate a term as *dysrhythmia,* because arrhythmia literally means _____ of a heart rhythm.

2. *Dysrhythmia* means _____ heart rhythm.

3. *Bradydysrhythmia* is the term for a heart rate that is _____ than normal.

4. *Tachydysrhythmia* is the term for a heart rate that is _____ than normal.

5. More rapid depolarization of Purkinje fibers results in rapid _____ contraction.

Matching

Match the electrolyte with the effect of blocking rapid potentials.

6. ____ Blocking this ion slows impulse conduction.
7. ____ Blocking this ion reduces myocardial contractility.
8. ____ Blocking this ion delays repolarization.

    a. Calcium
    b. Potassium
    c. Sodium

Match the antidysrhythmic drug with its action.

9. ____ Delay repolarization of fast potentials by blocking potassium (K^+) channels
10. ____ Reduce calcium (Ca^{++}) entry during fast and slow depolarization and depress phase 4 repolarization of slow potentials
11. ____ Slow impulse conduction in atria and ventricles by blocking sodium (Na^+) channels

    a. Class I
    b. Class II and IV
    c. Class III

CRITICAL THINKING, PRIORITIZATION, AND DELEGATION QUESTIONS

▶12. What is the priority nursing diagnosis for a patient with a dysrhythmia?
    a. Alteration in cardiac output
    b. Imbalance of fluid and electrolytes
    c. Inadequate peripheral tissue perfusion
    d. Ineffective breathing pattern

▶13. What do multiple P waves before the QRS complex on an ECG indicate?
    a. Atria are depolarizing faster than the ventricles.
    b. Atrial impulses to the ventricles are being slowed.
    c. Ventricles are depolarizing faster than the atria.
    d. Ventricular impulses to the atria are being slowed.

14. Ectopic foci can dominate the pace of the heart if the discharges of the ectopic stimuli are
    a. atrial in origin.
    b. faster than the SA node.
    c. from the ventricles.
    d. slower than the SA node.

▶15. A patient has been prescribed an antidysrhythmic drug that prolongs the QT interval on ECG. The nurse should teach the patient the importance of reporting which symptom that suggests that a dangerous adverse effect, torsades de pointes, may be occurring?
    a. Ankle edema
    b. Feeling faint
    c. Headache
    d. Shortness of breath

▶16. Instructing a patient on the Valsalva maneuver is asking the patient to do what?
    a. Bear down as if having a bowel movement
    b. Breathe through pursed lips
    c. Pant like a dog
    d. Tighten the pelvic floor muscles

▶17. A focused nursing assessment of a patient with atrial fibrillation should always include assessment of changes in what?
   a. Appetite
   b. Bowel pattern
   c. Deep tendon reflexes
   d. Mental status

▶18. Which laboratory result for international normalized ratio (INR), if identified in a patient with atrial fibrillation who is receiving warfarin (Coumadin), would indicate that warfarin therapy has achieved the desired effect?
   a. INR between 0.9-1.1
   b. INR between 2-3
   c. INR between 5-9
   d. INR greater than 10

19. The nurse responds quickly when a ventricular tachydysrhythmia is identified because this type of dysrhythmia impairs the ability of the heart
   a. to contract rapidly enough to meet body needs.
   b. to eject an adequate amount of blood.
   c. valves to close properly.
   d. valves to open properly.

20. A patient with a dysrhythmia, type 2 diabetes mellitus (T2DM), and heart failure (HF) is prescribed quinidine, metformin, furosemide, and digoxin. The nurse should be vigilant in monitoring for which early adverse effect of digitalis toxicity that may occur with this combination of drugs?
   a. Anorexia and nausea
   b. Cool, clammy skin
   c. Excessive urination and thirst
   d. Yellow-tinted blurred vision

▶21. Which of these assessment findings, if identified in a patient who is receiving quinidine, is of greatest priority to report to the prescriber?
   a. BP 150/88 mm Hg
   b. Tinnitus
   c. Sudden dyspnea
   d. Three soft stools in 8 hours

22. A patient asks the nurse why he was instructed to take quinidine with food. An appropriate response by the nurse is that taking the drug with food does what?
   a. Decreases the incidence of GI symptoms
   b. Increases absorption
   c. Prevents cinchonism
   d. Prevents ventricular tachycardia

▶23. The nurse is monitoring the ECG of a patient who received the first dose of quinidine 45 minutes ago. The nurse notes that the QRS complex was widened 25% from pre-drug therapy findings. What should the nurse do?
   a. Administer a beta-blocker.
   b. Continue nursing care.
   c. Discontinue monitoring the ECG.
   d. Notify the prescriber immediately.

24. The nurse should assess patients receiving long-term therapy with procainamide for which adverse effects? (Select all that apply.)
   a. Abdominal pain and nausea
   b. Chest pain and dyspnea
   c. Elevated antinuclear antibodies (ANA) and painful joint swelling
   d. Elevated platelet levels and increased venous thrombi formation
   e. Fever and chills

▶25. The prescriber writes an order to switch a patient from intravenous (IV) to oral procainamide. The IV drug was discontinued at 11:30 AM. What is the earliest that the nurse should administer the first dose of oral procainamide?
   a. Immediately
   b. 1:30 PM
   c. 2:30 PM
   d. 4:30 PM

26. Which anticholinergic effect of disopyramide (Norpace) would be of greatest priority to report to the prescriber?
   a. Blurred vision
   b. Dry mouth and thirst
   c. No BM × 2 days
   d. Postvoid residual of 350 mL

27. Because of extensive first-pass effect, the nurse expects to administer lidocaine in which way?
   a. Sustained-release formula
   b. Intravenously
   c. Orally on an empty stomach
   d. With a full glass of water

28. An appropriate nursing intervention to prevent adverse effects of gingival hyperplasia associated with long-term use of phenytoin (Dilantin) is teaching the importance of regular care with which health care professional?
   a. Dentist
   b. Ophthalmologist
   c. Podiatrist
   d. Pulmonologist

✱29. Which adverse effect of propafenone, if occurring for 3-4 days, would be of most concern to the nurse?
   a. Abdominal pain
   b. Anorexia
   c. Dizziness
   d. Vomiting

30. The nurse is preparing to administer the cardioselective beta-blocker acebutolol. Which assessment would indicate the need for immediate consultation with the prescriber?
   a. Apical pulse 105 beats/min
   b. Bronchial wheezes
   c. Capillary blood glucose 220 mg/dL
   d. 1+ pitting edema of the dorsal aspect of the foot

31. The patient must be informed of possible damage to the lungs when prescribed oral therapy with which drug?
   a. Amiodarone (Cordarone)
   b. Dofetilide (Tikosyn)
   c. Propafenone (Rythmol)
   d. Propranolol (Inderal)

32. In addition to monitoring the heart rate and rhythm, what assessment must the nurse continuously monitor when administering IV amiodarone (Cordarone)?
   a. Blood pressure
   b. Level of consciousness
   c. Intravenous site
   d. Respiratory effort

▶33. What is the most significant difference between amiodarone and dronedarone?
   a. Amiodarone does not increase thyroid hormone secretion.
   b. Amiodarone has a different effectiveness.
   c. Amiodarone has a different risk of death.
   d. Amiodarone has a shorter duration of significant adverse effects.

34. Which laboratory results would increase the risk of torsades de pointes when a patient is prescribed dofetilide?
   a. Potassium 3.2 mg/dL
   b. Potassium 5.3 mg/dL
   c. Sodium 132 mg/dL
   d. Sodium 148 mg/dL

▶35. Because verapamil (Calan) can cause blockade of calcium channels in vascular smooth muscle, a priority is for the nurse to teach a patient who is prescribed this drug to do what?
   a. Drink 2500 mL of fluid each day, especially water.
   b. Increase fiber in the diet.
   c. Take orthostatic BP precautions.
   d. Report bruising.

36. Which action is most appropriate when administering adenosine IV?
   a. Administer oxygen.
   b. Monitor vital signs.
   c. Have the patient perform the Valsalva maneuver.
   d. Administer dipyridamole concurrently.

37. In most cases, the need for antidysrhythmic drugs exceeds the risks of adverse effects when
   a. the dysrhythmia is prolonged.
   b. the QT interval is excessively long.
   c. ventricular pumping is ineffective.
   d. the SA node discharges at a rate exceeding 160 beats/min.

DOSE CALCULATION QUESTIONS

38. A patient who weighs 165 lb is prescribed IV diltiazem. The recommended initial bolus dose is 0.25 mg/kg. What is the recommended dose for this patient?

39. One gram of lidocaine in 250 mL of 5% dextrose in water at a rate of 2 mg/min is prescribed. The IV pump is calibrated in mL per hour. What rate should be programmed into the pump?

CASE STUDY

A 75-year-old man underwent open-heart surgery 5 days ago and postoperatively developed a cerebrovascular accident (CVA). His history includes hypertension, renal insufficiency, alcohol abuse, and a 2-pack-per-day smoking habit. He was progressing well postoperatively without any further complications. A physical therapist and nurse assisted the patient to transfer to a recliner. Following transfer, the patient complained to the physical therapist that his heart felt "like it was racing."

1. What assessments should the nurse perform at this time?

The monitor nurse walks in to check on the patient because the monitor revealed a heart rate of 185 beats/min. The nurse asks the patient to bear down to stimulate the vagus nerve and slow the heart rate. After obtaining a full set of vital signs, the nurse places a call to the attending physician. The physician orders a STAT 12-lead ECG. The attending physician arrives on the unit, examines the 12-lead ECG, and diagnoses ventricular tachycardia (v-tach). A bolus dose of lidocaine 100 mg is ordered.

2. What precautions must the nurse take before and during administration of the IV bolus dose?

3. The bolus dose is followed by an infusion of a solution of lidocaine. What patient data can the nurse provide to assist the prescriber with determining the amount of fluid with which to dilute the lidocaine?

4. One gram of lidocaine in 250 mL of 5% dextrose in water at a rate of 2 mg/min is prescribed. The IV pump is calibrated in mL per hour. Before infusing the drug, the nurse should examine the IV solution and not administer the drug if the solution contains what additives?

5. What should be included when the nurse reports to the prescriber the patient's response to lidocaine?

50

Prophylaxis of Coronary Heart Disease: Drugs That Help Normalize Cholesterol and Triglyceride Levels

STUDY QUESTIONS

Completion

1. Estrogen, progesterone, testosterone, and adrenal corticosteroids are _____ that require cholesterol for formation.

2. The _____ is the primary source of endogenous cholesterol in the body.

3. When trying to lower blood cholesterol, it is important to reduce intake of _____ fats.

4. _____ serve as carriers for transporting lipids in blood.

5. Literally, *hydrophilic* means _____ _____ and *hydrophobic* means _____ _____ _____.

6. Optimal LDL cholesterol is now defined in ATP III as less than _____ mg/dL.

7. Optimal HDL cholesterol is now defined in ATP III as at least _____ mg/dL.

8. The recommendation for regular physical activity is _____ to _____ minutes on most days.

CRITICAL THINKING, PRIORITIZATION, AND DELEGATION QUESTIONS

9. A 45-year-old female smoker with a family history of coronary heart disease (CHD) has been prescribed a lipid-lowering medication. Which outcome would be most important for this patient?
   a. Cholesterol total less than 200 mg/dL
   b. HDL greater than 40 mg/dL
   c. LDL less than 100 mg/dL
   d. Triglycerides less than 150 mg/dL

10. A patient has received instructions regarding cholesterol and the body. Which statement made by the patient would indicate the patient needs further teaching?
    a. "Drugs that decrease the liver's ability to produce cholesterol should be taken so that they peak during the night."
    b. "Drugs that prevent the absorption of cholesterol from food are more effective than drugs that limit the making of cholesterol by the liver."
    c. "It is more important to limit the amount of saturated fat in my diet than the total amount of cholesterol."
    d. "My cholesterol can be high even if I eat a low-fat diet and exercise regularly."

▶11. Recent laboratory results for a patient include HDL 85 mg/dL, LDL 145 mg/dL, and triglycerides 630 mg/dL. The nurse should assess the patient for what?
    a. Upper abdominal pain and nausea
    b. Chest pain and shortness of breath
    c. Rash and pruritus
    d. Tachycardia and diaphoresis

▶12. The nurse has reviewed the laboratory results for a patient who is scheduled to receive lovastatin (Mevacor) 40 mg. Results include AST 122 units/L, ALT 155 units/L, CK 250 units/L, HDL 45 mg/dL, and LDL 245 mg/dL. What should the nurse do?
    a. Administer the drug and continue nursing care.
    b. Hold the drug and assess for chest pain.
    c. Hold the drug and assess for abdominal pain.
    d. Hold the drug and notify the prescriber of the laboratory results.

▶13. A 38-year-old female patient has been diagnosed with hypercholesterolemia. The prescriber has ordered simvastatin (Zocor) 20 mg, once a day at hour of sleep, to be started after laboratory results are obtained. Which laboratory result would be of greatest priority to report to the prescriber?
    a. ALT 57 international units/L
    b. Creatinine 1.4 mg/international units/dL
    c. CRP 3 mg/dL
    d. hCG 287 international units/L

✳14. A patient who is receiving lovastatin experiences chest pain. CK level is 580 units/mL (CK-MM 99%) and troponin T 0.02 g/mL. It is of greatest priority for the nurse to monitor the functioning of which organ?
    a. Brain
    b. Heart
    c. Kidneys
    d. Lungs

15. A patient who is receiving nicotinic acid to elevate HDL and reduce triglycerides exhibits dry, hot, and flushed skin; thirst; hunger; and confusion. What is the appropriate next action?
    a. Assess for chest pain.
    b. Assess for abdominal pain.
    c. Continue nursing care.
    d. Notify the prescriber.

16. Which OTC drug is recommended to prevent the adverse effect of intense flushing that occurs with niacin?
    a. Acetaminophen (Tylenol)
    b. Acetylsalicylic acid (Aspirin)
    c. Diphenhydramine (Benadryl)
    d. Ranitidine (Zantac)

17. The nurse has been caring for a patient admitted with dehydration. The patient has been taking colesevelam and complains of nausea. Which assessment finding would be of most concern to the nurse?
    a. Bloating after medication administration
    b. Flatulence
    c. Hyperactive bowel sounds with rushes
    d. Indigestion

18. A patient has been prescribed cholestyramine in addition to hydrochlorothiazide. When should the cholestyramine be administered?
    a. 1 hour after other drugs
    b. 1 hour before other drugs
    c. 4 hours after other drugs
    d. 4 hours before other drugs

19. The nurse would be most concerned about which patient?
    a. A patient receiving lovastatin and experiencing a rash
    b. A patient receiving nicotinic acid and experiencing hot flashes with facial flushing
    c. A patient receiving colesevelam and experiencing nausea
    d. A patient receiving gemfibrozil and experiencing right upper quadrant pain

▶20. Which laboratory test result would be of greatest concern if noted in a patient who is prescribed ezetimibe (Zetia)?
    a. ALT 35 IU/L
    b. BUN 20 mg/dL
    c. Platelets 75,000/mm³
    d. WBC 10,000/mm³

21. A patient is prescribed gemfibrozil (Lopid) and warfarin. Which lab result suggests that the warfarin dose is therapeutic?
    a. INR 1
    b. INR 3
    c. INR 6
    d. INR 10

22. The nurse would teach the patient strategies to prevent constipation if the patient was prescribed which drug for dyslipidemia?
    a. Atorvastatin
    b. Colestipol
    c. Gemfibrozil
    d. Niacin

23. Which statement suggests that the patient who has been prescribed cholestyramine needs additional teaching?
    a. "I can mix the powder in applesauce."
    b. "I should not take this drug at the same time as other drugs."
    c. "I can take the powder dry."
    d. "It is a good idea to drink water after taking the drug to be sure that all of it went down."

DOSE CALCULATION QUESTIONS

24. Colesevelam (Welchol) is supplied as 625-mg tablets. How many tablets should the nurse administer if the prescribed dose is 1.9 g?

25. Gemfibrozil (Lofibra) 134 mg has been prescribed. Available are 67-mg capsules. How many capsules should be administered per dose?

CASE STUDY

A 46-year-old female Type 2 diabetes patient has been prescribed simvastatin because, despite good nutrition and exercise resulting in A1c within acceptable levels, her LDL cholesterol has not dropped below 150 mg/dL. The patient asks why she has to have additional bloodwork (LFT, CK, and hCG) before the doctor will prescribe the drug.

1. How should the nurse respond?

2. What teaching should the nurse provide about birth control?

3. The patient asks how she would know if liver or muscle cell damage was occurring. What should be included in the explanation?

4. Why is it important to teach the patient to report chest pain and to describe the characteristics and whether it is worsened by coughing or laughing?

5. The patient calls after getting the prescription filled. She states that the nurse told her to take the drug in the evening but the pharmacy information states that it can be taken at any time. How should the telephone triage nurse respond?

51

Drugs for Angina Pectoris

STUDY QUESTIONS

Completion

1. Angina pectoris occurs when the _____ supply to the _____ is inadequate.

2. Cardiac oxygen demand is determined by heart rate, contractility, _____, and _____.

3. Arterial blood flow to myocardial cells occurs during the _____ phase of a heartbeat.

4. The most common drug used to decrease platelet activity is _____.

CRITICAL THINKING, PRIORITIZATION, AND DELEGATION QUESTIONS

✻ 5. What is the priority nursing concern for a patient with angina pectoris?
   a. Decreased cardiac output
   b. Impaired gas exchange
   c. Ineffective tissue perfusion: cardiopulmonary
   d. Ineffective breathing pattern

6. What is the goal of drug therapy for chronic stable angina?
   a. Constrict coronary arteries to increase blood pressure during stress
   b. Decrease myocardial need for oxygen during stress
   c. Increase myocardial blood flow during systole
   d. Prevent coronary artery spasms

7. A patient asks the nurse why nitroglycerin can be administered in so many ways. What is the basis of the nurse's response?
   a. Nitroglycerin does not undergo first-pass effect in the liver.
   b. Nitroglycerin has few adverse effects, so varying doses can be administered via different routes.
   c. Nitroglycerin is an inactive compound, so it does not matter which route it is administered by.
   d. Nitroglycerin is lipid-soluble, so it is readily absorbed via different routes.

8. Nitroglycerin has myocardial vasodilation effects in variant (Prinzmetal's) angina but not in chronic stable angina, because in chronic stable angina myocardial arterioles are
   a. atherosclerotic.
   b. experiencing spastic vasoconstriction.
   c. occluded with thrombi.
   d. unable to diffuse oxygen into the cell.

9. A patient who has been using a nitroglycerin patch for angina has recently been prescribed diltiazem (Cardizem). Which statement, if made by this patient, would suggest that the patient understood teaching about the new drug?
   a. "I need to take this drug because nitroglycerin causes my blood pressure to go up."
   b. "If I take both of these drugs, I can use sildenafil (Viagra) if I experience erectile dysfunction."
   c. "This drug prevents my heart from racing, which can happen when people take nitroglycerin."
   d. "This drug will make the nitroglycerin work better."

► 10. A patient is prescribed a nitroglycerin patch that is to be applied at 0900 (9:00 AM) and removed at 2100 (9:00 PM). When preparing to administer the 0900 patch, the nurse notes that a nitroglycerin patch is still in place. What should the nurse do?
   a. Apply the new patch to a different site, but leave the old patch on until the nursing supervisor is contacted.
   b. Consult with the prescriber regarding application of a new patch.
   c. Remove the old patch and apply the new patch to a different site.
   d. Remove the old patch and change the timing of the medication so that the patch is removed at 0900 and applied at 2100.

11. When collecting data from a patient who is not obtaining relief from nitroglycerin tablets, the nurse should ask whether the patient allows the tablet to completely dissolve in her mouth. This is based on the nurse's understanding that swallowing sublingual nitroglycerin tablets
   a. allows the liver to inactivate the drug before it works.
   b. increases tolerance to the drug.
   c. prevents the small intestine from absorbing the drug.
   d. speeds excretion.

12. It is important for the nurse to teach a patient who has been prescribed nitroglycerin (NitroQuick) on an as-needed basis to do what?
   a. Discard unused tablets after 12 months.
   b. Store the tablets in a locked medicine cabinet in the bathroom.
   c. Take a few tablets from the bottle and keep them in her purse or pocket for emergency use.
   d. Write the date that the tablets are opened on the outside of the bottle.

► 13. When assessing a patient who is scheduled to receive the second dose of newly prescribed sustained-release nitroglycerin, the patient complains of a headache. What should the nurse do?
   a. Administer a prescribed PRN analgesic such as acetaminophen.
   b. Crush the medication to speed absorption through the oral mucosa.
   c. Notify the prescriber of the headache STAT.
   d. Withhold the drug and consult the prescriber.

14. The nurse is aware that which nitroglycerin preparation has a rapid onset?
   a. Sublingual tablets
   b. Sustained-release capsule
   c. Topical ointment
   d. Transdermal patch

► 15. How does cigarette smoking cause coronary artery disease?
   a. Damaging the heart valves
   b. Increasing the heart rate
   c. Promotes atherosclerosis
   d. Stretching the ventricles

16. The nurse recognizes that a drug is a beta blocker if the generic name of the drug ends in which suffix?
   a. -cillin
   b. -olol
   c. -pril
   d. -sartan

17. Beta blockers are useful to improve myocardial oxygen supply in angina because they slow the heart rate and force of contraction and
   a. dilate coronary arteries.
   b. dilate veins.
   c. increase the time that blood flows through coronary arteries.
   d. reduce blood return to the heart.

18. The nurse would withhold a beta$_1$ blocker and immediately contact the prescriber if it was discovered that the patient has a history of which condition?
   a. Asthma
   b. First-degree heart block
   c. Hyperglycemia
   d. Sick sinus syndrome

19. The nurse would assess for tachycardia when an anginal patient is receiving which drug(s) for angina? (Select all that apply.)
   a. Diltiazem
   b. Isosorbide
   c. Metoprolol
   d. Nifedipine
   e. Nitroglycerin

20. What would warrant notification of a prescriber when the nurse is caring for a patient who is receiving ranolazine?
   a. eGFR 95 mL/min
   b. Penicillin prescribed for upper respiratory infection
   c. Systolic BP decreases 8 mm Hg with position changes
   d. Unexplained fainting

DOSE CALCULATION QUESTIONS

21. Nitroglycerin ointment (2%) is dispensed from a tube, and the length of the ribbon squeezed from the tube determines dosage. (One inch contains about 15 mg of nitroglycerin.) How many inches would equal 30 mg?

22. Intravenous (IV) nitroglycerin is prescribed at a rate of 5 mcg/min. The drug is available in a pre-mixed glass bottle with 100 mg/L of 5% dextrose in water (D_5W). The IV pump is calibrated in mL/hr. At what rate should the nurse program the pump?

CASE STUDIES

Case Study 1

A 74-year-old man with a history of stable angina, asthma, and hypertension is admitted to the hospital with substernal chest pain that was not relieved by three sublingual nitroglycerin tablets. In the emergency department, the patient is prescribed diltiazem and an IV nitroglycerin drip.

1. What actions must the nurse take when administering IV nitroglycerin?

2. The patient's pain is relieved after receiving a dosage of 330 mcg/min. He is admitted to the coronary care unit. His vital signs are stable, and he is currently without pain. Cardiac enzyme levels do not suggest myocardial cell death. The ECG shows normal sinus rhythm. The physicians believe that the patient is having classic angina and not a myocardial infarction. The attending physician orders that the patient be weaned from the nitroglycerin drip and that nitroglycerin transdermal patches 10 mg/24 hr be started. He is also prescribed aspirin 81 mg, diltiazem-CD (30 mg), and ramipril (Altace) 2.5 mg, which he is to receive once a day. If the prescriber wants a continuous administration of nitroglycerin when changing the patient from the nitroglycerin drip to the patch, when, in relation to discontinuing the IV nitroglycerin, should the nurse apply the nitroglycerin patch?

3. What teaching should the nurse provide about administration of the nitroglycerin patch?

4. The patient has the nitroglycerin drip turned off, the nitroglycerin patch is applied, and the diltiazem-CD is administered. He asks the nurse what may have been the reason that his nitroglycerin sublingual tablets did not work. Based on knowledge of nitroglycerin sublingual tablets, what factors may have contributed to why the nitroglycerin tablets did not relieve his anginal pain?

5. The nurse asks the patient's spouse to bring the patient's supply of sublingual nitroglycerin tablets in to the hospital. The patient's spouse shows the nurse a small plastic pill container. "Heart pills" is handwritten on a masking-tape label. What teaching does the nurse need to provide?

6. The patient states that he guesses he will not need to get any more nitroglycerin sublingual tablets now that he is using the nitroglycerin patches. How should the nurse respond?

7. The nurse is reconciling medications during discharge instructions. The patient admits to adherence issues with taking his antihypertensive drug therapy because of experiencing erectile dysfunction. He asks what the nurse thinks about sildenafil (Viagra). What information should the nurse provide?

Case Study 2

A farmer who lives in a remote area was admitted with chest pain. He has been diagnosed with angina and is being discharged with a prescription for sublingual nitroglycerin tablets.

8. What teaching should the nurse provide about administration and storage of this drug?

9. The prescriber has written instructions that this patient should take the nitroglycerin before participating in stressful activity. What teaching should the nurse provide, considering that farm work includes operation of potentially dangerous equipment?

10. The prescriber has instructed this patient to continue to take nitroglycerin up to 3 tablets 5 minutes apart, take an aspirin, and to seek emergency medical care if relief is not obtained after administration of the first sublingual nitroglycerin tablet. The patient's spouse states that an older family member took nitroglycerin and had been instructed to seek medical care if relief was not experienced after taking 3 tablets. Why are the prescriber's instructions logical for this patient?

11. The patient has been instructed to take one baby aspirin tablet per day. The patient verbalizes that this seems silly because one baby aspirin tablet will not do much to relieve his chest pain. How should the nurse respond?

52

Anticoagulant, Antiplatelet, and Thrombolytic Drugs

STUDY QUESTIONS

True or False

For each of the following statements, enter T *for true or* F *for false.*

1. ____ Patients who take anticoagulant, antiplatelet, and thrombolytic drugs are at risk for bleeding.
2. ____ Pregnant or nursing patients should never be prescribed heparin.
3. ____ Anticoagulant and antiplatelet drugs only affect the formation of clots, not removal.
4. ____ When given at prescribed doses, anticoagulant and antiplatelet drugs can cause unintended bleeding.
5. ____ *Hemostasis* is a synonym for clot.
6. ____ *Aggregation* means clustering.

CRITICAL THINKING, PRIORITIZATION, AND DELEGATION QUESTIONS

7. A patient asks why heparin cannot be administered orally. What is the basis of the nurse's response?
   a. Heparin has a prolonged half-life when administered orally.
   b. Heparin can only be prepared as an oral solution and is bitter tasting.
   c. Heparin is destroyed by proteases in the gastrointestinal tract.
   d. Heparin is large and negatively charged, limiting absorption.

✻ 8. Which of these laboratory test results (which are flagged on the laboratory sheet as abnormal) would be a priority to report to the prescriber if a patient is prescribed heparin?
   a. aPTT 75 seconds
   b. BUN 22 mg/dL
   c. Platelet count 40,000/mm^3
   d. WBC 11,000/mm^3

9. What should the nurse do when a patient who has been receiving heparin tells the nurse that she thinks she could be pregnant?
   a. Administer the heparin as ordered and notify the prescriber of the possible pregnancy status.
   b. Withhold the heparin.
   c. Withhold the heparin until pregnancy status can be confirmed.
   d. Withhold the heparin and consult the prescriber regarding administration of the antidote protamine sulfate.

▶10. A patient has been receiving long-term high-dose heparin therapy. What nursing teaching would be best to prevent a common adverse effect of this type of therapy?
   a. Avoid crowds.
   b. Develop a plan for weight-bearing exercise as approved by the health care provider.
   c. Increase fluid and fiber in diet.
   d. Regular use of an over-the-counter antacid.

▶11. A patient is scheduled for a below-knee amputation at 1000 AM. Heparin 5000 units is scheduled to be administered subcutaneously (subQ) at 2100 the evening prior to surgery and 0900 the morning of surgery. Which action by the nurse is appropriate?
   a. Administer both doses of the medication as ordered.
   b. Administer the 0900 dose and contact the prescriber regarding the 2100 dose.
   c. Withhold the medication and contact the prescriber.
   d. Administer the 2100 dose and contact the prescriber regarding the 0900 dose.

12. A 110-lb (50-kg) patient who has just received a subcutaneous dose of 4000 units of heparin has developed hemoccult positive stool. A STAT aPTT is 155 seconds. The prescriber orders protamine sulfate. What is the recommended dose of protamine in this case?
   a. 10 mg of protamine
   b. 20 mg of protamine
   c. 40 mg of protamine
   d. 60 mg of protamine

13. Which aPTT result suggests that heparin therapy is in the therapeutic range?
   a. 30-40 seconds
   b. 40-50 seconds
   c. 60-80 seconds
   d. 90-120 seconds

14. Intravenous heparin 5000 units every 6 hours is prescribed today. Doses are scheduled at 1200, 1800, 2400, and 0600. If following monitoring recommendations, the nurse will enter a laboratory request for the aPTT specimen to be obtained at what times?
   a. 0800
   b. 0900 and 2100
   c. 1000, 1600, and 2200
   d. 1100, 1700, 2300, and 0500

▶15. An accident victim is prescribed heparin after open reduction and internal fixation (ORIF) of multiple fractures. Which symptom(s) would be of greatest concern to the nurse after beginning subcutaneous heparin therapy to prevent DVT?
   a. Bruising at the injection site
   b. Headache and faintness
   c. Pain and temperature 100° F (37.8° C)
   d. Pink saliva after brushing teeth

16. The nurse would consult the prescriber if which drug was prescribed with no order for monitoring of aPTT?
   a. Fragmin
   b. Heparin
   c. Warfarin
   d. Lovenox

17. Which statement applies to enoxaparin (Lovenox)? (Select all that apply.)
   a. Cost of treatment is more than cost of treatment with unfractionated heparin.
   b. Dosing may be based on patient's weight.
   c. May be used in combination with low-dose aspirin in patients with unstable angina.
   d. Protamine sulfate is an effective antidote.
   e. When ordered twice a day, should be administered every 12 hours.

＊18. A 79-year-old, 143-lb (65-kg) female patient was admitted with a hip fracture and is scheduled for an ORIF of the hip tomorrow. What would be a priority to report to the prescriber if the patient is prescribed enoxaparin (Lovenox)?
 a. A medical resident has ordered warfarin to be added in 2 days
 b. eGFR 85 mL/min
 c. INR 1.2
 d. Spinal anesthesia has been recommended for the surgery scheduled for tomorrow

19. Observations and research suggest that which OTC product(s) might increase the effects of warfarin (Coumadin) and increase the risk of bleeding? (Select all that apply.)
 a. Acetaminophen (Tylenol)
 b. Acetylsalicylic acid (aspirin)
 c. Cimetidine (Tagamet)
 d. Glucosamine/chondroitin
 e. Miconazole (Monistat intravaginal cream)

20. The nurse should teach patients who are prescribed warfarin (Coumadin) to eat consistent amounts of which food(s)? (Select all that apply.)
 a. Citrus fruits
 b. Liver
 c. Green, leafy vegetables
 d. Mayonnaise
 e. Red meat

▶21. What should the nurse teach a patient about precautions before dental surgery when the patient is prescribed long-term warfarin therapy?
 a. No action is needed.
 b. Inform the dentist of the most recent international normalized ratio (INR) results.
 c. Stop warfarin 3 days before dental surgery.
 d. Take half of the normal dose of warfarin for 3 days before dental surgery.

22. For how long after warfarin (Coumadin) therapy has been discontinued should the nurse maintain precautions to prevent bleeding,?
 a. 6 hours
 b. 8 to 12 hours
 c. 2.5 days
 d. 5 days

23. It would be of greatest priority to consult the prescriber if the nurse notes which laboratory test result for a patient who is prescribed dabigatran (Pradaxa)?
 a. ALT 65 IU/L
 b. eGFR (CrCL) 14 mL/min
 c. hCG 2 mIU/mL
 d. Na+ 140 mEq/L

24. Which assessment is of greatest priority when a patient is prescribed bivalirudin (Angiomax)?
 a. BP lying and sitting
 b. I&O
 c. Pain with movement
 d. Sleep

25. The nurse is teaching a male patient about rivaroxaban (Xarelto) prescribed after right knee replacement surgery. Which statement made by the patient suggests understanding of the teaching?
 a. "I should use a soft toothbrush and electric razor."
 b. "I should not touch the needle when injecting this drug."
 c. "I only need to have a blood test once a month when taking this drug."
 d. "If I have sudden shortness of breath, I should just sit down and rest."

26. While receiving an infusion of recombinant human AT (rhAT), the patient complains of tingling around the mouth and tightness in the chest. Which action by the nurse should be performed first?
 a. Assess lung sounds.
 b. Assess vital signs.
 c. Flush the IV line with normal saline solution.
 d. Stop the infusion of the drug.

27. Which statement, if made by a patient who has been prescribed low-dose aspirin therapy, would indicate a need for further teaching?
 a. "I need to inform my pharmacist that I am taking aspirin therapy."
 b. "I should quit smoking."
 c. "I should avoid using a drug that reduces stomach acid while on aspirin therapy."
 d. "If I use an enteric-coated aspirin, I don't need to worry about my stomach."

28. An acute coronary syndrome (ACS) patient who is prescribed clopidogrel (Plavix) vomits greenish-brown liquid with dark brown particles. Which action should the nurse take?
 a. Complete a head-to-toe assessment.
 b. Consult the prescriber to request emesis Hematest.
 c. Consult the prescriber regarding prescribing an antiemetic.
 d. Stop administration of the clopidogrel (Plavix).

29. The initial digoxin level of a patient who is pre-scribed digoxin (Lanoxin) 0.125 mg once a day and ticagrelor (Brilinta) 90 mg twice daily is 0.6 ng/mL. Both drugs are due to be administered. What action should the nurse take?
    a. Administer the digoxin as prescribed only.
    b. Administer the ticagrelor as prescribed only.
    c. Administer both drugs as prescribed.
    d. Withhold both drugs and contact the prescriber.

▶30. Which adverse effect, if noted in a patient who has recently been prescribed ticlopidine would be a reason for the nurse to contact the prescriber im-mediately?
    a. Change in level of consciousness
    b. Diarrhea
    c. Dyspepsia
    d. Itchy rash

▶31. The nurse is reviewing the laboratory tests of a patient who has been prescribed ticlopidine for the past week. The WBC count is 3000/mm^3, and the neutrophil count is 30%. What is a nursing priority for this patient?
    a. Assessing adequate cardiac output
    b. Evaluating effective airway clearance
    c. Maintaining skin integrity
    d. Preventing infection

32. A patient who received abciximab (ReoPro) as ad-junct to percutaneous coronary intervention (PCI) develops a hard lump at the access site and pain in the leg. Which nursing action would be appropri-ate at this time? (Select all that apply.)
    a. Administer oxygen.
    b. Apply pressure over the sheath insertion site.
    c. Maintain bedrest.
    d. Outline any bleeding on the dressing.
    e. Prepare for a CAT scan.

33. What is the most significant disadvantage of di-pyridamole/aspirin (Aggrenox)?
    a. Cost
    b. Dosing schedule
    c. Does not contain recommended dose of aspirin
    d. Does not contain recommended dose of dipyri-damole

34. The nurse teaches a patient who has been pre-scribed cilostazol (Pletal) that the risk of the bleeding is increased if the patient includes which food in the diet?
    a. Cabbage
    b. Dairy products
    c. Grapefruit juice
    d. Green vegetables

35. Which instruction is of greatest priority when teaching the family of a patient who is at risk for myocardial infarction?
    a. Drugs have been developed to open clogged circulation.
    b. It is important that they donate blood.
    c. They should seek immediate medical care when symptoms start.
    d. Thrombolytic drugs carry a significant risk of bleeding.

DOSE CALCULATION QUESTIONS

36. A patient who received 5000 units of heparin subQ at 0900 develops hematemesis at 1030. The pre-scriber orders 50 mg of protamine sulfate via slow intravenous (IV) push injection. Protamine sulfate is available as 10 mg/mL. How many mL will the nurse administer?

37. The nurse calculates the safe dose of tirofiban (Aggrastat) for a 220-lb patient undergoing bal-loon angioplasty. The drug comes in a solution of 12.5 mg/250 mL. The IV pump is calibrated in milliliters per hour. What rate will the nurse enter into the IV pump per hour?

CASE STUDY

A 36-year-old, 132-lb woman whose job requires frequent long airplane trips is admitted for treatment of a deep venous thrombosis (DVT) in the right thigh. The patient's spouse asks why the patient's primary care provider did not prescribe low-dose aspirin to prevent DVTs.

1. How should the nurse respond?

2. The patient is initially ordered a heparin drip by the emergency department physician. What is the most common adverse effect of heparin, and what symptoms of this adverse effect should be moni-tored by the nurse?

3. Heparin is pregnancy category C, which means that research studies suggest that risk to a developing fetus cannot be ruled out. If heparin does not cross the placenta, why is it not categorized as pregnancy class B?

4. The patient's primary care provider discontinues the IV heparin and orders enoxaparin 60 mg subQ every 12 hours. How much time should elapse between the nurse discontinuing the heparin drip and starting the subQ enoxaparin (Lovenox)? Why?

53

Management of ST-Elevation Myocardial Infarction

STUDY QUESTIONS

Completion

1. The medical term for a heart attack is _____ _____.

2. The abbreviation for an MI with complete blockage of the coronary artery is _____.

3. The "ST" in STEMI stands for elevation of the _____ _____ of the PQRST of the ECG.

4. Myocardial infarctions where there is partial blockage of the coronary artery are called non-_____ MI.

5. Risk factors for STEMI include _____, _____, _____, _____, _____, _____, and _____.

6. Almost all coronary occlusions occur at the site of a ruptured _____ _____.

7. Remodeling of the myocardium that occurs with MI is driven in part by local production of _____.

8. Intracellular proteins released when cardiac muscle cells are damaged are called _____ and _____.

9. Current recommendations for MI include administering oxygen if O_2 saturation is less than _____.

CRITICAL THINKING, PRIORITIZATION, AND DELEGATION QUESTIONS

10. Because of the impairment in blood flow and resulting acidosis with STEMI, the nurse would expect the patient to exhibit
    a. bradycardia.
    b. edema.
    c. flushing.
    d. rapid, deep respirations.

11. Research suggests which treatment(s) improve(s) outcomes in STEMI? (Select all that apply.)
    a. Administration of aspirin
    b. Administration of a beta-blocker
    c. Administration of ibuprofen (NSAID)
    d. Administration of morphine
    e. Administration of SL nitroglycerin
    f. Administration of oxygen

12. What is an expected response within minutes of administering IV morphine during a STEMI? (Select all that apply.)
    a. Decrease in pain
    b. Improved hemodynamics
    c. Increase in depth of respirations
    d. Inversion of T wave on ECG

13. A protocol in the emergency department (ED) is to administer four chewable 81-mg aspirin tablets (total 324 mg) to patients with suspected MI. A student nurse asks the nurse why four chewable aspirin tablets are administered instead of two regular aspirin tablets (650 mg). What is the most accurate explanation for this protocol for the first dose of aspirin?
    a. Aspirin is an acid, and acids are more readily absorbed in the acid environment of the stomach.
    b. Chewable forms of aspirin are rapidly absorbed through the buccal mucosa.
    c. Chewing breaks the tablet into smaller particles, which are more readily absorbed in the intestines.
    d. Exceeding 325-mg doses can offset the vasodilation and antiplatelet effects of lower doses.

＊14. A patient who is undergoing an acute STEMI is prescribed metoprolol 50 mg by mouth every 6 hours. It would be a priority to immediately contact the prescriber if which assessment finding was present?
    a. Altered taste
    b. Insomnia
    c. Rhinorrhea
    d. Wheezing

▶15. The ED triage nurse answers the call of a patient who has a history of angina pectoris and chronic obstructive pulmonary disease (COPD). The patient reports chest pain that has not been relieved by three doses of nitroglycerin. The patient had been told by his physician that he should take chewable aspirin should this occur, but he does not have any aspirin. What should the nurse tell the patient to do?
    a. Call 911.
    b. Call his physician for directions.
    c. Take ibuprofen and seek medical care.
    d. Turn on his home oxygen and rest.

16. Which drug prescribed for acute STEMI should be withheld and the prescriber consulted immediately if the patient's pulse is 118 beats/min?
    a. Aspirin
    b. Atenolol
    c. Morphine
    d. Nitroglycerin

17. The nurse knows that nitroglycerin decreases the workload of the heart by
    a. dissolving existing clots.
    b. preventing clot formation.
    c. slowing the heart rate.
    d. reducing venous return to the heart.

18. When caring for a patient during a STEMI who is prescribed alteplase, the nurse would question the prescriber if which drug was also prescribed?
    a. Abciximab (ReoPro)
    b. Clopidogrel (Plavix)
    c. Lisinopril (Zestril)
    d. Low molecular weight (LMW) heparin (Lovenox)

19. Which laboratory result in the history of a patient who is experiencing STEMI would be most important to report to the prescriber who has just ordered captopril (Capoten)?
    a. AST 120 international units/L
    b. BUN 15 mg/dL
    c. eGFR 38 mL/min
    d. Troponin T 0.8 ng/mL

DOSE CALCULATION QUESTIONS

20. Intravenous (IV) morphine 4 mg is prescribed for a STEMI patient. Available is 5 mg/mL. How many mL of morphine should be administered?

21. The drug book suggests diluting morphine to 4-5 mL and infusing over 4-5 minutes. To push a tenth of a mL every 5 seconds, the nurse would add how much sterile diluent to the 0.8 mL of morphine and push over what time?

CASE STUDY

A 57-year-old man who is vacationing locally is admitted to the ED with severe, crushing chest pain. The pain radiates into his left arm, and he is experiencing diaphoresis, weakness, and nausea. The ECG shows elevated ST segments in the inferior leads. Troponin T (TnT) is elevated three times above lower limits, and the total creatine kinase (CK) and the CK-MB isoenzyme are slightly elevated. The physician diagnoses STEMI. The physician decides to start thrombolytic therapy with alteplase (tPA).

1. What assessments should the nurse monitor related to the risk of intracranial bleeding?

2. The nurse is directed to interview the patient's spouse. What information does the nurse need to obtain to assist the physician with deciding if thrombolytic therapy is appropriate?

3. The following medications are ordered. What is the purpose of these drugs, and what assessment should the nurse perform relating to administration of these drugs?

   a. Aspirin (ASA) 81-mg chewable tablets, 4 tablets STAT

   b. Intravenous (IV) morphine 4 mg followed by 2 mg every 10 minutes as needed to control pain

   c. Metoprolol 5 mg IV every 2 minutes for 3 doses then 50 mg orally every 6 hours × 48 hours

   d. Nitroglycerin IV drip 10 mcg per minute

   e. Lisinopril 5 mg first two days followed by 10 mg daily

4. Why is it important for the nurse to assess if this patient has taken sildenafil in the past 24 hours?

5. The patient is being discharged with prescriptions for metoprolol (Lopressor) 100 mg once a day, captopril (Capoten) 25 mg every 8 hours, aspirin 81 mg once a day, and warfarin (Coumadin) 5 mg once a day. The patient's spouse asks why the patient must have bloodwork (INR) done every week. How should the nurse respond?

6. When explaining warfarin therapy, the nurse shares the patient's INR results, which most recently were 1.8. The laboratory result form lists the normal INR as 0.9 to 1.1. How can the nurse explain that the target INR is 3, which appears to be abnormal?

54

Drugs for Hemophilia

STUDY QUESTIONS

True or False

For each of the following statements, enter T for true or F for false.

1. ____ Hemophilia always produces a severe bleeding disorder.
2. ____ Hemophilia can result from a spontaneous gene mutation.
3. ____ Hemophilia interferes with the formation of a platelet plug.
4. ____ Hemophilia is inherited on the Y chromosome.
5. ____ Hemophilia has a risk factor of 50% for every boy born to a mother who is a carrier of the defective gene, no matter how many brothers have the disease.
6. ____ Hemophilia never occurs in females.
7. ____ 100% of daughters of hemophiliacs are carriers of the disease.
8. ____ Treatment with clotting factor replacement is costly.

CRITICAL THINKING, PRIORITIZATION, AND DELEGATION QUESTIONS

✳ 9. The nurse is caring for a 3-year-old patient who was admitted after a car accident. Laboratory tests indicate that the patient has 0.4% of the normal amount of clotting factor VIII. Which symptom would be of most concern to the nurse?
   a. Blood pressure 72/58 mm Hg
   b. Difficult to arouse
   c. Pulse 100 beats/min
   d. Swollen ankle

10. The nurse needs to give an intramuscular immunization to a patient with a history of mild hemophilia B. What should the nurse do?
   a. Administer the immunization as usual.
   b. Administer the immunization subcutaneously.
   c. Apply pressure to the site for 5 minutes after the injection.
   d. Administer only via an oral or nasal route.

11. The parent of a child with hemophilia calls the pediatrician's office. The parent has forgotten which medication can be given to the child for mild pain and fever. The telephone triage nurse follows protocol and explains that the safest choice for hemophiliacs is which drug?
   a. Acetaminophen (Tylenol)
   b. Acetylsalicylic acid (aspirin)
   c. Celecoxib (Celebrex)
   d. Ibuprofen (Motrin)

▶ 12. What nursing diagnosis would apply to all patients with hemophilia?
   a. Anxiety
   b. Ineffective coping
   c. Risk for altered growth
   d. Risk for injury

13. Calculations are available to predict patient response to infusion of factor concentrates. For each unit/kg of recombinant factor IX administered, the patient's normal factor IX should increase by what percentage?
   a. 0.1%
   b. 0.2%
   c. 1%
   d. 2%

14. Calculations are available to predict patient response to infusion of factor concentrates. For each unit/kg of recombinant factor VIII administered, the patient's normal factor VIII should increase by what percentage?
   a. 0.1%
   b. 0.2%
   c. 1%
   d. 2%

15. When the prescriber is determining the proper dose of factor concentrate, what is the most important patient factor to consider?
   a. Age
   b. Clinical response
   c. Target percentage of normal factor levels
   d. Weight

▶ 16. Desmopressin nasal spray 150 mcg is prescribed preoperatively for a 4-year-old patient with mild hemophilia A. The pharmacy only carries the spray that delivers 10 mcg/spray and is unable to obtain any other concentration. What should the nurse do?
   a. Administer 15 sprays of the medication.
   b. Administer 150 mcg intravenously.
   c. Consult with the prescriber regarding the fact that the pharmacy does not carry a needed drug.
   d. Consult with the prescriber regarding an oral dose order.

✳ 17. The nurse is administering factor concentrate to a child who begins to experience swelling around the face. What is of greatest priority and should be performed first?
   a. Administer diphenhydramine (Benadryl).
   b. Administer prescribed epinephrine (EpiPen).
   c. Slow the infusion.
   d. Stop the infusion.

18. Aminocaproic acid solution may be prescribed to prevent bleeding from dental care for patients with what condition(s)?
   a. Hemophilia A and B
   b. Hemophilia A only
   c. Hemophilia B only
   d. Severe hemophilia A and B only

19. The nurse knows that inhibitor antibodies to factor concentrate are most likely to occur in hemophiliacs of which descent? (Select all that apply.)
   a. African American
   b. Asian
   c. Hispanic
   d. Middle Eastern
   e. Native American

20. When a patient is receiving factor VIIa (NovoSeven), the patient should be carefully assessed for what?
    a. Allergy to pork
    b. Anorexia and nausea
    c. Chest pain and shortness of breath
    d. Muscle weakness and fatigue

DOSE CALCULATION QUESTIONS

21. A nurse in the perioperative area is caring for a 12-year-old child with hemophilia A who weighs 99 lb. What is the recommended number of units of recombinant factor VIII concentrate to raise the child's level to 50%?

22. Desmopressin [DDAVP] 0.3 micrograms/kg is prescribed for a 66-lb child. The drug is available in a solution of 4 mcg/mL to be further diluted in 0.9% normal saline and infused over 30 minutes. How many mL will be drawn up to further dilute? What rate will be programmed into the IV pump if the solution of desmopressin was further diluted in 50 mL of 0.9% normal saline?

CASE STUDY

A 17-month-old child has been newly diagnosed with hemophilia A. Review of the chart indicates that the patient has not been immunized for hepatitis A.

1. What teaching needs to be provided relating to hepatitis immunization, and what information relating to immunizations does the nurse need to obtain regarding caregivers?

2. The patient's parents ask why aspirin should not be given to their child. What should the nurse explain?

3. The nurse provides a comprehensive list of over-the-counter drugs that contain salicylate. Which of these drugs would the nurse include on the list? Alka Seltzer, Anacin, Aspergum, Arthropan, Ascriptin, Disalcid, Doan's original, Dolobid, Empirin, Keygesic, Kaopectate, Momentum, Pepto-Bismol, St. Joseph's baby aspirin, Trilisate.

4. The home health nurse goes to the patient's home to teach the parents how to administer recombinant factor VIII concentrate via a central venous catheter. What are the nursing diagnoses that the nurse should consider when developing the plan of care for this family?

5. Administering factor concentrate carries a risk of complications. What should the nurse teach the caregiver to prepare for possible complications?

55

Drugs for Deficiency Anemias

STUDY QUESTIONS

Matching

Match the term with its definition.

1. ___ Developing red blood cell (RBC) in marrow after incorporating hemoglobin

2. ___ Developing RBC in bone marrow before incorporating hemoglobin

3. ___ Immature erythrocytes

4. ___ Oxygen-storing molecule of muscle

5. ___ Measures color of RBCs

6. ___ Measures size of RBCs

7. ___ Oxygen-carrying protein of RBCs

8. ___ Percentage of RBCs in a volume of blood

9. ___ Saturation capacity of transferrin with iron

10. ___ Storage form of iron within mucosal cells

11. ___ Storage form of iron in bone marrow

12. ___ Transports absorbed iron to bone marrow

13. ___ Variation in size of RBC

a. Erythroblast
b. Ferritin
c. Hematocrit
d. Hemoglobin
e. Hemosiderin
f. Iron-binding capacity (IBC) [total IBC (TIBC)]
g. Mean corpuscular hemoglobin concentration (MCHC)
h. Mean corpuscular volume (MCV)
i. Myoglobin
j. Proerythroblast
k. Red blood cell distribution width (RDW)
l. Reticulocyte
m. Transferrin

Match the term with its definition.

14. ___ Excessive color
15. ___ Large erythroblast
16. ___ Large erythrocyte
17. ___ Pale
18. ___ Small-size cell

a. Hyperchromic
b. Hypochromic
c. Macrocyte
d. Megaloblast
e. Microcytic

CRITICAL THINKING, PRIORITIZATION, AND DELEGATION QUESTIONS

▶19. The nurse is caring for a cancer patient who is anemic who is receiving chemotherapy that prevents the reproduction of rapidly dividing cells, including the cancer cells, hair, RBCs, and epithelium of the gastrointestinal (GI) tract. Which laboratory result suggests that the anemia is getting worse?
a. Hemoglobin 10 mg/dL
b. Hematocrit 26%
c. RBC 3.8×10^{12}/L
d. Reticulocyte count 0.002%

∗20. It is a priority for the nurse to assess for symptoms of anemia in a patient who has a history of what condition?
a. Chronic obstructive pulmonary disease
b. Chronic kidney disease
c. Diabetes insipidus
d. Hypertension

21. Normally the body prevents excessive buildup of iron in the body by
a. decreasing intestinal absorption of iron.
b. increasing metabolism of RBCs.
c. increasing excretion of RBCs in bile.
d. increasing excretion of RBCs in urine.

22. Which food(s) should the nurse include in dietary teaching for pregnant women regarding prevention of iron-deficiency anemia? (Select all that apply.)
    a. Carrots, red peppers, squash
    b. Cheese, milk, yogurt
    c. Chicken, fish, red meat
    d. Egg yolk, legumes
    e. Oranges, apples, pears

23. In iron-deficiency anemia, the nurse would expect which test to be elevated from normal levels?
    a. Hematocrit (Hct)
    b. Hemoglobin (Hgb or Hb)
    c. (Total) iron-binding capacity (IBC or TIBC)
    d. Mean corpuscular volume (MCV)

24. What is a common nursing diagnosis for patients with iron-deficiency anemia?
    a. Body image disturbance
    b. Breathing pattern, ineffective
    c. Cardiac output, decreased
    d. Fatigue

▶25. The school nurse has been consulted by a fifth-grade teacher regarding a student who is pale and tires excessively as the day progresses, and whose academic performance has been declining. What action would be appropriate at this time?
    a. Contact the child's parents and inform them that their child is anemic.
    b. Contact the child's parents and tell them their child needs to be seen by their pediatrician.
    c. Make an appointment, along with the teacher, to speak with the parents about noted concerns.
    d. Tell the child that you think he/she is anemic and should tell his/her parents.

26. What is the most common adverse effect of administration of ferrous sulfate?
    a. Discoloration of teeth
    b. Heartburn
    c. Hypotension
    d. Weak, rapid pulse

27. A patient complains of intolerable nausea and heartburn from taking an oral iron preparation. What should the nurse instruct the patient to do?
    a. Consult with the prescriber.
    b. Take a calcium carbonate antacid with the iron.
    c. Take the iron with milk.
    d. Take the iron with orange juice.

▶28. The nurse is providing care to a patient who is receiving an oral iron preparation. The patient's stool is greenish-black. What should the nurse do?
    a. Administer a dose of the iron preparation.
    b. Consult the prescriber.
    c. Determine if this stool is usual or a change for this patient.
    d. Hold the iron preparation.

✳29. A patient with peptic ulcer disease has developed severe anemia. Iron dextran (DexFerrum) has just been prescribed. The nurse has administered a test dose. It is a priority for the nurse to observe the patient for what adverse effect?
    a. Edema of the face and throat
    b. Hives
    c. Phlebitis at the site of injection
    d. Tissue damage from extravasation

30. When iron must be administered by injection, which method of administration should be used?
    a. Intradermal
    b. Intrathecal
    c. Subcutaneous
    d. Z-track intramuscular

✳31. The dialysis nurse has administered iron dextran and erythropoietin. What is a priority nursing concern relating to adverse effects?
    a. Gastrointestinal cramping
    b. Infusion site discomfort
    c. Tissue perfusion
    d. Taste alterations

✳32. A patient with chronic kidney disease is prescribed ferumoxytol (Feraheme). It would be a priority to inform the consulting physician of this drug if he or she orders which diagnostic test?
    a. Computed tomography (CT)
    b. Magnetic resonance imaging (MRI)
    c. Positron emission tomography (PET)
    d. Ultrasound

33. Which foods are good sources of vitamin B_{12}?
    a. Organ meats
    b. Fruits
    c. Grains
    d. Vegetables

✳34. It is a priority to teach the patient with pernicious anemia to report which issue?
    a. Fatigue
    b. Joint pain
    c. Paresthesias
    d. Temperature >100.4° F (38° C)

▶35. A patient with pernicious anemia complains of numbness and tingling of the hands and feet. What data relating to possible neurologic damage should the nurse collect before notifying the prescriber of the patient's complaint?
   a. Blood pressure
   b. Deep tendon reflex
   c. Capillary glucose
   d. Skin color

36. To prevent damage to the developing neural tube of a fetus, it is important for women of child-bearing age to have adequate daily intake of folate, which can be found in which foods? (Select all that apply.)
   a. Asparagus and spinach
   b. Egg yolks and red meat
   c. Enriched cereals and whole-wheat breads
   d. Lentils and okra
   e. Liver and chicken

37. When a patient is prescribed drugs that increase the production of RBCs, it is a priority to monitor the effect of changes in serum potassium on which system?
   a. Cardiovascular system
   b. Endocrine system
   c. Gastrointestinal system
   d. Pulmonary system

DOSE CALCULATION QUESTIONS

38. The pediatrician prescribes ferrous sulfate drops 25 mg twice a day. The child weighs 22 lb, and the recommended dose is 5 mg/kg/day. Is the dose safe and effective?

39. Ferrous sulfate drops are available as 75 mg in 0.6 mL. How much should the parents administer with each dose?

CASE STUDIES

Case Study 1

An 11-month-old child, who drinks 8-ounce bottles of whole milk 5-6 times a day, is diagnosed with iron-deficiency anemia.

1. What can the nurse teach the parents about factors that could be contributing to the anemia and measures to change the factors that can be altered?

2. What should the nurse teach the parents about ferrous sulfate therapy?

Case Study 2

A 28-year-old woman has had gastric bypass surgery. She has lost 25 lb in the past 2 months. She comes to her primary care provider (PCP) with complaints of fatigue and glossitis (smooth, beefy, red tongue).

3. Because of a history of this surgery, the patient is at risk for what type of anemia? Why?

4. The patient is prescribed parenteral injections of vitamin B_{12} (30 mcg) and folic acid 200 mcg daily for 1 week. She then will receive oral cyanocobalamin 10,000 mcg/day and folic acid 400 mcg/day. The patient tells the nurse that she had learned that oral administration of cyanocobalamin is ineffective. How should the nurse respond?

5. The patient discusses concerns about taking "all of these pills" every day. The prescriber discontinues the oral cyanocobalamin and prescribes intranasal cyanocobalamin (Nascobal) one spray in one nostril once a week. What teaching will the nurse provide about intranasal administration of the drug?

6. The nurse teaches the patient to report which symptoms that suggest the adverse effect of hypokalemia that is possible when taking cyanocobalamin (vitamin B_{12})?

56
Hematopoietic Agents

STUDY QUESTIONS

Completion

1. In addition to the kidneys, erythropoietin is secreted by cells of many organs including

   _____, _____,

   _____, _____,

   _____, _____, and

   _____.

2. Erythropoiesis-stimulating agents (ESAs) can shorten life in certain _____ patients.

3. Epoetin has been associated with an increase in _____ and _____ when hemoglobin levels rise higher than 11 g/dL.

4. Dosage of epoetin alfa should be reduced when hemoglobin increases by more than _____ g/dL in two weeks.

5. When administering filgrastim (Neupogen), the nurse should review the WBC count _____ times per week.

6. Allergy to _____ would be a contraindication to administration of sargramostim (Leukine).

7. Romiplostim (Nplate)'s action is to _____ platelet production.

8. The nurse needs to assess for shortness of breath, chest pain, and change in level of consciousness when a patient is prescribed the thrombopoietin receptor agonists (TRAs) because these drugs increase the risk of _____.

CRITICAL THINKING, PRIORITIZATION, AND DELEGATION QUESTIONS

9. Which new assessment finding would be of greatest priority to report to the prescriber when a patient is receiving epoetin alpha (Procrit)?
   a. Chest pain
   b. Fatigue
   c. Pallor
   d. Weak dorsalis pedis pulse

10. A patient with a history of type 2 diabetes mellitus (T2DM) and chronic kidney disease (CDK) is receiving epoetin alpha (Procrit) because her failing kidneys do not produce adequate amounts of erythropoietin, and she has become anemic. What would be a realistic goal for therapy?
    a. Hgb 8 g/dL; transferrin 25%; ferritin 90 ng/mL
    b. Hgb 10 g/dL; transferrin 20%; ferritin 125 ng/mL
    c. Hgb 12 g/dL; transferrin 10%; ferritin 80 ng/dL
    d. Hgb14 g/dL; transferrin 15%; ferritin 100 ng/mL

11. When darbepoetin alfa is administered preoperatively to reduce the need for blood transfusion postoperatively, the nurse would question the prescriber if which drug was not also prescribed?
    a. Ferrous sulfate
    b. Folate
    c. Furosemide
    d. Heparin

✳12. It would be a priority to report to the prescriber of darbepoetin alpha (Aranesp) which assessment finding?
    a. Blood pressure 170/98 mm Hg
    b. Pulse 100 beats/min
    c. Respirations 24
    d. Temperature 101.4° F (38° C)

▶13. A chemotherapy patient who has received three injections in the past week of epoetin alpha (Procrit) is due for the next dose. The patient's hemoglobin has not increased. What should the nurse do?
a. Hold the next dose.
b. Administer the medication as ordered.
c. Consult the prescriber regarding assessing for renal failure.
d. Consult the prescriber regarding assessing for neutralizing antibodies.

▶14. Epoetin alpha (Procrit) 4000 units subcutaneous is ordered at 0900 pending endogenous erythropoietin levels for an anemic HIV-infected patient receiving zidovudine (AZT). Lab results arrived at 0830, including endogenous erythropoietin level of 578 milliunits/mL. What should the nurse do?
a. Administer the epoetin alpha (Procrit) STAT.
b. Administer the epoetin alpha (Procrit) with the 0900 medications.
c. Hold the medication and consult the prescriber.
d. Hold the medication.

＊15. Elevation of uric acid is an adverse effect of filgrastim (Neupogen) therapy. What is the priority assessment for the nurse to evaluate relating to possible elevations of uric acid?
a. Edema
b. Elevated temperature
c. Joint redness and swelling
d. Tachycardia

▶16. The nurse is teaching administration of filgrastim (Neupogen) to the parent of a child with congenital neutropenia who weighs 88 lb. The prescribed dose is 240 mcg (6 mcg/kg). The medication is available in a concentration of 300 mcg/mL in 1.6-mL vials. The nurse should teach the parent to administer which dosage?
a. 0.6 mL, discarding the vial after the first dose
b. 0.6 mL, obtaining 2 doses from each vial
c. 0.8 mL, discarding the vial after the first dose
d. 0.8 mL, obtaining 2 doses from each vial

17. Administration directives for filgrastim (Neupogen) for a patient receiving chemotherapy include which directive?
a. Administering after each dose of chemotherapy
b. Consulting the prescriber once absolute neutrophil count has reached 10,000/mm^3
c. Keeping the drug refrigerated at all times
d. Wiping the rubber stopper with alcohol when reentering the vial

18. Advantages of using pegfilgrastim (Neulasta) instead of filgrastim (Neupogen) include what?
a. It can be administered immediately before or after chemotherapy.
b. The course of therapy is one injection lasting 2 weeks.
c. It does not cause bone pain.
d. There is less elevation of LDH, alkaline phosphatase, and uric acid.

＊19. What would be a symptom of an extremely rare but significant adverse reaction to massive doses of sargramostim (Leukine)?
a. Crackles (rales)
b. Gurgles (rhonchi)
c. Pleural friction rub
d. Wheezes

20. If the final concentration of sargramostim (Leukine) is to be less than 10 mcg/mL, the drug should be diluted in
a. 0.9% sodium chloride.
b. 0.9% sodium chloride with 20 mEq KCl.
c. 0.9% sodium chloride with 0.1% albumin.
d. 0.9% sodium chloride with 5% dextrose in water.

21. What is true about oprelvekin (Neumega)? (Select all that apply.)
a. It decreases count of abnormal platelets.
b. It increases production and maturity of megakaryocytes.
c. It is eliminated more rapidly in children than adults.
d. It is excreted in active form in the urine.
e. It peaks in action in 24 hours.

＊22. Which of these adverse effects of oprelvekin (Neumega) would be of greatest priority to report to the prescriber?
a. Dyspnea
b. Peripheral edema
c. Rash
d. Red eyes

＊23. What is a priority nursing concern for a patient with idiopathic thrombocytopenic purpura (ITP) who is prescribed eltrombopag (Promacta)?
a. Fluid volume
b. Impaired mobility
c. Nutritional needs
d. Safety

24. It is important to ask a patient who has just been prescribed eltrombopag (Promacta) about use of which over-the-counter products? (Select all that apply.)
    a. Analgesics
    b. Antacids
    c. Cough medicines
    d. Decongestants
    e. Laxatives

DOSE CALCULATION QUESTIONS

25. A patient is prescribed sargramostim (Leukine) 250 mcg/m² after a bone marrow transplant. The patient weighs 50 kg and is 163 cm tall. The pharmacy delivers sargramostim (Leukine) 500 mcg/mL, which the nurse dilutes to a concentration of 10 mcg/mL. How much sargramostim (Leukine) should be administered?

26. The intravenous pumps are calibrated at mL/hr. The sargramostim (Leukine) above is to be infused over 4 hours. What rate should the nurse program into the pump?

CASE STUDIES

Case Study 1

A 65-year-old male patient has had T2DM for 40 years and CKD managed with hemodialysis for 5 years. He is anemic, and has been prescribed epoetin alfa (Procrit) three times a week to help maintain his erythrocyte count. The prescriber has ordered his periodic laboratory tests, including BUN, creatinine, phosphorus, potassium, RBC indices, hemoglobin, transferrin saturation, ferritin, and uric acid. The patient is tired of "being jabbed" and asks the nurse why these tests have to be done.

1. Describe the rationale for each test in a way the patient can understand.
    a. BUN/creatinine

    b. Phosphorus

    c. Potassium

    d. Hemoglobin

    e. RBC indices

    f. Ferritin

    g. Transferrin saturation

    h. Uric acid

2. What adverse effects should the nurse assess in this patient?

3. The nurse is reviewing laboratory results for this patient. Hemoglobin is 13.5 g/dL. What should the nurse do?

Case Study 2

A patient is prescribed sargramostim (Leukine) 250 mcg/m² after a bone marrow transplant.

4. What is the rationale for this therapy?

5. What should the nurse do or not do if the patient experiences these adverse effects?

    a. Diarrhea

    b. Weakness

    c. Rash

    d. Bone pain

57

Drugs for Diabetes Mellitus

STUDY QUESTIONS

True or False

For each of the following statements, enter T *for true or* F *for false.*

1. ____ Glycemic control involves metabolism of carbohydrates, proteins, and fats.
2. ____ Diabetes affects blood flow to all organs.
3. ____ Foods with a low glycemic index have fewer carbohydrates than those with a high glycemic index.
4. ____ Blood sugar control will best be achieved if the patient follows a plan created by the health care providers.
5. ____ Exercise improves cellular response to insulin.
6. ____ Clear insulin is always short-acting.
7. ____ Insulin therapy with one long-acting agent that mimics the body's basal insulin secretion and another short-acting agent to cover eating most closely mimics normal functioning.
8. ____ Once the patient's blood sugar is stabilized, the patient will be able to maintain control with oral drugs.
9. ____ Saturated fats should be limited to less than 10% of the total calories.
10. ____ Administering insulin or sulfonylurea drugs and not eating can cause serious effects from the blood sugar going too low.
11. ____ Tight glucose control decreases the incidence of kidney failure.
12. ____ Treatment can be monitored by blood or urine.
13. ____ Weight loss is always needed to decrease the patient's insulin requirements.

CRITICAL THINKING, PRIORITIZATION, AND DELEGATION QUESTIONS

14. Which complication of diabetes causes the most deaths?
    a. Cardiovascular effects
    b. Hypoglycemia
    c. Ketoacidosis
    d. Kidney damage

15. Which antihypertensive drug might be prescribed for a patient with DM who does not have hypertension?
    a. Benazepril (Lotensin)
    b. Carvedilol (Coreg)
    c. Diltiazem (Cardizem)
    d. Furosemide (Lasix)

▶16. What is an appropriate outcome for drug therapy with metoclopramide (Reglan) for a patient with DM?
    a. Alert and oriented ×3
    b. No adventitious lung sounds
    c. Palpable peripheral pulse
    d. Soft, nondistended abdomen

17. What would be the most appropriate nursing intervention for a 23-year-old patient who, for the first time, has a fasting plasma glucose level of 145 mg/dL?
    a. Advise the patient to include 30 minutes of vigorous exercise in his daily activities.
    b. Discuss possible diet changes with the patient.
    c. Explain the need for oral antidiabetic medication to the patient.
    d. Teach the patient how to do a urine dip for glucose and ketones.

18. Which type of diabetes often exists for years before diagnosis, but fasting blood glucose is not elevated because of hyperinsulinemia?
    a. Gestational diabetes
    b. Juvenile diabetes
    c. Type 1 diabetes
    d. Type 2 diabetes

✳19. It would be a priority for the nurse to respond to which symptoms if exhibited by a patient who is receiving insulin therapy for diabetes?
    a. Fatigue and blurred vision
    b. Perineal itching and copious urine
    c. Profuse sweating and difficult to arouse
    d. Thirst and constant hunger

20. A patient who has type 2 DM has been unable to follow the recommended diet and exercise regimen. He tries to alter his laboratory test results by eating less than usual before having blood testing performed. Which test would be most accurate for this patient because it evaluates his glucose control over the past 3 months?
    a. Fasting glucose
    b. A1c
    c. Postprandial glucose
    d. Two-hour glucose tolerance

21. A patient with diabetes who has been using traditional insulin therapy has been prescribed intensive insulin therapy to achieve tighter glucose control. Which information should be included in the teaching?
    a. An insulin pump is used to provide the best glucose control and requires about the same amount of attention as intensive insulin therapy.
    b. Intensive insulin therapy usually requires four injections of a rapid-acting insulin each day in addition to an injection of a basal insulin.
    c. Intensive insulin therapy is indicated only for newly diagnosed type 1 diabetics who have never experienced ketoacidosis.
    d. Studies have shown that intensive insulin therapy is most effective in preventing the macrovascular complications characteristic of type 2 DM.

►22. The nurse assesses for which symptom of the electrolyte imbalance that is most likely when a patient is receiving large doses of insulin?
    a. Muscle weakness and constipation
    b. Restlessness and irritability
    c. Spasm of the wrist and fingers when circulation of the upper arm is constricted for several minutes
    d. Twitching of the facial nerve when the face is tapped over the nerve

23. A nurse administered 30 units of glargine (Lantus) insulin in the same syringe as 8 units of aspart (Humalog) insulin coverage so that the patient would need only one injection. The nurse contacts the prescriber and monitors the patient for which symptom caused by the effects of this combination on the absorption of the insulin?
    a. Profuse sweating
    b. Itching
    c. Thirst
    d. Vomiting

►24. When obtaining a new vial of NPH insulin from the refrigerator, the nurse notes that the suspension is partially frozen. What should the nurse do?
    a. Discard the vial and obtain a new one from the pharmacy.
    b. Shake the vial vigorously to produce heat.
    c. Warm the suspension in warm water.
    d. Withdraw the unfrozen portion then discard the rest.

►25. A patient is admitted in a state of diabetic ketoacidosis. The resident orders insulin detemir 0.1 mg/kg/hr to be administered by intravenous (IV) drip. What should the nurse do?
    a. Calculate the insulin dose and mix it with 100 mL of normal saline.
    b. Calculate the insulin dose and mix it with 100 mL of D_5W.
    c. Calculate the insulin dose and infuse the solution prepared by the pharmacy.
    d. Consult the prescriber STAT.

►26. The nurse has done an initial assessment on assigned patients and is preparing to administer prescribed insulin. All patients are alert and oriented. It is 8:07 AM, and breakfast trays are scheduled to arrive at 8:45 AM. The nurse should administer the insulin first to the patient who has
    a. 8:00 AM SMBG 100 mg/dL; prescribed insulin aspart (NovoLog) 5 units
    b. 8:00 AM SMBG 110 mg/dL; prescribed insulin glulisine (Apidra) 7 units
    c. 8:00 AM SMBG 80 mg/dL; prescribed NPH insulin (Novolin N) 34 units
    d. 8:00 AM SMBG 90 mg/dL; prescribed regular insulin (Humulin R) 5 units

27. A patient has been prescribed 5 units of insulin aspart (NovoLog) and 25 units of insulin detemir (Levemir) to be administered at 0800. What should the nurse do?
    a. Draw up the two insulins in different syringes.
    b. Draw up 5 units of aspart insulin first, then 25 units of detemir insulin in the same syringe.
    c. Draw up the clear insulin, then the cloudy insulin, in the same syringe.
    d. Draw up 25 units of detemir insulin first, than 5 units aspart insulin in the same syringe.

28. What special administration techniques must the nurse use when administering NPH insulin?
    a. Never mix with another insulin.
    b. Administer this insulin only at bedtime.
    c. Roll the vial gently to mix particles in solution.
    d. When mixing with another insulin, draw the NPH into the syringe first.

29. The nurse is caring for a patient who is NPO for a diagnostic test. Which dose of insulin should be administered, if ordered, even if the patient is not eating?
    a. 8:00 AM SMBG 100 mg/dL; prescribed insulin aspart (NovoLog) 5 units and NPH (NovoLog) 34 units
    b. 8:00 AM SMBG 190 mg/dL; prescribed regular insulin (Humulin R) 4 units per sliding scale coverage
    c. 8:00 AM SMBG 110 mg/dL; prescribed insulin detemir 26 units
    d. 8:00 AM SMBG 80 mg/dL; prescribed NPH insulin (Novolin N) 34 units

30. A patient is prescribed 4 units of insulin aspart (NovoLog) based on a sliding scale relating to SMBG. Available syringes are marked 50 units in 0.5 mL or 100 units in 1 mL. Why should the nurse choose the 50 units in a 0.5-mL syringe to administer this dose?
    a. It is the only syringe that can accurately measure this dose.
    b. It is the only syringe that has the correct needle for administering this dose.
    c. It is easier to administer the insulin using this syringe.
    d. It is easier to see the line indicating the 4 units on this syringe.

31. Research suggests that intensive insulin therapy (tight control) in type 1 and 2 DM is most effective in preventing
    a. cerebrovascular accidents (CVAs).
    b. neuropathic pain.
    c. peripheral vascular disease requiring amputation.
    d. ophthalmic complications.

✳32. When performing the initial morning assessment on a patient with diabetes, the nurse notes that the patient is diaphoretic and confused. The nurse checks the SMBG, which is 37 mg/dL. What is the priority assessment before administering orange juice?
    a. Blood pressure
    b. Deep tendon reflexes
    c. Swallowing reflex
    d. Temperature

33. A patient with type 2 DM that is controlled with diet and metformin (Glucophage) also has severe rheumatoid arthritis (RA) and has been prescribed prednisone (Deltasone) to control inflammation. What is most likely to occur?
    a. Development of acute hypoglycemia because of the RA exacerbation
    b. Development of a rash caused by metformin-prednisone interactions
    c. Needing a diet higher in calories while receiving prednisone
    d. Prescription of insulin on a sliding scale while on prednisone

▶34. The college health nurse is caring for a college student who has type 2 DM who was brought to the health clinic after getting intoxicated at a party. The student is prescribed metformin (Glucophage) 850 mg once a day. The nurse assesses the student. What assessment would be of most concern to the nurse?
    a. Dorsalis pedis pulse difficult to palpate
    b. Respirations 32 breaths per minute and deep
    c. Pulse 100 beats/min
    d. Severe frontal headache

35. After receiving teaching about the drug glipizide (Glucotrol), which statement, if made by the patient, would suggest that the patient understood the teaching?
    a. "I need to notify my doctor if I have episodes of sweating and shakiness."
    b. "I should not have low blood sugar with this drug because it does not stimulate the release of insulin."
    c. "It is all right to eat what I want as long as I take enough of the drug."
    d. "This drug is less potent than the newer drugs."

36. A patient with type 2 DM who is prescribed glipizide has just been prescribed carvedilol (Coreg). Which statement suggests that the patient needs additional teaching?
    a. "I should check my SMBG before meals and bedtime and any time I don't feel right."
    b. "This drug can make my low blood sugar worse."
    c. "I should not assume that my blood sugar is OK if I don't feel the palpitations that I usually get when my SMBG is low."
    d. "I should take my pulse before taking the carvedilol and consult my doctor if it is less than 60 beats/min."

37. Which laboratory test result increases the risk that a patient who is prescribed glyburide might experience hypoglycemia?
    a. Alk Phos 142 international units/L
    b. BUN 24 mg/dL
    c. eGFR 42 mL/min
    d. G6PD 2.4 U/g of hemoglobin

38. Which assessment change from yesterday morning in a patient who is prescribed pioglitazone (Actos) would be of most concern to the nurse?
    a. Abdominal pain and two loose stools this morning
    b. Crackles throughout lung fields and 2½-lb weight gain
    c. Decrease in BP from 130/82 to 118/78 mm Hg and pulse drop from 82 to 74 beats/min
    d. Temperature 102.4° F and cough

▶39. What would warrant the nurse not administering repaglinide (Prandin) and consulting the prescriber?
    a. Fasting blood glucose 95 mg/dL
    b. Glycosylated hemoglobin (A1c) 5.5%
    c. Patient is NPO for a colonoscopy
    d. Patient is scheduled for hemodialysis at 1000

40. Which nursing outcome would be most appropriate for a patient who is prescribed acarbose (Precose) or nateglinide (Starlix)?
    a. Bedtime SMBG 160 mg/dL
    b. Fasting blood glucose less than 90 mg/dL
    c. Glycosylated hemoglobin (A1c) 7%
    d. Two-hour postprandial blood sugar less than 150 mg/dL

41. A hospitalized patient who has diabetes and who is blind is receiving acarbose (Precose) 50 mg 3 times a day with meals. Because of possible adverse effects of the drug, the patient is most likely at risk for which nursing problem?
    a. Activity intolerance
    b. Ineffective coping
    c. Injury
    d. Powerlessness

42. A patient with diabetes who receives glipizide and miglitol (Glyset) is diaphoretic, tachycardic, and anxious. The SMBG is 43 mg/dL. What product would be most effective to quickly raise the patient's blood sugar?
    a. Glucose tablet
    b. Honey
    c. Orange juice
    d. Sugar cube

43. Which nursing action is appropriate when a patient is prescribed bromocriptine (Cycloset) for type 2 DM?
    a. Change positions slowly.
    b. Elevate the head of the bed for 30 minutes after eating.
    c. Monitor fluid intake and output.
    d. Weigh daily.

44. What are the only drugs currently used to treat type 2 DM during pregnancy and lactation? (Select all that apply.)
    a. Acarbose (Precose)
    b. Glipizide (Glucotrol)
    c. Insulin
    d. Metformin (Glucophage)
    e. Pioglitazone (Actos)

45. After administration of glucagon for severe hypoglycemia, what is the priority goal of therapy?
    a. Correct acidosis.
    b. Correct cachexia.
    c. Restore stores of glycogen in the liver.
    d. Treat the adverse effect of diarrhea.

46. The nurse is preparing to perform the last assessment of the 1900 to 0700 shift at 0600. Several assigned patients have diabetes. The patient receiving which drug should be assessed for hypoglycemia first?
    a. Acarbose (Precose) 50 mg 3 times a day with meals
    b. Glargine (Lispro) insulin units every evening plus insulin aspart (NovoLog) according to dietary intake and SMBG
    c. Metformin (Glucophage) 500 mg before breakfast and supper
    d. Neutral protamine Hagedorn (NPH) (Humulin N) 35 units every morning

DOSE CALCULATION QUESTIONS

47. A 132-pound patient is prescribed an intravenous infusion of regular insulin at 0.1 units/kg/hr, which calculates to 6 units per hour. The insulin comes mixed as a solution of 25 units in 100 mL of normal saline. The IV pump calibration is in milliliters per hour. What rate should the nurse program for the continuous IV insulin drip?

CASE STUDY

The nurse educator is presenting a seminar on insulin to nursing students. What would be the best response to these questions?

1. Why are regular and rapid-acting insulins the only insulins administered intravenously?

2. If regular insulin is most like human insulin, why do doctors prescribe rapid-acting insulins such as insulin aspart (NovoLog) and insulin glulisine (Apidra)?

3. How is using detemir (Levemir) or glargine (Lantus) insulin better than using NPH insulin?

4. What is the disadvantage of using basal glargine (Lantus) insulin?

5. Some prescribers order basal glargine (Lantus) insulin in the morning rather than in the evening as the literature recommends. Why would they do this?

6. Patients sometimes need both basal and bolus doses of insulin at the same time. What could happen if the basal detemir (Levemir) or glargine (Lantus) insulin is mixed with a bolus of insulin aspart (NovoLog) or other rapid- or fast-acting insulins?

7. What should the patient or nurse do if a vial of insulin aspart is cloudy?

58
Drugs for Thyroid Disorders

STUDY QUESTIONS

True or False

For each of the following statements, enter T for true or F for false.

1. ____ The 3 and 4 in T_3 and T_4 indicate the number of atoms of iodine in the molecule.
2. ____ Liver impairment could prolong the effect of thyroid hormones.
3. ____ Free T_4 is the count of T_4 hormone not bound by protein.
4. ____ Maternal hypothyroidism has the most significant effects on the fetus in the third trimester when most fetal weight is gained.
5. ____ Assessment for congenital hypothyroidism (cretinism) should be done at the infant's 2-month checkup.
6. ____ Exophthalmos is not seen in all cases of hyperthyroidism.
7. ____ Natural thyroid hormone products from animals are more likely to contain the exact amount of thyroid hormone than synthetic hormone replacement products.

8. ___ It is more important to take thyroid hormone replacement at the same time each day than with or without food.

9. ___ Because TSH would decrease if thyroid hormone replacement is taken by a euthyroid person who is trying to lose weight, a dose that produces the adverse effects of hyperthyroidism would be needed to achieve weight loss.

CRITICAL THINKING, PRIORITIZATION, AND DELEGATION QUESTIONS

▶10. The nurse is preparing to administer synthetic levothyroxine (Synthroid). Which laboratory value, if significantly low, would be a reason for the nurse to withhold the medication and consult the prescriber?
a. Free T_3
b. Free T_4
c. TSH
d. T_3

✳11. It is a priority for the nurse to teach a hypothyroid pregnant woman that adequate thyroid hormone replacement therapy is critical during which stage of the pregnancy?
a. First trimester
b. Second trimester
c. Third trimester
d. Postpartum period

✳12. Which would be of greatest priority when a patient is admitted in thyrotoxicosis?
a. Lowering the heart rate
b. Providing adequate nutrition
c. Raising the secretion of TSH
d. Suppressing thyroid hormone secretion

13. Which statement, if made by a patient receiving the antithyroid drug propylthiouracil (PTU), would indicate a need for further teaching?
a. "After this drug gets to a therapeutic level, it should help my heart to stop feeling like it is racing."
b. "I should gain weight while eating less when I am on this drug."
c. "This drug should help decrease the bulging appearance of my eyes."
d. "This drug should stop the feeling that I am always too hot."

✳14. Which assessment finding would be most critical for the nurse to report to the prescriber immediately if noted in a patient admitted with urosepsis who has a history of Graves' disease treated by an antithyroid drug?
a. Blood in urine on urinalysis
b. Burning when urinating
c. Flank pain
d. Temperature 104° F (40° C)

15. The nurse is caring for a patient who receives levothyroxine. Which OTC drugs should not be administered within hours of the administration of levothyroxine? (Select all that apply.)
a. Aluminum hydroxide (Maalox)
b. Calcium carbonate (OsCal)
c. Cimetidine (Tagamet HB)
d. Ferrous sulfate (iron supplement)
e. Milk of magnesia (MOM)

▶16. Because of drug interactions, the nurse should monitor a patient who is taking warfarin and levothyroxine for which condition?
a. Bleeding
b. Dysrhythmias
c. Insomnia
d. Tachycardia

17. Which statement, if made by a patient who has type 1 diabetes mellitus and was recently diagnosed with hypothyroidism and prescribed levothyroxine (Synthroid), would indicate a need for further teaching?
a. "I should check my blood sugar if I get really thirsty and hot and feel flushed."
b. "I will not need as much insulin when I am taking Synthroid."
c. "It is very important to check my blood sugar before meals and at bedtime."
d. "It will be weeks before the Synthroid levels off in my blood and my basal insulin dose can be adjusted accordingly."

18. A patient who has hypothyroidism tells the nurse that her insurance company now requires that she use a generic drug if one is available. Up to now, she has been taking brand-name Synthroid. The nurse should advise the patient to
a. ask the pharmacist what is best.
b. discuss this change with her prescriber.
c. pay for the brand name.
d. use the generic brand; there is no difference.

19. A patient has received instructions regarding administration of levothyroxine (Synthroid). Which of these statements made by the patient would indicate that the patient understood the directions?
    a. "I should take the drug in the morning with breakfast."
    b. "Stomach upset occurs if the drug is taken with an antacid."
    c. "Taking the drug on an empty stomach 30-60 minutes before breakfast increases drug absorption."
    d. "Taking the drug with orange juice increases drug absorption."

✱20. It would be a priority to report which laboratory test result to the prescriber of methimazole (Tapazole)?
    a. ALT 50 IU/L
    b. BUN 24 mg/dL
    c. FBG 138 mg/dL
    d. hCG 425 mIU/mL

▶21. Because of the risk of agranulocytosis, the nurse should teach the patient who has been prescribed methimazole (Tapazole) to report which symptom?
    a. Anorexia
    b. Bleeding gums
    c. Pale conjunctiva
    d. Sore throat

22. A 34-year-old female patient is prescribed iodine[131] for toxic nodular goiter. Which statement, if made by this patient, would indicate a need for further teaching?
    a. "I can develop inadequate thyroid hormone secretion from this therapy."
    b. "I must stay at home during therapy to avoid exposing others to radiation."
    c. "I need to use two reliable methods of birth control."
    d. "This drug takes months before it is fully effective."

23. Which of these factors, if identified in a patient receiving Lugol's solution, would be a concern to the nurse?
    a. Decrease in free T_3
    b. Weight gain of 2 lb in 2 weeks
    c. Beverages having a brassy taste
    d. Drug taken with grapefruit juice

▶24. Propranolol (Inderal) has been prescribed for a patient in thyrotoxicosis. Which outcome is appropriate for this therapy?
    a. BP 110/80-90/60 mm Hg
    b. Free T_4 0.8-2.3 ng/dL
    c. Pulse 60-80 beats/min
    d. TSH 0.4-4 mU/L

DOSE CALCULATION QUESTIONS

25. Levothyroxine (Synthroid) 50 mcg is prescribed for a 4-month-old child with congenital hypothyroidism who weighs 9 lb. Is this a safe dosage?

26. Levothyroxine (Synthroid) 0.2 mg tablets are available. The patient has been prescribed 100 mcg. How many tablets should the nurse administer?

CASE STUDIES

Case Study 1

A 30-year-old woman visits her family physician complaining that she has been experiencing unusual fatigue, lethargy, intolerance to cold, and weight gain. At the visit, her vital signs are BP 100/58 mm Hg, P 62, R 16, and T 97.8° F.

1. What thyroid disorder do these symptoms suggest?

2. What laboratory test results would the nurse expect to see for this patient if she is hypothyroid?

3. After appropriate history, physical examination, and laboratory studies, the patient is diagnosed with primary hypothyroidism and started on levothyroxine (Synthroid) 112 mcg once a day. What teaching should the nurse provide about expected timing for relief of symptoms?

4. What teaching should the nurse provide to this patient about administration of levothyroxine (Synthroid)?

5. The nurse should teach about possible adverse effects of levothyroxine. What adverse effects warrant notifying the prescriber?

6. The patient tells the nurse that her sister has asked for some of her thyroid pills to help her lose weight. She wants to know if this would be a problem. How should the nurse respond?

7. The patient returns for her 1-year checkup. She wonders if she still needs the medication because she sometimes forgets to take the drug and does not feel any different on those days. How should the nurse respond?

Case Study 2

Propranolol (Inderal) 10 mg and propylthiouracil (PTU) 100 mg 3 times a day are prescribed for a 25-year-old woman who was recently diagnosed with Graves' disease.

8. What laboratory results would the nurse expect to see when reviewing this patient's chart?

9. The patient asks the nurse why two drugs have been prescribed. What information should the nurse provide regarding the need for both drugs?

10. The drug methimazole (Tapazole) is less toxic than PTU. What would be a possible reason why the prescriber chose PTU for this patient?

11. What assessments should the nurse teach the patient to monitor, and what findings should be reported to the prescriber?

12. Six months later, the patient's heart rate, blood pressure, TSH, and free T_3 levels are within normal limits. The prescriber provides a plan for gradual decrease, then discontinuation of propranolol (Inderal). Why was this drug dose tapered rather than discontinued if vital signs are normal?

59

Drugs Related to Hypothalamic and Pituitary Function

STUDY QUESTIONS

Matching

Match the hormones (abbreviations) with their functions.

1. ____ Helps regulate GH release.
2. ____ Acts on the adrenal cortex to promote synthesis and release of adrenocortical hormones.
3. ____ Acts on the ovaries to promote ovulation and development of the corpus luteum, and acts on the testes to promote androgen production.
4. ____ Acts on the ovaries to promote follicular growth and development, and acts on the testes to promote spermatogenesis.
5. ____ Stimulates milk production after childbirth.
6. ____ Stimulates growth in practically all tissues and organs.
7. ____ Acts on the thyroid gland to promote synthesis and release of thyroid hormones.

8. ___ Promotes uterine contractions during labor and stimulates milk ejection during breast-feeding.

9. ___ Acts on the kidney to cause reabsorption of water.

    a. ACTH
    b. ADH
    c. FSH
    d. GH
    e. LH
    f. Oxytocin
    g. Prolactin
    h. Somatostatin
    i. TSH

CRITICAL THINKING, PRIORITIZATION, AND DELEGATION QUESTIONS

10. Which finding would the nurse expect in a child who has a deficiency in secretion of growth hormone (GH)?
    a. Cognitive deficiency
    b. Long trunk and short extremities
    c. Profuse sweating
    d. Short stature but normal proportions

▶11. Which assessment of a 7-year-old child indicates increased risk for severe adverse effects of somatropin?
    a. Anterior cervical lymphadenopathy
    b. BMI 35
    c. Dry, flaky skin on elbows
    d. Pulse 100 beats/min

✶12. It would be a priority to teach a child who has been prescribed mecasermin, and the child's parents, to seek medical care if the child experiences
    a. diaphoresis and tremor.
    b. dry skin and itching.
    c. nausea and vomiting.
    d. sore throat and fever.

▶13. Which of these assessment findings, if identified in a patient who is receiving pegvisomant (Somavert), most likely suggests possible liver injury and should be reported to the prescriber?
    a. Headache
    b. Nasal congestion
    c. Malaise
    d. Tea-colored urine

▶14. Which assessment finding would be a reason to consult the prescriber regarding administration of vasopressin? (Select all that apply.)
    a. BP 82/60 mm Hg
    b. Chest pain
    c. eGFR 45 mL/min
    d. Fluid intake 2000 mL/day

15. The nurse is teaching a patient how to administer intranasal desmopressin. What is the proper way to administer a dose to ensure accuracy?
    a. While lying down with the head turned toward the side of administration
    b. Upon arising in the morning
    c. Tilt bottle so tube draws from deepest portion of medication
    d. When inhaling

16. A patient who was recently diagnosed with hypothalamic diabetes insipidus and prescribed vasopressin reports weight gain of 1 to 2 lb per day for the past week. The nurse should recognize that this may indicate
    a. failure to comply with directions for administration of the drug.
    b. failure to limit water intake.
    c. improper diagnosis.
    d. inadequate drug dosage.

▶17. When administering vasopressin to a patient with diabetes insipidus, which urine specific gravity results would indicate that therapy has achieved the desired effect?
    a. 1.0002
    b. 1.002
    c. 1.02
    d. 1.2

18. It is a priority to monitor which electrolyte when a patient is prescribed tolvaptan?
    a. Calcium
    b. Phosphate
    c. Magnesium
    d. Sodium

19. Which laboratory result would be a priority to report to the prescriber when a patient is prescribed pegvisomant for acromegaly?
    a. Amylase 150 IU/L
    b. ALT 275 IU/L
    c. A1c 6.8%
    d. Hemoglobin 13 g/dL

DOSE CALCULATION QUESTIONS

20. A child is prescribed somatropin (Humatrope) 0.2 mg/kg/wk SubQ to be divided into three doses to be administered every other day. The nurse teaches the parents of the child, who weighs 30 kg, to administer how much somatropin (Humatrope) at each dose?

21. Mecasermin 800 micrograms is prescribed for a 44-lb child. The drug is available as 10 mg/mL. How much drug will the nurse administer?

CASE STUDIES

Case Study 1

The nurse works in an endocrine clinic at a major pediatric center that sees children with short stature. When GH therapy with somatropin (Humatrope) is prescribed, the nurse must teach the patient and parents self-administration of the drug.

1. What should the nurse include in the teaching of the technique of subcutaneous injection of this drug?

2. What will the nurse include when explaining the importance of monitoring weight while on this drug?

3. Some parents want therapy with GH for their child, but the prescriber decides that the risks are greater than benefits. What information can the nurse provide to reinforce prescriber teaching about why therapy with GH may not be advisable for children with the following conditions?
   a. Prader-Willi syndrome

   b. Diabetes mellitus

   c. Uncontrolled asthma

Case Study 2

Intramuscular vasopressin, 5 units now and 5 units every 4 hours as needed, are prescribed for a patient with post-operative abdominal distention.

4. What should the nurse assess before administering this drug?

5. What assessment findings would be a reason to withhold the drug and contact the prescriber?

Case Study 3

A child who has become unresponsive to somatropin (Humatrope) has been prescribed mecasermin (insulin-like growth factor-1). The nurse is teaching the patient and parents about possible adverse effects and management.

6. What would the nurse include in teaching about the following?
   a. Hypoglycemia

   b. Tonsillar hypertrophy

   c. Local and systemic allergic reactions

60

Drugs for Disorders of the Adrenal Cortex

STUDY QUESTIONS

Matching

Match the term with its description.

1. ___ Androgens
2. ___ Glucocorticoids
3. ___ Mineralocorticoids

   a. Influence carbohydrate metabolism and other processes
   b. Modulate salt and water balance
   c. Contribute to expression of sexual characteristics

True or False

For each of the following statements, enter T for true or F for false.

4. ___ The terms *adrenocorticoid, corticosteroid,* and *corticoid* only refer to glucocorticoids.
5. ___ Normal secretion of glucocorticoids should not cause hyperglycemia unless the patient is a diabetic.
6. ___ Thin extremities from muscle wasting is a symptom of glucocorticoid excess such as is seen in Cushing's syndrome.
7. ___ Glucocorticoid excess prevents the breakdown of fat for energy.
8. ___ Glucocorticoids raise BP by allowing blood vessels to constrict and limiting capillary permeability and loss of fluid into tissues.
9. ___ Excess glucocorticoid secretion is associated with depression.
10. ___ Adverse effects of water retention and muscle wasting are expected when a patient takes glucocorticoid therapy because of insufficient secretion by the adrenals.
11. ___ Patients who take glucocorticoid therapy because of insufficient secretion by the adrenals are at risk for hypotension and hypoglycemia any time they experience elevated levels of physical or emotional stress.
12. ___ A patient who takes multiple drugs that block/decrease the release of aldosterone is at risk for metabolic acidosis.

13. ___ Addison's disease involves insufficient secretion of adrenocorticoids and Cushing's syndrome is excessive production of adrenocorticoids.
14. ___ Cushing's syndrome is usually treated by administration of drugs that suppress adrenal secretion of hormones.

CRITICAL THINKING, PRIORITIZATION, AND DELEGATION QUESTIONS

15. The adrenals of the full-term fetus release a burst of glucocorticoids during labor and delivery. These steroids act to:
    a. accelerate maturation of the fetal lungs.
    b. lower maternal blood pressure.
    c. prevent uterine contractions.
    d. stimulate fetal weight gain.

16. Ideally, to follow the normal circadian pattern of glucocorticoid release, glucocorticoid replacement therapy would be administered at what time?
    a. Midmorning
    b. Just after the patient wakes
    c. Midafternoon
    d. Just before the patient falls asleep

∗17. It would be a priority to report which finding when caring for a patient with Cushing's syndrome?
    a. Fasting blood sugar 235 mg/dL
    b. pH 7.44, HCO_3 28 mEq/L, pco_2 45 mm Hg
    c. Peaked T waves on electrocardiogram (ECG)
    d. Sinus rhythm on ECG

▶18. Untreated Cushing's syndrome would be most dangerous if a patient had a history of what condition?
    a. Aspiration pneumonia
    b. Bowel obstruction
    c. Cerebral palsy
    d. Heart failure

19. Eplerenone and spironolactone are prescribed for a patients with adrenal hyperplasia because these drugs
    a. cause greater excretion of water than other diuretics.
    b. increase renal reabsorption of hydrogen.
    c. influence the normalization of potassium levels.
    d. protect the heart.

20. What is the priority teaching for a patient who has been prescribed hydrocortisone for adrenal insufficiency?
    a. Importance of adequate sodium in the diet
    b. Importance of taking extra doses of corticoids when ill
    c. Importance of including fresh vegetables and fruits in the diet
    d. Importance of orthostatic BP precautions

✳21. Which of these findings would be a priority to report to the prescriber if a patient was prescribed fludrocortisone?
    a. Blood pressure 135/88 mm Hg
    b. Flushed, dry skin
    c. Nausea and vomiting
    d. Weight gain of 2 lb in 24 hours

22. The nurse is caring for a patient who is scheduled for an adrenalectomy for adrenal adenoma. During the night, the nurse should assess the patient for which symptom of the hyperaldosteronism?
    a. Blood pressure that is difficult to control
    b. Postural hypotension when getting up to the bathroom
    c. Tremor and cool, clammy skin from hypoglycemia
    d. Vomiting, diarrhea, and subsequent electrolyte imbalances

▶23. Which of these laboratory results, if identified in a patient with Cushing's syndrome who is receiving 800 mg of ketoconazole to inhibit corticosteroid synthesis, should the nurse report to the prescriber immediately?
    a. ALT 150 international units/L
    b. BUN 15 mg/dL
    c. Creatinine 1.5 mg/dL
    d. Glucose 150 mg/dL

DOSE CALCULATION QUESTIONS

24. Fludrocortisone acetate is available in 0.1-mg tablets. The patient is prescribed 0.05 mg once a day. How many tablets should the nurse administer for one dose?

25. The recommended dose of hydrocortisone for a patient with adrenal insufficiency is 12-15 mg/m². A patient who is 5 feet 11 inches tall and weighs 176 lb has been prescribed 25 mg. Is the dose safe?

CASE STUDY

A 32-year-old man has been admitted with severe episodic right upper quadrant (RUQ) pain, anorexia, and nausea. Oral cholecystography reveals acute cholecystitis, and an open cholecystectomy is planned. When gathering data regarding medical history, the patient reveals he has been experiencing extreme fatigue, dizziness when changing position, and muscle weakness. He has felt this way for a long time, but thought the symptoms were caused by his stressful job. He also states that he loves every kind of salty food and eats at least one bag of potato chips daily. He states that he has experienced impotence on occasion. The nurse notes that he has increased pigmentation around the face and hands and a decrease in body hair. Bloodwork includes fasting glucose 62 mg/dL, sodium 132 mEq/L, potassium 53 mEq/L, and blood urea nitrogen (BUN) 28 mg/dL. Synthetic adrenocorticotropic hormone (ACTH) is administered IV, and plasma cortisol levels were checked. Levels failed to rise from the ACTH stimulation. He is diagnosed with Addison's disease. He asks the nurse how this causes his symptoms.

1. Describe how the nurse relates current and possible symptoms to decreased levels of adrenal cortex hormones.

2. The patient is prescribed hydrocortisone 50 mg IV every 8 hours. Text states that daily doses of hydrocortisone should mimic normal daily secretion (20-30 mg per day). Why is this patient receiving such a high dose?

3. Because the patient is ill with cholecystitis and adrenal insufficiency, what is the most critical concern of the nurse? What should be included in the nursing plan of care to address this concern?

4. The patient is prescribed hydrocortisone 20 mg/day. What administration regimen would be used for the hydrocortisone if the prescriber wanted to mimic the body's natural basal secretion of glucocorticoids?

5. What teaching should the nurse provide to a patient who has been prescribed oral glucocorticoids?

61

Estrogens and Progestins: Basic Pharmacology and Noncontraceptive Applications

STUDY QUESTIONS

Matching

Match the hormone with its actions during the menstrual cycle.

1. ____ Causes the dominant follicle to swell rapidly, burst, and release its ovum
2. ____ Following menstruation, promotes endometrial restoration
3. ____ Occurs when progesterone levels are insufficient to balance the stimulatory influence of estrogen on the endometrium
4. ____ Converts the endometrium from a proliferative state into a secretory state
5. ____ Acts on the developing ovarian follicles, causing them to mature and secrete estrogens

    a. Dysfunctional uterine bleeding
    b. Estrogen
    c. FSH
    d. LH
    e. Progesterone

CRITICAL THINKING, PRIORITIZATION, AND DELEGATION QUESTIONS

6. Which site is not acceptable for application of transdermal formulations of estrogen?
   a. Breast
   b. Calf
   c. Forearm
   d. Thigh

7. What is not a function of progesterone during pregnancy?
   a. Promotes growth and proliferation of breast structures that produce milk
   b. Prevention of immune rejection of the fetus
   c. Promotes follicular maturation and ovulation
   d. Suppression of uterine contractions

8. A 45-year-old patient has not had a menstrual period for 2 months. The nurse is reviewing laboratory tests. Which result suggests that the patient may be entering menopause (perimenopause)?
   a. Elevated estradiol
   b. Elevated human chorionic gonadotropin
   c. Elevated luteinizing hormone
   d. Elevated progesterone

9. The nurse is caring for a 56-year-old patient who is post–total knee replacement. The patient has been taking estrogen to relieve menopausal symptoms and increase bone mineral density. Which new assessment finding would be of most concern to the nurse?
   a. Dizziness with position changes
   b. Dyspnea while resting
   c. Nausea and vomiting
   d. Vaginal spotting of sanguineous discharge

10. Research suggests that hormone replacement does not provide which benefits? (Select all that apply.)
    a. Cardiovascular protection
    b. Increase in bone density
    c. Prevention of vaginal atrophy
    d. Protection from dementia
    e. Relief of insomnia and hot flushes (hot flashes)

11. Which symptom, if exhibited by a patient who is receiving estrogen therapy (ET), is most likely to be an effect of this therapy?
    a. Constipation
    b. Nausea
    c. Profuse vaginal drainage
    d. Orthostatic hypotension

*12. The nurse is assessing a 62-year-old female patient who is post–knee arthroplasty. The patient is prescribed raloxifene (Evista) to treat osteopenia. What would be of greatest priority to report to the surgeon?
    a. Capillary refill 3 seconds
    b. Difficulty passing hard stool
    c. Dry mucous membranes
    d. Pain and increased circumference of the right calf

*13. The nurse is reviewing laboratory test results for a 42-year-old patient who has been taking medroxy-progesterone acetate (Provera) for dysfunctional uterine bleeding. Which test result would be a priority to report to the prescriber?
    a. hCG 2225 international units/mL
    b. LDL 102 mg/dL
    c. INR 1.1
    d. WBC 8,765/mm^3

14. Research suggests that which natural strategy is most effective in relieving symptoms of premenstrual syndrome (PMS)?
    a. Taking black cohosh every other day
    b. Taking evening primrose oil every day
    c. Taking red clover twice a week
    d. Eating whole-grain foods every day

15. A patient with premenstrual syndrome (PMS) has been prescribed fluoxetine (Prozac) for PMS. Which statement, if made by the patient, would suggest that the patient understands the potential benefits of this drug therapy for PMS?
    a. "I must take this drug every day even though my symptoms are present only part of the month."
    b. "It takes 2 to 4 weeks of daily therapy before I should notice improvement in how I feel."
    c. "This drug may help reduce my breast tenderness, bloating, and headache."
    d. "This drug should improve my depression and irritability."

CASE STUDY

A 46-year-old patient has just received the recommendation that she undergo a total hysterectomy and bilateral salpingo-oophorectomy for uterine fibroids.

1. The patient should be informed that which symptoms should be expected postoperatively relating to the removal of both ovaries (surgical menopause)?

2. The prescriber orders laboratory tests, including a lipid panel, mammogram, and DEXA scan, and tells the patient that results are needed before they can discuss options to prevent surgically induced menopausal symptoms. The patient asks the nurse why these tests have been ordered. What information can the nurse provide?

3. Lab results include bone mineral density 1.5 standard deviations below normal, LDL 150 mg/dL, HDL 55 mg/dL, and no evidence of lesions on mammogram. The patient is interested in postoperative hormone replacement. What additional information must be obtained before the prescriber considers ordering hormone replacement?

4. There are no contraindications for estrogen replacement therapy. The woman states that her mother received relief of menopausal symptoms by taking estrogen-progesterone combination (Prempro). Why would this particular drug not be prescribed for this patient?

5. After discussing risks and benefits, the prescriber orders Climara, a transdermal estrogen patch, and asks the nurse to teach administration directives. What should the nurse include?

6. What teaching should the nurse provide that can help reduce the risk of cardiovascular events?

7. The patient asks if there are any alternative treatments for menopausal symptoms. What information can the nurse provide?

62

Birth Control

STUDY QUESTIONS

True or False

For each of the following statements, enter T *for true or* F *for false.*

1. ___ Abortion is a common approach to deal with unplanned pregnancies.
2. ___ Unplanned pregnancy rarely occurs after age 20 years.
3. ___ Tubal ligation and vasectomy are the most commonly used form of birth control in the USA.
4. ___ The most effective pharmacologic forms of birth control have the most adverse effects.
5. ___ Oral and transdermal contraceptives are the most effective forms of birth control.
6. ___ Most oral contraceptives (OCs) cause spontaneous abortion of a fertilized ovum.
7. ___ Smoking and migraine headache history increases the risk of serious blood clot events when a woman uses OCs.
8. ___ Estrogen in OCs, but not progesterone, increases the risk of developing a thrombus.
9. ___ Combination OCs are not associated with an increased risk of ovarian and endometrial cancer.

10. ___ Combination OCs do not increase the risk of breast cancer for most women.
11. ___ OCs can speed the growth of existing breast cancer.
12. ___ OCs are contraindicated during pregnancy.
13. ___ Progestin-only OCs are safer and more effective than combination OCs.
14. ___ Newer progestins in combination OCs are not more effective but they have different adverse effects.
15. ___ OC use can prevent anemia in some patients.
16. ___ When using a continuous-cycle OC, once the pills have been taken daily for at least 3 weeks, up to 7 days can be missed with little or no increased risk of pregnancy.
17. ___ Cervical caps are more effective in women who have already had babies.
18. ___ IUDs are only recommended for persons at low risk for STI.
19. ___ A diaphragm with spermicide is more effective than male condoms with actual and theoretical use.
20. ___ Nonoxynol-9 may increase the risk of HIV transmission through promotion of vaginal, cervical, anal, and rectal lesions that facilitate HIV penetration to cells.

CRITICAL THINKING, PRIORITIZATION, AND DELEGATION QUESTIONS

✳21. What would be the priority nursing teaching when a woman is prescribed an OC containing the progestin drospirenone?
   a. "Do not eat too many bananas while you're taking this drug."
   b. "Seek medical care if you have chest pain or unexplained shortness of breath."
   c. "You should have less bloating with this drug than with other OCs."
   d. "You should have your blood pressure checked at every health visit."

22. What is a potential cause of OC failure?
   a. FBG > 125 mg/dL
   b. Hypertension
   c. Multiple sexual partners
   d. Shift work that makes a routine challenging

✳23. It would be of greatest priority for the patient to report which symptom if she is prescribed an OC containing drospirenone and naproxen for osteoarthritis?
   a. Bleeding between menstrual periods
   b. Fatigue
   c. Chest pain
   d. Skin discoloration

24. Which supplement can decrease the effectiveness of OCs?
   a. Echinacea
   b. Garlic
   c. Ginkgo biloba
   d. St. John's wort

✳25. A patient who has been using OCs for birth control has been prescribed warfarin (Coumadin) to prevent DVTs during a period of prolonged impaired mobility. Which action by the patient is of greatest priority in this situation?
   a. Consuming adequate calcium in the diet
   b. Complying with scheduled blood tests
   c. Increasing fluid intake to 2000 mL/day
   d. Using a soft toothbrush

▶26. A patient who has epilepsy that is managed with phenytoin comes to the college health center requesting OCs for birth control and menorrhagia. She has no contraindications for OC use. Phenytoin decreases the effectiveness of OCs. What is the best strategy in this situation?
   a. Teach the patient to use a barrier (condom) in addition to prescribed OCs.
   b. Tell the patient to start OCs and stop taking phenytoin and see if seizures resume.
   c. Teach the patient that abstinence is the only alternative in this situation.
   d. Teach the patient how to predict the times when she is most fertile.

▶27. Which patient would be at greatest risk for pregnancy when using the contraceptive patch (Ortho Evra) as a contraceptive?
   a. 19-year-old with multiple sexual partners
   b. 25-year-old who weighs 210 pounds
   c. 37-year-old who is anemic
   d. 40-year-old who smokes 2 packs of cigarettes per day

✳28. A 19-year-old healthy patient who has been taking a combination OC for 2 years is involved in an automobile accident and undergoes surgical reduction and fixation of multiple fractures of both lower extremities. What assessment finding is of greatest priority to report to the prescriber?
   a. Capillary refill of 2 seconds
   b. Diaphoresis
   c. Sudden dyspnea
   d. Temperature 100° F (37.8° C)

✳29. The nurse is working in a women's health clinic. Several walk-in patients who take OCs arrive at the same time. Which patient should be given the highest priority for seeing the APRN?
   a. 17-year-old who is experiencing a migraine headache with aura
   b. 26-year-old who is experiencing breakthrough bleeding
   c. 35-year-old who smokes and needs her prescription refilled
   d. 42-year-old who has had episodes of severe right upper quadrant pain

▶30. Which sign, if present, suggests that a patient who is prescribed ethinyl estradiol and drospirenone (Yaz) oral contraceptives may be experiencing hyperkalemia?
   a. Confusion
   b. Tachycardia
   c. Positive Trousseau's sign
   d. Restlessness

▶31. How should the nurse respond to a patient's concern that she has not had a period since starting low-dose oral contraceptives 3 months ago?
a. "Some women do not have periods when taking oral contraceptives."
b. "You should see a gynecologist to decide if another oral contraceptive should be used."
c. "You should have a biopsy to test for uterine malignancy."
d. "You should have a pregnancy test immediately."

▶32. Because of the effect of oral contraceptives on glucose levels of diabetics, it is most important for the nurse to assess for
a. anorexia.
b. diaphoresis.
c. flushed skin.
d. tachycardia.

33. A nullipara patient, who plans to get pregnant after 1 year of using contraceptives, is discussing different pharmacologic agents for birth control with the nurse. What should be included in the teaching?
a. Alternative forms of birth control should be used for 3 months after stopping oral contraceptives if the patient wants to minimize the risk of multiple births.
b. When medroxyprogesterone injections are discontinued, return of fertility is delayed by an average of 9 months.
c. Contraception usually continues for 2 to 3 months after subdermal implanted contraceptive capsules are removed.
d. The Mirena IUD is probably the best choice for this patient.

▶34. A patient taking an oral contraceptive containing mestranol complains of right upper quadrant discomfort. Because of the possibility of a highly vascular benign hepatic adenoma, which assessment technique should the nurse use for assessment of the liver after inspection?
a. Deep palpation
b. Light palpation
c. Percussion
d. Auscultation

35. What is the best way to evaluate teaching regarding administration directives, including what to do if a dose of OC is missed?
a. Demonstrate taking the pill from the blister pack.
b. Have the patient read the directions to you.
c. Have the patient repeat the directions.
d. Have the patient write the directions in her own words.

36. The nurse instructs the patient who is prescribed the transdermal contraceptive patch, Ortho Evra, to apply the patch to the (Select all that apply.)
a. breasts.
b. buttocks.
c. lower abdomen.
d. upper torso.
e. upper inner arm.

37. What nutritional strategy could prevent adverse effects of depot medroxyprogesterone (Depo-Provera)?
a. Decreasing intake of bananas and other foods high in potassium
b. Decreasing intake of red meat and other foods high in iron
c. Increasing intake of dairy products and other foods high in calcium
d. Increasing intake of green, leafy vegetables and other foods high in vitamin K

38. When a patient has an IUD in place, the nurse should assess for which symptom of a common adverse effect?
a. Breast tenderness
b. Dull pelvic pain
c. Dysmenorrhea
d. Edema

39. Which method of birth control is contraindicated when a patient has a pattern of multiple partners?
a. Etonogestrel subdermal implant (Implanon)
b. Intramuscular medroxyprogesterone acetate (Depo-Provera)
c. Progesterone T (Progestasert) IUD
d. Vaginal contraceptive ring (NuvaRing)

40. What are advantages of polyurethane condoms over latex condoms? (Select all that apply.)
a. Cause fewer allergic reactions
b. Do not have increased risk of failure with lubricant use
c. Are more effective in preventing pregnancies
d. Prevent transmission of genital herpes
e. Are thinner and more pleasurable to use

CASE STUDY

A 17-year-old sexually active female patient has used condoms as a form of birth control and prevention of STIs. She is monogamous and has decided to start on an OC. The patient's history includes asthma that is controlled with Theo-Dur, dysmenorrhea, and irregular menses. Her last normal menstrual period was 2 months ago, but she says she is not concerned because this is a common occurrence for her. The patient is anxious and asks the nurse about the medical exam and what procedures will be performed.

1. Briefly describe what will be included in the pre-administration assessment and how frequently the patient will need to have it repeated.

2. The patient asks the nurse, "How do oral contraceptives prevent pregnancy?" How does the nurse respond?

3. When educating the patient in the use of OCs, it is important to stress the need to take them every day at the same time as prescribed. The patient is started on a triphasic OC and is concerned that she may forget to take the pills consistently. If she does forget, what procedures should she take to minimize the risk of pregnancy?

4. The patient asks about using an alternative form of contraception. What teaching should the nurse provide about the use of condoms and spermicides?

5. Knowing that the patient has asthma and is presently taking Theo-Dur (a form of theophylline), what assessments relating to interaction of OCs and theophylline need to be taken and why?

6. What possible adverse effects warrant discontinuation of the OC, and what symptoms of these conditions should the nurse teach the patient to report to her prescriber?

63
Drug Therapy of Infertility

STUDY QUESTIONS

Matching

Match the hormone with its function.

1. ___ Hormone that stimulates testicular cells to produce testosterone and the corpus luteum to secrete progesterone
2. ___ Hormone that stimulates maturation of ovarian follicles
3. ___ Stimulating hormone produced by the hypothalamus that affects the anterior pituitary

a. Follicle-stimulating hormone (FSH)
b. Gonadotropin-releasing hormone (GnRH)
c. Luteinizing hormone (LH)

True or False

For each of the following statements, enter T *for true or* F *for false.*

4. ___ *Infertility* is defined as being unable to reproduce.
5. ___ Treatment for low sperm count is more successful than treating female causes of infertility.

6. ___ *Nidation* is the medical term for implantation of the products of conception.

7. ___ The drug clomiphene has similar effects as the hormone GnRH.

8. ___ Menotropins and follitropins act on mature follicles to cause ovulation.

9. ___ Human chorionic gonadotropin (hCG) stimulates ovarian follicles to mature.

10. ___ Scant or thick mucus produced by the glands at the neck of the uterus can impair motility of sperm into the uterus.

11. ___ Symptoms of excessive prolactin include secretion of milk when not breast-feeding.

12. ___ Leuprolide and nafarelin are drugs used for infertility associated with endometriosis.

13. ___ The priority reason for using drugs to treat polycystic ovary syndrome (PCOS) is to decrease the number of ovarian cysts.

14. ___ Urofollitropin (Bravelle) is a highly purified preparation of FSH extracted from the urine of pregnant women.

15. ___ hCG is similar in structure and identical in action to luteinizing hormone.

CRITICAL THINKING, PRIORITIZATION, AND DELEGATION QUESTIONS

∗16. The nurse is explaining possible adverse effects of clomiphene (Clomid). Which adverse effect, if experienced by the patient, would be a priority for the patient to report to the prescriber?
 a. Breast engorgement
 b. Hot flushes (hot flashes)
 c. Low abdominal pain
 d. Nausea

17. Which laboratory test result would be an absolute contraindication to the administration of clomiphene (Clomid)?
 a. AST 41 international units/L
 b. Creatinine 1.4 mg/dL
 c. hCG 800 milli-international units/mL
 d. Sperm motility 70%

18. Patients who are prescribed clomiphene (Clomid) may experience increased viscosity of cervical mucus, hindering sperm motility. Estrogen is a possible treatment to thin the cervical mucus. Estrogen therapy would be of particular concern if the patient also has which chronic condition?
 a. Asthma causing bronchoconstriction when exposed to mold
 b. Hypertension requiring diuretic therapy
 c. Type 2 diabetes mellitus with peripheral neuropathy
 d. Venous stasis resulting in thrombophlebitis

▶19. For early detection of the serious adverse effect of ovarian hyperstimulation syndrome from therapy with menotropins (Repronex, and Menopur), the nurse would be most concerned if, after starting therapy, the patient reported
 a. a fever higher than 100.4° F.
 b. a gain of 2 lb in 24 hours.
 c. a pulse rate higher than 80 beats/min.
 d. redness across cheeks and nose.

▶20. The nurse is caring for a patient who experienced ovarian hyperstimulation syndrome after infertility therapy with hCG. It is a priority to assess for which possible effect of this syndrome?
 a. Abdominal distention
 b. Dyspnea
 c. Edema in ankles
 d. Weight gain

21. The nurse is explaining drug therapy to a patient who is prescribed cetrorelix. Which statement, if made by the patient, indicates a need for further teaching?
 a. "I should have someone else perform the injection because it must go into a muscle."
 b. "I should inject the drug into the fat below my skin about 2 inches away from my belly button."
 c. "I must stop taking the drug when instructed or I will not ovulate."
 d. "This drug prevents immature eggs from being released."

22. Bromocriptine (Parlodel) inhibits prolactin secretion by activating receptors for which neurotransmitter?
 a. Acetylcholine
 b. Dopamine
 c. Nicotine
 d. Norepinephrine

DOSE CALCULATION QUESTIONS

23. Cabergoline is supplied in 0.5-mg tablets. The initial dosage is 0.25 mg. How many tablets should be administered?

24. Human chorionic gonadotropin (hCG) (Pregnyl), 8000 USP units, is prescribed intramuscularly. Available is 20,000 units in 10 mL. How many mL should be administered at each site?

CASE STUDY

A heterosexual married couple has no children. Both the husband and the wife are in their late thirties. They have been trying to conceive for the past 2 years but have not been successful. During a lengthy diagnostic work-up for infertility, the wife was found to have no increase in her basal body temperature throughout her menstrual cycle. The husband has a normal sperm count and no health issues. The physician diagnoses primary infertility and decides to induce ovulation. Clomiphene (Serophene) and hCG (Pregnyl) are prescribed to promote ovarian follicular maturation and ovulation.

1. What organ functioning must be present for this drug to work?

2. One year later, the couple has not conceived. Menotropins—specifically, hMG (Repronex) 1 ampule intramuscularly for days 9 through 12 of the menstrual cycle, followed by hCG 5000 units—are prescribed for the wife. The nurse provides counseling relevant to the need for follow-up and early detection of ovarian hyperstimulation syndrome. What symptoms should the nurse teach the patient to report immediately?

3. What will the nurse teach the patient about the timing of administration of hCG?

4. The couple asks whether a multiple pregnancy (i.e., more than one fetus) is more likely with this drug regimen. How should the nurse respond?

64
Drugs that Affect Uterine Function

STUDY QUESTIONS

True or False

For each of the following statements, enter T for true or F for false.

1. ____ Tocolytic drugs are used to induce and strengthen uterine contractions and to control postpartum bleeding.
2. ____ Magnesium sulfate is the most effective drug available to suppress preterm labor.
3. ____ Ergot alkaloids are not normally used to induce contractions during labor because they can cause prolonged uterine contractions.
4. ____ It is common for patients to have elevated temperature after receiving a dose of carboprost tromethamine (Hemabate) to control postpartum hemorrhage.
5. ____ The best way to administer carboprost tromethamine (Hemabate) is subcutaneously.

CRITICAL THINKING, PRIORITIZATION, AND DELEGATION QUESTIONS

✳ 6. What should women be taught to decrease the incidence of the most common risk factors for preterm labor? (Select all that apply.)
   a. Teaching the patient to avoid the use of alcohol during pregnancy.
   b. Teaching the patient to eat nutritious foods and exercise during pregnancy.
   c. Promoting patient behaviors that decrease the incidence of sexually transmitted infection.
   d. Counseling the patient on smoking cessation.

✳ 7. Which new assessment finding would be a priority to report to the obstetrician when the nurse is caring for a patient who is 35 weeks pregnant and receiving terbutaline to suppress preterm labor?
a. Patient is experiencing diaphoresis.
b. Patient's heart rate is 90 beats/min between contractions.
c. Patient is very thirsty.
d. Patient is short of breath, and her sputum is foamy.

✳ 8. The priority nursing focus when caring for the neonate immediately after birth, relating to recent administration of nifedipine to the neonate's mother, is to provide adequate
a. hydration.
b. nourishment.
c. ventilation.
d. warmth.

9. Based on adverse effects of nitroglycerin on the pregnant patient, when this drug is being administered, the nurse needs to closely monitor the patient's
a. blood pressure.
b. blood glucose.
c. respiratory status.
d. urine output.

▶ 10. If a patient is receiving magnesium sulfate to suppress preterm labor, which of these laboratory test results will be of most concern to the nurse?
a. ALT 50 international units/L
b. Calcium 11 mg/dL
c. Creatinine 4 mg/dL
d. Magnesium 1.2 mEq/L

11. What nursing outcome best indicates that intravenous (IV) oxytocin (Pitocin) therapy has achieved the desired effect during the first hour after delivery of the placenta?
a. Blood pressure is 120/80 mm Hg.
b. Pulse is 80 beats/min.
c. Saturation of a perineal pad takes longer than 20 minutes.
d. Skin is warm and dry.

12. Which assessment(s) would be reason to hold the infusion of oxytocin (Pitocin)? (Select all that apply.)
a. Contractions lasting longer than 1 minute
b. Contractions occurring more frequently than every 4-5 minutes
c. Late decelerations of fetal heart rate
d. Intrauterine pressure exceeds 20 mm Hg during contractions
e. Umbilical cord palpable in cervix

✳ 13. The labor and delivery nurse is preparing to administer methylergonovine to a woman who has just delivered the placenta. Before administering the medication, it is a priority for the nurse to assess the patient for what?
a. Elevated BP
b. Lochia flow
c. Respiratory depression
d. Uterine firmness

14. Dinoprostone for cervical softening is contraindicated in patients with a history of what condition(s)? (Select all that apply.)
a. Acute pelvic inflammatory disease
b. Blood sugar greater than 200 mg/dL
c. Asthma
d. Hypertension
e. Hypotension
f. Previous cesarean section
g. Wheezing

15. What are the responsibilities relating to dinoprostone gel (Prepidil) for obstetric nurses working at most hospitals? (Select all that apply.)
a. Calculating the proper dose of the drug
b. Determining the number of doses needed
c. Ordering the correct number of doses for the patient
d. Positioning the patient during and after administration
e. Storing the drug at the proper temperature

✳ 16. The dinoprostone (Cervidil) vaginal insert pouch has been inserted in a patient's posterior fornix. Monitoring indicates that moderate contractions lasting 15 seconds have begun. What is the nurse's priority nursing action?
a. Immediately begin infusion of oxytocin (Pitocin).
b. Instruct the patient that she must lie on her back for at least 2 hours.
c. Place the patient on a fetal monitor.
d. Remove the dinoprostone pouch.

CASE STUDY

A 25-year-old multipara (gravida 2, para 1) is admitted to the labor and delivery unit for induction of labor. She is at 41 weeks gestation. Vital signs and fetal heart rate are stable. Dinoprostone gel (Prepidil) is ordered for cervical ripening.

1. What will the nurse teach the patient about this therapy?

2. The cervix has softened and is 50% effaced. The fetal head was at 0 station in a left occiput anterior position. The medication order reads: "oxytocin (Pitocin) 10 mU. May increase 1 to 2 mU/ min every 30 minutes until normal pattern of uterine contractions are established." What is a normal pattern of uterine contractions?

3. When is oxytocin augmentation of labor contraindicated?

4. An IV infusion of 1000 units of oxytocin in 100 mL of 5% dextrose and 0.45% normal saline is infusing via a secondary line into a primary infusion line. The oxytocin infusion was regulated by an infusion pump and was initiated at 1 mU/ min. Why is the oxytocin infusion "piggybacked" into the primary infusion line rather than added to the primary infusion solution?

5. The patient has suddenly started having contractions lasting 90 seconds every 2 minutes. What should the nurse do?

6. When reporting the patient's response to oxytocin therapy to the obstetrician, what should the nurse include?

7. The patient has delivered her 6-lb 4-oz baby. She received one dose of carboprost tromethamine (Hemabate) 250 mg IM to control postpartum hemorrhage. The next day she spiked a temperature of 101.6° F. Acetaminophen (Tylenol) 650 mg every 4 hours as needed is included in the postpartum orders. Fever is a common adverse effect of carboprost. Why is it important to notify the obstetrician rather than just administer the antipyretic?

65

Androgens

STUDY QUESTIONS

Completion

1. The body responds to increased testosterone levels by suppressing the release of _____ and _____ from the anterior pituitary.

2. Androgens increase absorption of iron from the gastrointestinal (GI) tract and may be used to treat refractory_____.

3. Because methyltestosterone can cause cholestatic hepatitis, the nurse should monitor _____, _____, and _____ lab tests when a patient is receiving this drug.

4. A weight gain of 2 lb in 24 hours suggests that a patient who is receiving androgen therapy may be experiencing the adverse effect of retention of _____ and _____.

5. When taken by women in high doses, androgens can cause clitoral growth, hair loss, and lowering of the voice that may be _____.

CRITICAL THINKING, PRIORITIZATION, AND DELEGATION QUESTIONS

6. Laboratory test results for a patient who is prescribed androgen therapy include ALT 45 mg/dL; calcium 9 mg/dL; FBG 82 mg/dL; Hgb 14.2; Hct 45%; and HDL 22 mg/dL. It would be a priority to teach this patient the importance of
   a. eating a cardio-healthy diet.
   b. increasing protein in the diet.
   c. limiting refined carbohydrates in diet.
   d. performing weight-bearing exercise.

✳ 7. When a patient is prescribed an androgen, which adverse effect would be a priority for the nurse to report to the prescriber?
   a. Breast enlargement
   b. Change in menstrual pattern
   c. Edema in lower extremities
   d. Increased libido

✳ 8. Which adverse effect of testosterone is a medical emergency?
   a. Closure of epiphyses before age 12 years
   b. Elevated LDL higher than 200 mg/dL
   c. 1+ pitting edema of ankles
   d. Priapism lasting longer than 4 hours

9. A patient has received instructions regarding administration of testosterone buccal tablets (Striant). Which of these statements made by the patient would indicate the need for further teaching?
   a. "I should apply the tablet to my gum above an incisor."
   b. "I should alternate sides of my mouth with each dose."
   c. "I should hold the tablet in place by pressing over the tablet from the outside of my mouth for 30 seconds to ensure adhesion."
   d. "I should remove the tablet when drinking hot fluids."

10. The pediatrician's triage nurse receives a call at 2:00 PM (1400) from a 14-year-old patient who was recently prescribed testosterone buccal tablets. The patient applied the buccal tablet at 7:00 AM (0700), and it fell out during lunch. He asks what he should do. The nurse should direct the patient to do what?
   a. Do not replace the tablet until the next dose is due at 7:00 PM.
   b. Replace the tablet with a new one and remove it as scheduled for the original tablet at 7:00 PM (1900).
   c. Replace the tablet with a new one and remove it 12 hours later (at 0200).
   d. Replace the tablet with a new one and remove it the following morning at 7:00 AM (0700).

11. Which behaviors, if occurring when topical androgens are applied, would be of most concern?
   a. Chewing tobacco
   b. Drinking hot tea
   c. Showering before application
   d. Smoking cigarettes

12. The high school nurse is planning a teaching presentation on the use of anabolic steroids. Developmentally, discussion of which effects of anabolic steroid use would most likely discourage their use by male high school athletes?
   a. Atherosclerosis
   b. Hypertension
   c. Liver damage
   d. Testicular shrinkage

✳ 13. Which of these assessment findings, if identified in a patient who is receiving oxandrolone for muscle wasting associated with advanced HIV disease, would be a priority to report to the prescriber?
   a. Acne
   b. Fatigue, jaundice, and nausea
   c. Loss of hair
   d. Weight gain of ½ lb per week

✳ 14. During admission history, a patient who has a history of androgen deficiency describes symptoms of dark-colored urine and clay-colored stool. What is the greatest priority for the nurse to do at this time?
   a. Assess the patient's abdomen.
   b. Contact the prescriber and ask for an order for a complete metabolic panel.
   c. Continue obtaining all admission data and review liver function tests.
   d. Notify the pharmacy and tell them not to deliver any androgenic drugs.

DOSE CALCULATION QUESTIONS

15. Testosterone cypionate (Depo-Testosterone) 50 mg IM is prescribed. 200 mg/mL is available. How much should be administered?

16. Testosterone pellets (Testopel) 75 mg are available. Prescribed is 300 mg. How many pellets will the nurse have available for insertion into the patient's abdomen?

CASE STUDY

A 16-year-old male patient has come to the health care provider because of his small testes and penis. The nurse notes that the patient is very tall (6 feet 10 inches) and thin (160 lb). His legs are unusually long for his trunk. He tells the nurse that he has frequently been in trouble in school, and he will finally be a freshman in high school this year. He is considering dropping out of school. Laboratory test results reveal the absence of sperm in the semen and the presence of two more X chromosomes than would be expected for a male. The diagnosis of Klinefelter's syndrome is made. The nurse knows that this is not extremely rare, occurring in 1 of every 500 live male births, but is often not discovered until the male patient comes in for an infertility workup. Therapy will be directed toward administration of the male hormone testosterone. The patient is prescribed 1% testosterone transdermal gel (Androgel). He asks, "Why can't I take a pill?"

1. How should the nurse respond?

2. The patient's mother is 36 years old and may wish to have another child. What precautions does the nurse need to teach the patient's mother and the patient?

3. What teaching should the nurse provide to the patient about administration of the gel?

4. The patient asks if there are any alternative routes of administration of testosterone. How should the nurse respond?

5. What information does the patient need regarding the adverse effects of testosterone?

66

Drugs for Erectile Dysfunction and Benign Prostatic Hyperplasia

STUDY QUESTIONS

True or False

For each of the following statements, enter T for true or F for false.

1. ____ Phosphodiesterase type 5 (PDE-5) inhibitors are contraindicated if the patient has a history of hypertension or diabetes mellitus.

2. ____ Phosphodiesterase type 5 (PDE-5) inhibitors are most effective if the cause of the sexual dysfunction is depression.

3. ____ Sexual activity can be more dangerous than the drugs for ED for patients taking nitrates.

4. ____ Phosphodiesterase type 5 (PDE-5) inhibitors activate the parasympathetic nervous system.

5. ____ Intestinal absorption of phosphodiesterase type 5 (PDE-5) inhibitor drugs can be impaired for 3 days if the patient regularly ingests grapefruit juice.

6. ____ Patients who are prescribed sildenafil (Viagra) should be warned of possible loss of vision and/or hearing.

7. ____ Vardenafil (Levitra) works faster, longer, and better than sildenafil.

8. ____ Tadalafil (Cialis) is approved for daily use at lower than an as-needed dose if the patient anticipates sexual activity at least once a week.

9. ____ Finasteride is protective against high-grade prostate cancer.

10. ____ Finasteride can interfere with the laboratory test for prostate cancer.

11. ____ Patients should not donate blood while taking dutasteride.

12. ____ There are no concerns for patients taking phosphodiesterase type 5 (PDE-5) inhibitors if they are also prescribed the alpha$_{1a}$ blockers silodosin (Rapaflo) or tamsulosin (Flomax).

13. ____ Tolterodine, a muscarinic antagonist developed for urge incontinence, is contraindicated in patients with benign prostatic hyperplasia (BPH).

CRITICAL THINKING, PRIORITIZATION, AND DELEGATION QUESTIONS

14. The nurse who works in a reproduction clinic counsels patients who are experiencing sexual dysfunction. Many patients ask if sildenafil (Viagra) will help. The nurse knows that this drug will be effective if the basis of the male's problem is (Select all that apply.)
    a. desire for a more intense experience in a normally functioning male.
    b. improvement of erection quality in a patient with impaired blood flow.
    c. lack of desire for sexual activity.
    d. improved duration of erection in a patient with erectile dysfunction.
    e. premature ejaculation.

▶15. Which of these findings, occurring 4 hours after sexual activity, would be an emergency situation for a patient who uses sildenafil (Viagra)?
    a. Blood pressure 160/80 mm Hg
    b. Diarrhea
    c. Persistence of erection
    d. Headache

＊16. It is a priority to assess if a male patient has taken sildenafil (Viagra) within the past 24 hours if the nurse is preparing to administer which medication?
    a. Cimetidine (Tagamet)
    b. Doxazosin (Cardura)
    c. Finasteride (Proscar)
    d. Isosorbide (Imdur)

＊17. It is a priority for the nurse to immediately report to the prescriber which of these findings, if identified in a patient who has been prescribed sildenafil (Viagra)?
    a. Chest pain when engaging in any moderate physical activity
    b. Facial flushing within 1 hour of taking the drug
    c. Rhinorrhea in the spring season
    d. Urinary frequency or difficulty starting the stream of urine

18. Which sudden change in a patient taking sildenafil (Viagra) should be monitored, but does not warrant consulting the prescriber before continuing to use the drug for ED?
    a. Blurring of vision
    b. Chest pain during sexual activity
    c. Difficulty hearing out of one ear
    d. Dizziness with position changes that resolves in less than 1 minute

＊19. A patient who took vardenafil (Levitra) this evening comes to the emergency department complaining of palpitations and dizziness. Assessment findings include heart rate of 122 beats/min and BP of 80/46 mm Hg. The triage nurse recognizes that the priority is to report this information and consult the emergency department physician regarding the need for which procedure, STAT?
    a. Echocardiogram
    b. Electrocardiogram
    c. Stress test
    d. Serum drug level

20. Why is tadalafil (Cialis) not contraindicated for use with the alpha-blocker tamsulosin (Flomax)?
    a. Tamsulosin does not significantly lower BP.
    b. Tamsulosin is a short-acting drug.
    c. Tamsulosin is taken in the morning.
    d. Tamsulosin levels are not reduced by tadalafil.

21. What is an effect of injection of papaverine plus phentolamine that differs from the effects of oral drugs for ED?
    a. An erection occurs without sexual stimulation.
    b. Arterial inflow is increased.
    c. Hypotension will not occur.
    d. Outflow of venous blood is decreased.

22. What is true about BPH? (Select all that apply.)
    a. It can cause kidney damage.
    b. It can involve restriction of urine outflow from the bladder without significant increase in the size of the gland.
    c. It is not associated with risk for prostate cancer.
    d. Its symptoms are directly related to the size of the gland.
    e. Its treatment is based on the presence of subjective symptoms, not objective findings.

▶ 23. When administering finasteride (Proscar), which nursing outcome would be appropriate?
    a. The erection lasts long enough to achieve sexual satisfaction.
    b. The prostate-specific antigen (PSA) level is less than 4 ng/mL.
    c. Postvoid residual urine is less than 50 mL on bladder scan.
    d. The size of the prostate gland is reduced by 50%.

✳ 24. Which action is a priority when a female nurse is administering dutasteride (Avodart)?
    a. Administering on an empty stomach.
    b. Administering with food.
    c. Delaying blood donation for at least 6 months.
    d. Avoiding touching the capsule.

✳ 25. It is a priority to perform and evaluate which assessment before the nurse administers terazosin (Hytrin) to a patient who has been diagnosed with BPH?
    a. Bladder distention
    b. Blood pressure
    c. Respirations
    d. Temperature

✳ 26. What is the priority teaching regarding effects of doxazosin (Cardura) prescribed for BPH?
    a. Nasal congestion is possible.
    b. Orthostatic blood pressure precautions must be taken.
    c. Quantity of ejaculate may decrease.
    d. Symptoms may be relieved soon after starting the drug.

27. What is a disadvantage of the herbal preparation saw palmetto?
    a. It is often toxic.
    b. It is available only in specialized stores.
    c. Research suggests that it is not effective.
    d. It has significant adverse effects.

CASE STUDY

The nurse is providing medication teaching for a 45-year-old male patient who was admitted with cellulitis of the left lower leg. The patient has a history of type 2 diabetes mellitus and hypertension. During the discussion, the patient's wife mentions that he has been experiencing "difficulties with sex" since he started taking medication for his high blood pressure.

1. Why is it particularly important to address sensitive adverse effects, such as ED, especially when they occur as a result of antihypertensive medications?

2. The nurse notifies the prescriber of the patient's and wife's concerns. After discussing the problem with the patient, the prescriber orders sildenafil (Viagra) 50 mg as directed and asks the nurse to explain administration of the drug. What should be included in this explanation?

3. Why is it important for the patient to have information on his person stating that he takes sildenafil (Viagra) and to share this information with all prescribers?

67

Review of the Immune System

STUDY QUESTIONS

Matching

Match the term with its primary action.

1. ___ Antigen-presenting cells found in lymph nodes and other lymphoid tissues
2. ___ Attack and kill target cells directly
3. ___ Attack and destroy foreign particles that have been coated with antibodies of the IgE class
4. ___ Devour cells that have been tagged with antibodies of the IgG class
5. ___ Mediate immediate hypersensitivity reactions
6. ___ The principal scavengers of the body
7. ___ Produce all antibodies
8. ___ Promote delayed-type hypersensitivity
9. ___ Molecule that binds to a bacterium, thereby promoting phagocytosis
10. ___ Makes possible the discrimination between self and nonself

a. B lymphocytes (B cells)
b. Basophils and mast cells
c. Cytotoxic T cell (CD8)
d. Dendritic cells
e. Eosinophils
f. Helper T cells (CD4 cells)
g. Macrophages
h. Major histocompatibility complex (MHC)
i. Neutrophils
j. Opsonin

Match the immunoglobulin with its descriptor.

11. ___ Stimulates release of histamine, heparin, and other mediators from the mast cells, thereby causing symptoms of allergy
12. ___ First antibody produced in response to an antigen
13. ___ First line of defense against microbes entering the body via gastrointestinal (GI) tract and lungs

14. ___ The major antibody in blood
15. ___ Found only on the surface of mature B cells

a. IgA
b. IgD
c. IgE
d. IgG
e. IgM

Completion

16. Antibodies are also known as _____ and _____.

17. Specific immune responses are possible because _____ and _____ possess receptors that can recognize individual antigens.

CRITICAL THINKING, PRIORITIZATION, AND DELEGATION QUESTIONS

18. What is true about natural immunity?
    a. It intensifies with each exposure to an antigen.
    b. It involves lymphocyte receptors that recognize individual antigens.
    c. It is specific to a particular antigen.
    d. Its protection includes the skin.

19. The nurse assesses for declining immune status of patients who are infected with human immunodeficiency virus (HIV) by monitoring for declining levels of
    a. basophils.
    b. CD4 cells (helper T cells).
    c. CD8 cells (cytotoxic T lymphocytes).
    d. macrophages.

20. What is true about breast-feeding?
    a. It does not affect the infant's immunity.
    b. It produces lifelong immunity for the diseases for which the mother has immunity.
    c. It transfers maternal IgA to the infant's GI tract.
    d. It triggers the release of mediators from mast cells.

21. When do autoimmune diseases occur?
   a. A new antigen is introduced to the body, and the immune system does not recognize the antigen.
   b. A person has an inflammatory reaction to an antigen.
   c. An antigen is introduced, and the immune response fades too quickly.
   d. There is a failure in MHC molecules' ability to identify self.

22. A person who is allergic to penicillin could expect a more severe reaction with exposure to penicillin in the future. Why?
   a. Helper T cells attack the penicillin molecule.
   b. Higher doses of penicillin would have to be used.
   c. Memory cells that identified the penicillin as an antigen allow for a more rapid, intense, and prolonged response.
   d. The immune system cannot eliminate the penicillin.

23. What is an immunologic reason for the fact that red blood cells (RBCs) can be transfused from one person to another?
   a. Human RBCs do not have class I MHC molecules.
   b. Human blood is exactly the same in all individuals.
   c. Human blood does not respond to class II MHC molecules.
   d. There is no reason because the above statement is not true.

24. The nurse is reviewing the laboratory tests for a patient who is jaundiced. Laboratory results include an elevated tumor necrosis factor (TNF). This suggests the patient has what condition?
   a. Cirrhosis or hepatitis
   b. Diabetes mellitus or insipidus
   c. Inflammation or a tumor
   d. Kidney cancer or renal failure

25. Cells that provide signals to regulate cell proliferation and function during immune responses are called
   a. antigen-presenting cells.
   b. cytokines.
   c. MHC molecules.
   d. opsonins.

26. Activation of the complement pathway occurs when the first component of the complement system (C1) encounters
   a. a free antibody.
   b. a free antigen.
   c. an antibody-antigen complex.
   d. phagocytic cell

CASE STUDY

The nurse is preparing to perform allergy testing by intradermal injection of house dust, molds, foods, and other common allergens.

1. Why are injected extracts called *antigens*?

2. The allergic reaction causes degranulation of mast cells. What cells respond in the skin, what do they release, and what dermal symptoms will the patient have if allergic to the antigen?

3. The patient is required to remain in the office for 20 minutes after injection of any antigen because that is the usual time frame for an immediate hypersensitivity reaction. Describe what the nurse should do if the following reactions occur.

   a. Itching and redness at the site of injection

   b. Tingling around the mouth

4. Why is it important to teach this patient about possible anaphylaxis?

68

Childhood Immunization

STUDY QUESTIONS

Matching

Match the term with its description.

1. ____ Refers to production of both active immunity and passive immunity
2. ____ Giving a patient preformed antibodies
3. ____ Substance that stimulates the immune system to produce antibodies
4. ____ Not pathogenic
5. ____ Documents that describe the benefits and risks of specific vaccines
6. ____ A mercury-based preservative found in some vaccines
7. ____ Preparations made from donated blood which contain a high concentration of antibodies directed against a specific antigen
8. ____ Preparation containing whole or fractionated microorganisms, causing the recipient's immune system to manufacture antibodies directed against the microbe
9. ____ Giving any vaccine or toxoid
10. ____ Protein produced by the body's immune system in response to a specific antigen
11. ____ Develops in response to infection or to administration of a vaccine or toxoid
12. ____ Bacterial toxin that has been changed to a nontoxic form, causing the recipient's immune system to manufacture antitoxins

   a. Active immunity
   b. Antibody
   c. Antigen
   d. Avirulent
   e. Immune globulin
   f. Immunization
   g. Passive immunity
   h. Thimerosal
   i. Toxoid
   j. Vaccine
   k. Vaccination
   l. Vaccine information statements (VIS)

CRITICAL THINKING, PRIORITIZATION, AND DELEGATION QUESTIONS

13. The pediatric office nurse is responsible for obtaining vaccine information sheets to be provided to parents before they consent to vaccinations for their children. What is the best source of this information?
    a. www.cdc.gov
    b. www.immunize.org
    c. pubmedcentral.nih.gov
    d. www.webmd.com

14. Because cases of anaphylaxis associated with MMR can be severe, the nurse should ensure immediate access within the office to which drug before administering any immunization?
    a. Albuterol (Proventil)
    b. Cetirizine (Zyrtec)
    c. Diphenhydramine (Benadryl)
    d. Epinephrine (Adrenaline)

▶15. What is the appropriate immunization strategy for a child who is behind in getting immunizations and is being seen at the pediatric office for a temperature of 100.6° F (38.1° C) and uncomplicated acute otitis media that is treated with amoxicillin?
    a. Administer needed immunizations at the next scheduled well-child visit.
    b. Administer needed immunizations during this visit.
    c. Do not administer immunizations until the child is afebrile.
    d. Do not administer immunizations until the child has finished the antibiotic.

✳16. It would be of greatest priority for the parent to contact the prescriber if a child experienced which symptom after administration of a DTaP immunization?
    a. Drowsiness
    b. Refusal to eat
    c. Swelling around lips
    d. Temperature of 100.4° F (38° C)

17. When should the nurse provide parents or legal guardians with vaccine information sheets?
    a. Before the first dose of a particular vaccine is to be administered
    b. Before each dose of each vaccine
    c. Once, before any vaccines are administered
    d. Only when requested

►18. The nurse would consult with the prescriber if
＊ which immunization was prescribed for a child who is receiving long-term high doses of predniso-lone? (Select all that apply.)
    a. DTaP
    b. Hib
    c. IPV
    d. MMR
    e. Varicella vaccine

19. Foster parents bring a 14-month-old child in for the first visit at the pediatrician's office. The Child Protective Agency is unable to obtain any immunization records. The child has no contraindications to vaccination. What approach to immunizations is appropriate?
    a. Administer immunizations as if the child has not received any vaccines per the catch-up schedule.
    b. Administer the immunizations regularly scheduled for 12-14 months of age.
    c. Delay immunizations until the records can be found.
    d. Immunize the child with the immunizations scheduled for 2 months of age.

20. What are appropriate measures to decrease discomfort associated with immunizations? (Select all that apply.)
    a. Administer the appropriate dose of acetaminophen or ibuprofen 30-60 minutes before the immunization.
    b. Apply topical anesthetic to the injection site prior to administering the injection.
    c. Aspirate before injecting an intramuscular vaccine.
    d. Tell the child when the nurse is done with administration of the immunization.
    e. Use 25- to 26-gauge needles when administering the injection.

＊21. It would be of greatest priority to consult the prescriber if MMR was ordered in which situation?
    a. The child's mother is receiving chemotherapy for breast cancer.
    b. The child has had a positive Monospot test (EBV infection).
    c. The child is being treated with chemotherapy for leukemia.
    d. The child is asymptomatic, but HIV positive.

►22. The nurse is preparing to administer Gardasil to an 18-year-old college-bound female patient. The nurse tells the patient, "You cannot get pregnant for 2 months if I give you this shot." Why is this not a good statement for the nurse to make to this adolescent?
    a. Pregnancy is not contraindicated after MMR vaccination.
    b. The statement assumes that the patient is sexually active.
    c. The statement is a communication blocker.
    d. The patient may interpret the statement as meaning that the injection prevents pregnancy.

23. Which nursing actions would be critical when the office nurse is discussing a scheduled MMR vaccination with the parents of a 12-month-old boy? (Select all that apply.)
    a. Determining whether the child has allergies to gelatin
    b. Teaching that any adverse effects from receiving the vaccine should occur within 48 hours
    c. Asking whether the child has received blood or blood products in the past 6 months
    d. Instructing the parents to contact the office if they notice unusual bleeding or bruising
    e. Instructing the parents to prevent the child from having close contact with anyone who is pregnant for 3 weeks after receiving the vaccine

►24. The triage nurse receives a call from parents who are concerned about their 2-month-old son, who received a DTaP vaccination 5 days ago. Which symptoms would be of most concern to the nurse?
    a. Crying inconsolably for the past 24 hours
    b. Breast-feeding for 20 minutes every 3-4 hours
    c. Redness and swelling at the injection site
    d. Temperature of 103° F for 12 hours

25. Why does the CDC currently recommend administration of the inactivated poliovirus vaccine (IPV[IPOL], or Salk) instead of the oral polio vaccine (OPV/Sabin)?
    a. OPV can cause vaccine-induced polio.
    b. IPV is less expensive than OPV.
    c. OPV has not been studied long enough.
    d. OPV is less effective than IPV.

26. Which information would be a reason to consult the prescriber before administering the varicella vaccine to a 15-month-old child?
    a. The child had a severe reaction to the MMR vaccine.
    b. The child is allergic to eggs.
    c. The child's aunt and her newborn are temporarily staying with the family.
    d. The office has used all of the syringes with 1-inch needles.

▶27. The triage office nurse receives a call from the father of a 16-year-old who received a varicella vaccine 10 days prior. The teenager experienced a fever after the injection, which was treated with aspirin. Yesterday he stayed home from school with stomach flu. He has not vomited today, but the father is having difficulty awakening him. What directions should the nurse provide to the father?
    a. Allow the teenager to rest and encourage fluid intake.
    b. Make an appointment for his son to be seen in the office as soon as possible.
    c. Reassess the teenager's temperature after administering acetaminophen and call back in the afternoon.
    d. Seek emergency medical care for his son immediately.

28. Which child should return for a booster dose of varicella vaccine 1 month after the first dose?
    a. A 12-year-old who did not experience a vesicular rash after the first dose
    b. A child who was 12 years old when receiving the first dose who has not had chickenpox
    c. A child younger than 13 years old at the time of the first dose who has had chickenpox
    d. A child who is younger than 18 months

29. The nursery nurse would expect to administer which vaccination(s) to the neonate within 12 hours of birth if the neonate's mother is HBsAg-positive? (Select all that apply.)
    a. Hepatitis B immunoglobulin (HBIG)
    b. Havrix
    c. Influenza vaccine
    d. Pneumovax
    e. Recombivax HB
    f. Twinrix

30. What are indications for hepatitis A vaccine? (Select all that apply.)
    a. All children age 1 to 12 years
    b. Children with hemophilia that requires clotting factor infusions
    c. Children with renal failure
    d. Children who will be traveling to the Caribbean
    e. Children who will be traveling to Japan

▶31. Parents of a child with asthma were reluctant to have their 3-year-old receive the flu vaccine because they were afraid that she would get the disease from the injection. The pediatrician convinced them to allow immunization in January of this year. When should the child receive the next annual flu vaccine?
    a. As soon as the new vaccine is available
    b. September of this year
    c. November of this year
    d. January of next year

✳32. The nurse administers Rotarix rotavirus vaccine to an infant at a medical clinic in the Dominican Republic. It is of greatest priority for the nurse to teach the child's caregivers to seek immediate emergency care if within the next month the infant exhibits which symptom?
    a. Loose stool × 2 in 24 hours
    b. Runny nose for 3 days
    c. Sore throat and cough
    d. Stool that looks like jelly

33. A patient who has had a splenectomy asks why he needs to get a meningitis vaccine. What is the basis of the nurse's response?
    a. The spleen destroys old red blood cells.
    b. The spleen forms blood cells.
    c. The spleen is a critical defense whenever a patient has a fever.
    d. The spleen helps fight bacteria causing pneumonia and meningitis.

CASE STUDIES

Case Study 1

Parents bring their 7-month-old child to the clinic. They state that they were told by an emergency department (ED) physician of the local hospital to bring their child in for "baby shots." The parents are concerned, stating that they have heard that children can die from these shots.

1. What teaching can the nurse provide about the safety and benefits of the immunizations?

2. The parents have difficulty understanding complex concepts. How can the nurse explain reactions to immunizations?

3. How would the nurse explain the laws requiring children to have immunizations before they can attend school and, in some cases, day care?

4. What subjective data and medical history does the nurse need to review before administering an immunization?

Case Study 2

Parents of an elementary school child in Lancaster, Pennsylvania have verbalized to the school nurse that their children have never been "contaminated" with immunizations. The parents state that their unimmunized child has not contracted the measles, mumps, diphtheria, or other illness for which immunizations are routinely administered.

5. How should the school nurse respond?

6. The parents state that they are particularly concerned about MMR because of its association with autism. What has research suggested about the association of MMR and autism?

7. The school nurse is aware that exposure to certain populations or situations puts unvaccinated children at risk for contracting vaccine-preventable disease. What are possible populations and situations that would put children at risk in this school and geographic area?

Case Study 3

During pharmacology class, a nursing student remarks that he would not have his 11-year-old daughter vaccinated with Gardasil because "she is a good girl."

8. What should be included in the discussion about this parent's reaction?

9. The concerned parent/nursing student agrees with the explanation but states that his daughter has heard that the injection is painful. What might the parent discuss with the pediatrician about this concern?

10. The literature reports a number of adolescent patients fainting when given the human papillomavirus (HPV) vaccine. What might contribute to this reaction, and what can the office nurse do to prepare for this possible reaction?

11. Another nursing student states that she will have her daughter vaccinated because the adolescent will not have to have Pap smears and pelvic examinations until she is ready to get pregnant. What should be included in response to this statement?

69
Immunosuppressants

STUDY QUESTIONS

Completion

1. Because of the possible adverse effect of prednisone on blood glucose, the nurse should assess the patient for symptoms of _____.

2. Unexplained bleeding is a possible adverse effect of _____.

3. A liver transplant patient's orders include discontinuation of IV tacrolimus (Prograf) and starting oral tacrolimus. The last IV dose was administered at 10:00 AM. The first oral dose should be administered no sooner than _____.

4. Because sirolimus has a half-life of 2.5 days and it is categorized as pregnancy category C, the nurse teaches women of child-bearing years to continue using birth control for _____ after discontinuing use of sirolimus.

5. The nurse should teach patients who take sirolimus to take the medication consistently either without food or with consistent amounts of _____ in foods.

6. The nurse should teach a patient who is prescribed mycophenolate mofetil (Cell-Cept) not to take over-the-counter (OTC) _____.

CRITICAL THINKING, PRIORITIZATION, AND DELEGATION QUESTIONS

∗ 7. The nurse is providing postoperative teaching for a patient who has had carpal tunnel release surgery and who is receiving immunosuppressant therapy for rheumatoid arthritis. Based on the surgery and medication, the priority nursing concern in this case would be preventing
   a. airway constriction.
   b. impaired tissue perfusion.
   c. infection.
   d. pain.

8. Which symptom should the nurse teach a patient who has been prescribed immunosuppressant drugs to report because it is an early sign of infection?
   a. Chills and rigor
   b. Cough
   c. Rash
   d. Sore throat

9. A 16-month-old child receives a heart-lung transplant. What teaching should the nurse provide about immunizations relating to immunosuppressant therapy?
   a. The child may need more than the usual recommended doses of inactivated vaccines.
   b. The child may need more than the usual recommended doses of live vaccines.
   c. The child should not receive any inactivated vaccines.
   d. The child should not receive any live vaccines.
   e. The child should not receive any vaccines.

10. Body image is developmentally important to many patients. It is important for the nurse to discuss body image when cyclosporine has been prescribed to a young woman, because the drug can cause
   a. acne.
   b. facial hair.
   c. rash.
   d. weight gain.

∗11. Because of the risk of nephrotoxicity with administration of cyclosporine (Sandimmune), a priority nursing assessment is
   a. intake and output.
   b. pulse.
   c. temperature.
   d. weight.

✳12. The nurse is administering intravenous (IV) cyclosporine (Sandimmune). Within 15 minutes after beginning the infusion, the patient complains of feeling hot and says her chest feels tight. Which action would be of greatest priority?
   a. Administer prescribed epinephrine (Adrenalin).
   b. Assess vital signs.
   c. Assess lung sounds.
   d. Stop the infusion of cyclosporine.

13. When reviewing the laboratory results of patients receiving cyclosporine (Sandimmune) or tacrolimus (Prograf), which result(s) would be a reason to contact the prescriber? (Select all that apply.)
   a. ALT 28 international units
   b. BUN 17 mg/dL
   c. Creatinine 3.2 mg/dL
   d. Potassium 5.4 mEq/L
   e. WBC 3800/mm^3

14. The nurse is providing discharge teaching regarding prescribed oral cyclosporine to prevent rejection of a transplanted kidney. Which statement, if made by the patient, suggests understanding of the teaching? (Select all that apply.)
   a. "I should make an appointment to see the doctor if I have episodes of nausea and abdominal pain or if my BM changes color."
   b. "I should use the same pharmacy for all of my prescriptions."
   c. "I should dress in layers in case I feel hot when taking this drug."
   d. "It is important to see my dentist regularly."

15. A liver transplant patient who is prescribed tacrolimus (Prograf) reveals that he has been drinking grapefruit juice, but he has made sure it has been at least 4 hours between the juice and the medication. Which lab result, if a change from recent findings, suggests a drug-food interaction?
   a. Blood pressure 88/47 mm Hg
   b. eGFR 50 mL/hr
   c. Fasting blood sugar 235 mg/dL
   d. Temperature 102° F

✳16. It is a priority for the nurse to teach a patient who is prescribed tacrolimus (Prograf) to read labels of over-the-counter drugs and not take drugs that contain
   a. acetaminophen.
   b. acetylsalicylic acid.
   c. diphenhydramine.
   d. ibuprofen.

17. Trough levels of tacrolimus are 10 ng/mL. What should the nurse do?
   a. Repeat the trough level.
   b. Consult the prescriber before doing anything else.
   c. Administer the drug.
   d. Withhold the drug.

✳18. Which symptom, if reported by a patient receiving sirolimus (Rapamune), would be a priority to report to the prescriber or attending physician?
   a. Productive cough
   b. Fatigue
   c. Joint pain
   d. Tinnitus

19. Which drug, if taken with everolimus (Zortress), is most likely to cause toxicity?
   a. Erythromycin
   b. Phenobarbital
   c. Phenytoin
   d. Rifamycin

20. Due to the adverse effect on bone density, it would be a priority to protect the patient from falls when taking which drug?
   a. Azathioprine
   b. Prednisone
   c. Sirolimus
   d. Tacrolimus

21. Which laboratory results should be immediately reported to the prescriber when a patient is administered azathioprine (Imuran)?
   a. ALT 65 IU/L
   b. hCG 328 mIU/mL
   c. Platelets 145,000/mm^3
   d. WBC 4900/mm^3

22. Which technique(s) should be employed when administering antilymphocyte globulin (Atgam)? (Select all that apply.)
   a. Administer via a central line using an inline filter.
   b. Assess for flushing, dyspnea, and generalized anxiety.
   c. Dilute in 5% dextrose in water.
   d. Infuse slowly—over 4 hours or more.

DOSE CALCULATION QUESTIONS

23. A patient is prescribed oral cyclosporine (Gengraf) 9 mg/kg/day divided into 2 doses 12 hours apart. The patient weighs 132 lb, and the medication is available as a solution of 100 mg/mL. How much medication should the nurse administer?

24. Mycophenolate mofetil 1 g IV over 2 hours is prescribed before renal transplant surgery. The drug is diluted in 5% dextrose in water at a concentration of 1000 mg/28 mL. The intravenous pump is programmed in mL/hr. What rate should the nurse program into the pump?

CASE STUDIES

Case Study 1

A 4-year-old girl received an allogenic heart transplant at age 16 months for transposition of the great vessels and only one ventricle, which resulted in cardiac failure.

1. What is an allogenic transplant?

The patient was discharged on cyclosporine, azathioprine (Imuran), and prednisone. She is brought back to the transplant hospital monthly for bloodwork to monitor rejection status and performance of her new heart. During the past year, she has shown no sign of rejection or limitation of her activities. Her growth has more closely followed normal growth charts, and outwardly she appears to be a healthy 4-year-old. Recently, following a trip to a national park, she developed fatigue and appeared tired. Bloodwork indicated evidence of macrophages and monocytes beginning the rejection process. She was hospitalized and diagnosed with evidence of transplant rejection.

2. What are nursing priorities for this patient?

3. Intravenous muromonab-CD3 is added to the patient's medication regimen to prevent rejection of the transplanted heart. What actions should the nurse take in the hospital to prevent the patient from contracting an infection?

4. What special steps must be taken when administering this drug IV?

5. Four hours after the patient receives the first dose of muromonab-CD3, the patient's parents tells the nurse that the patient is shivering. Her temperature is 102.6° F. These symptoms could be indicative of further organ rejection or adverse effects of the drug. What should the nurse do?

Case Study 2

A 38-year-old kidney transplant recipient is prescribed immunosuppressant therapy with IV cyclosporine (Sandimmune), prednisone, and ketoconazole.

6. The patient asks why she is prescribed ketoconazole in addition to cyclosporine. What should the nurse explain is the main reason these two drugs are administered concurrently?

7. It is important for the nurse to teach the patient about the cyclosporine's possible effects on a developing fetus and that current contraceptive recommendations include use of which type of birth control?

8. What teaching should the nurse provide relating to the adverse effect of increased risk of neoplasms from taking cyclosporine?

9. The prescriber of cyclosporine (Sandimmune) has ordered a trough level after the fourth dose. When should the trough level be drawn?

10. The patient's cyclosporine orders are changed to oral cyclosporine (Gengraf). The hospital pharmacy sends the Sandimmune formulation (100 mg/mL). What should the nurse do?

11. The patient has a history of osteoarthritis and a seizure disorder. What should be included in the plan of nursing care relating to immunosuppressant therapy that she is receiving and her medical history?

70
Antihistamines

STUDY QUESTIONS

True or False

For each of the following statements, enter T for true or F for false.

H_1-blocking drugs for allergic reactions

1. ___ are the active ingredient in most over-the-counter (OTC) drugs to induce sleep.
2. ___ can cause excitement, nervousness, and tremors.
3. ___ can cause urinary retention.
4. ___ cause the skin to become red and warm.
5. ___ decrease release of histamine present in high levels in the skin.
6. ___ decrease pruritus.
7. ___ elevate the pH of stomach secretions.
8. ___ have sedation as the most common adverse effect.
9. ___ prevent local edema.
10. ___ prevent the release of histamine from mast cells and basophils.

CRITICAL THINKING, PRIORITIZATION, AND DELEGATION QUESTIONS

11. A patient is scheduled to receive a radiocontrast media for a CAT scan. The patient has never received any radiocontrast media. Why must the radiology nurse carefully assess for an allergic reaction?
    a. Allergic reactions are common because patients often are unaware if they have had radiocontrast media in the past.
    b. Allergic reactions can occur even without prior exposure to radiocontrast media.
    c. Allergic reactions occur in more than 30% of patients.
    d. Allergic reactions to contrast media are usually asymptomatic until anaphylaxis occurs.

12. The parent of a 3-year-old child who was recently diagnosed with asthma calls during phone hour at the pediatrician's office. The child has a cold, which often triggers an asthma attack. The parent has forgotten which drug the child should be given when he starts wheezing. Which drug would be safe and effective?
    a. Diphenhydramine (Benadryl)—first-generation H_1 antagonist
    b. Loratadine (Claritin)—second-generation H_1 antagonist
    c. Fexofenadine (Allegra)—second-generation H_1 antagonist
    d. No antihistamines are safe and effective for wheezing of asthma

13. Why is it important to teach patients to be prepared for possible allergic reactions every time they take a certain drug?
    a. Because allergic reactions are common.
    b. Because allergic reactions are most likely to occur on the third or fourth day of taking a drug.
    c. Because allergic reactions frequently occur even if a patient has never been exposed to the drug or its components.
    d. Because allergic reactions usually occur after previous exposure to a drug or its components.

14. On admission, the nurse is reviewing all of the drugs that a 78-year-old patient takes at home. The patient has a history of hypertension and diabetes. The patient takes OTC diphenhydramine (Benadryl) when she has a cold. That nurse explains the effect of first-generation histamine blockers on the body and on a cold. Which statement, if made by the patient after the teaching, suggests a need for additional teaching?
    a. "Benadryl does not prevent colds but it can make my cold go away faster."
    b. "Benadryl can make mucus from a cold hard to expel because it thickens the mucus."
    c. "Benadryl can make my constipation worse."
    d. "My 3-year-old granddaughter could have convulsions if she took some of my Benadryl."

15. The term *antihistamine* is used to refer to drugs that block
    a. H_1 receptors.
    b. H_2 receptors.
    c. H_1 and H_2 receptors.

16. Why do second-generation H_1 blockers cause less sedation than first-generation H_1 blockers?
    a. They are less potent.
    b. They bind reversibly to histamine receptors.
    c. They do not cross the blood-brain barrier.
    d. They are rapidly metabolized.

∗17. Which of these assessment findings, if identified by the delivery room nurse in a full-term neonate whose mother has taken diphenhydramine (Benadryl) just before going into labor, would be a priority to immediately report to the pediatrician?
    a. Systolic BP 60 mm Hg
    b. Temperature 37.2° C (99° F)
    c. Pulse 180 beats/min
    d. Respirations 25 breaths per minute

18. The nurse is teaching a patient who has a history of benign prostatic hyperplasia (BPH) and allergic rhinitis about taking desloratadine (Clarinex). What should teaching include? (Select all that apply.)
    a. Avoid alcohol and other CNS depressants.
    b. Avoid any activity that requires coordination or alertness.
    c. High doses are more likely to cause sedation.
    d. Taking doses higher than recommended does not help the drug work better.
    e. The drug may aggravate urinary retention from the enlarged prostate.

▶19. The nurse is administering 6 AM medications, including chlorpheniramine (Chlor-Trimeton) 4 mg every 6 hours for urticaria. The patient complains of nausea associated with the medication. What should the nurse do?
    a. Change the timing of the medication to 8 AM (0800), 12 noon (1200), 5 PM (1700), and 8 PM (2000) to correspond to meals and bedtime snack.
    b. Decrease the dose of the medication.
    c. Hold the medication and consult the prescriber.
    d. Provide a snack with each dose of medication.

DOSE CALCULATION QUESTIONS

20. Fexofenadine, 30 mg twice a day, is prescribed for a 4-year-old with allergy-induced asthma. It is available as a suspension containing 6 mg/mL. How many mL should be administered at each dose?

21. Promethazine (Phenergan) 25 mg is prescribed for a patient with nausea and vomiting. The drug is available as 25 mg/mL. Would it be safe to administer 0.1 mL every 5 seconds IV push if the drug is to infused no faster than 25 mg/minute?

CASE STUDY

A 25-year-old taxi driver has come to his health care provider to obtain information and help for his "hay fever." He says he doesn't know what to take because OTC drugs seem so confusing. His condition is diagnosed as allergic rhinitis and is seasonal, with reactions lasting from May until the end of June each year. He also says that he is occasionally bothered by dust during the rest of the year. He complains of headache; congestion; sneezing; rhinorrhea (runny nose); and itchy, burning, watery eyes. He asks how allergies cause these symptoms.

1. What information could be included in the explanation?

2. What are the disadvantages to antihistamines for those who drive or use heavy equipment at work?

3. The patient is concerned about cost. He asks if prescription antihistamines are more effective than OTC diphenhydramine (Benadryl). How should the nurse respond?

4. How do second-generation antihistamines work but not cause sedation?

5. The prescriber orders azelastine (Astelin) 2 sprays of 250 micrograms in each nostril twice a day. Why is this medication appropriate for this patient?

6. What suggestions can the nurse make if the patient chooses to use one of the antihistamines that cause sedation?

71

Cyclooxygenase Inhibitors: Nonsteroidal Anti-inflammatory Drugs and Acetaminophen

STUDY QUESTIONS

Completion

1. The half-life of aspirin is 15-20 minutes, but the antiplatelet effects last _____ _____.

2. Preoperative teaching for knee replacement surgery should include that the patient should discontinue high-dose aspirin therapy for _____ before surgery.

3. When taking aspirin for antiplatelet action, other NSAIDs should be separated from the aspirin dose by at least _____ hours.

4. Aspirin should not be taken by children, especially for symptoms of viral illness, because of the risk of _____ _____.

5. The nurse should instruct patients to dispose of aspirin tablets if they develop an odor that smells like _____.

6. Chronic alcohol use interferes with the metabolism of large doses of _____.

7. _____ is the antidote for acetaminophen overdose.

8. The recommended maximum dose of acetaminophen for individuals who regularly consume alcohol is _____.

CRITICAL THINKING, PRIORITIZATION, AND DELEGATION QUESTIONS

✶ 9. The following information was included in the change of shift report on a patient who is prescribed aspirin for its anticoagulant effects. Which patient symptom, if present, would be a priority for the nurse to report to the attending physician?
    a. Abdominal bloating
    b. Emesis of dark-brown particles
    c. Heartburn when recumbent
    d. Two liquid stools in the past 24 hours

▶ 10. Which would not be an appropriate reason for the nurse to administer an as-needed dose of 650 mg of aspirin?
    a. Hand pain and stiffness when arising
    b. Knee pain with ambulation
    c. Right temporal headache associated with a tense neck
    d. Abdominal pain with distension

11. What should the nurse do to prevent the most common adverse effect of long-term aspirin therapy?
    a. Administer the drug with fluids and food.
    b. Assess lung sounds for wheezing before administering the drug.
    c. Monitor urine output.
    d. Teach the patient to report tarry-colored stool.

12. Which statements, if made by a patient who is receiving aspirin therapy for rheumatoid arthritis, suggests that the patient needs further teaching?
    a. "Drinking a full glass of water with my aspirin can help prevent pill particles from getting trapped in the inside folds of my stomach."
    b. "I will know if aspirin is causing ulcers because it will cause abdominal pain."
    c. "If I drink alcohol, it can irritate my stomach and make it easier for aspirin to cause it to bleed."
    d. "I should stop taking aspirin and consult with my physician if I experience a sudden watery runny nose."

13. Which diagnostic test is performed before starting long-term aspirin therapy to identify an increased risk for gastric ulceration?
    a. Colonoscopy
    b. Complete blood count and differential
    c. Esophagogastroduodenoscopy
    d. Test for *H. pylori*

✳14. It is of greatest priority for the nurse to communicate self-prescribed aspirin use to the primary care provider if the patient has which history?
    a. Genetic hypercoagulability disorder
    b. Sexually active woman not using any form of birth control
    c. Smoking two packs of cigarettes per day
    d. Type 2 diabetes mellitus

✳15. A patient brought into the emergency department (ED) after taking aspirin for a headache exhibits the following symptoms. Which symptom would be of greatest priority for the nurse to address?
    a. Bronchospasm
    b. Profuse, watery nasal discharge
    c. Tachycardia
    d. Urticaria

16. Which symptom suggest that blood levels of a salicylate such as aspirin are too high?
    a. Fatigue
    b. Heartburn after meals
    c. Ringing in the ears
    d. Vomiting

▶17. The nurse notes a respiratory rate of 14 breaths per minute when assessing an 18-month-old child with suspected salicylate poisoning. Which laboratory results support this diagnosis?
    a. pH 7.32; $Paco_2$ 40 mm Hg; HCO_3^- -20 mEq/L
    b. pH 7.35; $Paco_2$ 37 mm Hg; HCO_3^- 22 mEq/L
    c. pH 7.41; $Paco_2$ 35 mm Hg; HCO_3^- 20 mEq/L
    d. pH 7.46; $Paco_2$ 31 mm Hg; HCO_3^- 18 mEq/L

18. A patient has been prescribed aspirin 81 mg once a day after undergoing angioplasty. It is important for the nurse to teach this patient to avoid using which over-the-counter (OTC) medication?
    a. Acetaminophen (Tylenol)
    b. Calcium carbonate (TUMS)
    c. Guaifenesin (Robitussin)
    d. Ibuprofen (Motrin, Advil)

19. Which aspirin preparation is the least irritating to the stomach?
    a. Buffered aspirin solution
    b. Enteric-coated aspirin
    c. Four chewable children's aspirin
    d. Timed-release aspirin

20. It is a priority to assess for which symptom if a patient has taken aspirin before delivery of a neonate?
    a. Boggy uterus
    b. Fatigue
    c. Perineal discomfort
    d. Sedation

▶21. Which condition would be of greatest concern when a patient reports regular use of sodium salicylate for joint pain?
    a. Chronic obstructive pulmonary disease
    b. Heart failure
    c. Diabetes mellitus
    d. Excessive bleeding with dental procedures

22. A patient has been prescribed naproxen/esomeprazole (Vimovo). Which statement suggests that patient teaching regarding administration of this drug has been successful?
    a. "Taking this drug combination is better than taking the two drugs separately."
    b. "This drug combination will protect my kidneys."
    c. "The additional drug decreases acid production in my stomach."
    d. "The addition of the second drug will make the naproxen more effective."

23. Indomethacin (Indocin) is prescribed for premature neonates to promote closure of the duct located between the
    a. inner ear and cochlea.
    b. liver and the duodenum.
    c. pulmonary artery and the aorta.
    d. umbilical vein and the neonate's abdomen.

►24. A medical resident has prescribed ketorolac 15 mg intramuscular (IM) for a woman who is requesting pain relief during labor. Which nursing action is most appropriate at this time?
   a. Administer the drug and monitor the neonate's respirations for depression after delivery.
   b. Assess the patient's stage of labor and question the order if the patient is in transition.
   c. Question administering an IM injection for a woman in labor.
   d. Withhold the drug and question the prescriber.

►25. The prescriber orders celecoxib (Celebrex) 100 mg to be administered twice a day. The nurse would consult the prescriber before administering the drug if the patient is allergic to
   a. amoxicillin.
   b. Bactrim.
   c. Ceftin.
   d. Zithromax.

＊26. Which assessment finding would be a priority for the nurse to report if a patient was receiving celecoxib (Celebrex)?
   a. Bruising of arms and shins
   b. A weight gain of 1 lb each day for 3 days
   c. Heartburn at night
   d. Inadequate joint pain relief after taking for 1 week

＊27. It is of greatest priority to report which change when a 65-year-old female patient is prescribed celecoxib (Celebrex)?
   a. Belching
   b. Bruise on left arm
   c. Difficulty speaking
   d. Headache
   e. Nausea

►28. A patient is admitted to an extended-care facility for rehabilitation after an open reduction and internal fixation (ORIF) of a hip fracture. She requests Percocet (acetaminophen 325 mg-oxycodone 5 mg) 1 tablet, ordered every 4 hours as needed, before going to physical therapy. The patient states that her pain is 2/10 currently but that she experiences unbearable pain if she does not take the Percocet before therapy. The patient has not received a dose of this drug in the last 4 hours. What should the nurse do?
   a. Administer the drug.
   b. Encourage the patient to wait until after therapy to take the drug so that it is longer between doses.
   c. Withhold the drug and question the prescriber.
   d. Withhold the drug because the patient's pain does not warrant administration of a narcotic.

►29. What nursing action is appropriate when a parent calls the pediatrician's office stating that his 15-month-old child just ingested an unknown quantity of children's chewable Tylenol tablets?
   a. Assess for the presence of nausea, vomiting, abdominal pain, or diaphoresis.
   b. Direct the parent to seek immediate medical care for the child.
   c. Make an appointment for the child to be seen as soon as possible.
   d. Take the opportunity to teach the parent about childproofing his home.

＊30. While infusing acetylcysteine (Acetadote) for acetaminophen overdose, the nurse notes that the patient is scratching her arms. Which action is of greatest priority at this time?
   a. Assess respirations, breath sounds, and vital signs.
   b. Consult the prescriber regarding changing to an oral formula.
   c. Report the itching to the prescriber.
   d. Stop the infusion and contact the prescriber STAT.

►31. A 3-year-old child is brought to the ED. The child's mother states that he had a rash and fever over a week ago. He vomited several times last night. This morning he was so drowsy that she could not rouse him. The child is lethargic and does not resist examination. It is of greatest priority to ask the mother if she administered which of the OTC drugs to her child during his illness?
   a. Bayer low-dose aspirin
   b. Robitussin cough syrup
   c. Sudafed decongestant
   d. Tylenol elixir

DOSE CALCULATION QUESTIONS

32. Acetylcysteine (Acetadote) 2250 mg intravenous is to be infused over 30 minutes. The drug is diluted in 200 mL of 5% dextrose. The infusion pump is calibrated in mL/hr. What rate should the nurse enter as the infusion rate?

33. The nurse is teaching parents about use of infant acetaminophen drops (80 mg/0.8 mL) and age-appropriate dose. How many mL should be administered per dose to a 13-month-old child?

CASE STUDIES

Case Study 1

The nurse is assisting a 58-year-old science teacher who is postoperative total abdominal hysterectomy and bilateral salpingo-oophorectomy (TAH-BSO) with ambulation in the hallway when the patient complains of knee pain and stiffness. The patient has a history of hypertension and osteoarthritis (degenerative joint disease, DJD). The patient states she was prescribed a COX-2 inhibitor for a short period of time several years ago. She tells the nurse that the drug really helped her knee pain and did not cause stomach distress like other NSAID drugs. She asks the if she could have the medication again.

1. What could the nurse tell the patient?

2. The patient says, "I am glad there is still one drug that I can take for my arthritis that does not cause side effects." How should the nurse respond?

3. What nonpharmacologic teaching can the nurse provide this patient?

Case Study 2

A 21-year-old patient comes to the family planning clinic to determine what she can do for relief of moderate dysmenorrhea. She states that the pain is not incapacitating, but creates discomfort during the first day of her menses. She says she does not want anything that makes her sleepy and that she has tried acetaminophen without relief. After further assessment, the nurse practitioner suggests that she try ibuprofen as a beginning drug to see how she responds. She is told to take 2 ibuprofen (200-mg tablets) every 4 hours for the first 2-3 days of her menstrual period, starting with the first symptom of menses or cramping.

4. Why is this schedule appropriate in this situation?

5. What information should be provided to this patient about possible adverse effects of this drug therapy?

6. Based on the developmental stage of this patient, what teaching should the nurse provide about use of ibuprofen and other over-the-counter NSAID drugs?

72

Glucocorticoids in Nonendocrine Disorders

STUDY QUESTIONS

Matching

Match the possible glucocorticoid-drug interactions.

1. ____ May require increased dose
2. ____ Increased risk of hypokalemia
3. ____ Can decrease antibody response
4. ____ Increased risk of ulceration
5. ____ Can help prevent osteoporosis

a. Bisphosphonates
b. Insulin
c. Loop diuretics
d. NSAIDs
e. Vaccines

CRITICAL THINKING, PRIORITIZATION, AND DELEGATION QUESTIONS

6. Which possible effect of glucocorticoid therapy in the doses used for nonendocrine disorders would be a priority to report to the prescriber?
   a. Calcium 9 mg/dL
   b. Chloride 95 mg/dL
   c. Potassium 3.1 mg/dL
   d. Sodium 145 mg/dL

＊ 7. It would be a priority to report which laboratory test result to the prescriber if a patient is receiving therapeutic doses of glucocorticoids?
   a. ALT 30 international units/L
   b. BUN 20 mg/dL
   c. A1c 5.9%
   d. WBC 2000/mm^3

8. The school nurse would notify the parents of a fourth-grade child who is receiving oral glucocorticoids to control asthma symptoms if height and weight screening findings included a
   a. change from the 35th to 75th percentile in height.
   b. change from the 75th to 35th percentile in height.
   c. gain of 2 lb in the last year.
   d. gain of 5 lb in the last year.

9. The nurse should be especially vigilant in assessing for adverse systemic effects of a topical glucocorticoid therapy when administering the preparation (Select all that apply.)
   a. to intertriginous areas.
   b. to mucous membranes.
   c. to well-hydrated skin.
   d. to infants.
   e. under an occlusive barrier.

▶10. A child would be at risk of contracting the disease if which immunization was administered when the child is receiving glucocorticoid therapy? (Select all that apply.)
   a. Inhaled influenza
   b. Injected influenza
   c. Measles, mumps, and rubella (MMR)
   d. Pneumococcal
   e. Varicella

▶11. Patients on long-term glucocorticoid therapy may minimize a common complication of therapy by having adequate servings of which foods in their diet?
   a. Broccoli and cauliflower
   b. Citrus fruits
   c. Legumes
   d. Whole grains

12. Which are common symptoms of hypokalemia caused by glucocorticoids with high mineralocorticoid activity?
   a. Anxiety and flushed skin
   b. Hypotension and cool, clammy skin
   c. Muscle weakness and fatigue
   d. Tingling around the mouth and fingers

13. Alternate-day glucocorticoid therapy is most appropriate for a patient who is
   a. 9 years old.
   b. 29 years old.
   c. 45 years old.
   d. 65 years old.

▶14. A patient who has been receiving glucocorticoid therapy for 2 months is being tapered off the glucocorticoids. Which symptom suggests a withdrawal syndrome?
   a. BP 84/47 mm Hg
   b. Fasting glucose 255 mg/dL
   c. Potassium 3.5 mEq/L
   d. Pulse 55 beats/min

▶15. A patient is taking dexamethasone for chronic obstructive pulmonary disease (COPD) and digoxin for heart failure (HF). Because of the increased risk for digoxin toxicity, the nurse should assess for what effect(s)? (Select all that apply.)
   a. Loss of appetite
   b. Positive Chvostek's sign
   c. Flushed skin
   d. Confusion
   e. Visual changes

DOSE CALCULATION QUESTIONS

16. A patient is prescribed dexamethasone 8 mg intravenous (IV) push. The drug is available as an injectable solution of 10 mg/mL. Instructions are to administer the dose over 1 minute. How many mL should the nurse administer every 15 seconds?

17. Dexamethasone 5 mg orally every 12 hours is prescribed for a 10-year-old child who weighs 82.5 lb. The recommended maximum safe dose for children is 0.3mg/kg/day. Is the dose safe?

CASE STUDY

A 43-year-old man with severe persistent asthma is admitted with an acute exacerbation. After the crisis is averted, the patient is prescribed dexamethasone sodium succinate 4 mg IV push. The pharmacy sends dexamethasone acetate 16 mg/mL.

1. How much should the nurse administer?

2. The patient is switched to oral glucocorticoid therapy. Because of the severity of the patient's asthma, the prescriber explains that long-term oral glucocorticoids will probably be necessary in addition to an inhaled glucocorticoid and bronchodilators. What instructions should the nurse provide this patient regarding minimizing the following adverse effects of glucocorticoid therapy?

   a. Adrenal insufficiency

   b. Osteoporosis

   c. Infection: suppresses immune response and phagocytic activity of neutrophils and macrophages

   d. Glucose intolerance

   e. Myopathy

   f. Edema, hypernatremia, and hypokalemia

   g. Mood

   h. Cataracts and glaucoma

   i. Peptic ulcer disease

73

Drug Therapy of Rheumatoid Arthritis

STUDY QUESTIONS

Matching

Match the drug to its action.

1. ____ Provide rapid relief of symptoms and can slow disease progression; with long-term use they can cause serious toxicity.
2. ____ Provide rapid relief of symptoms, but do not prevent joint damage and do not slow disease progression.
3. ____ Drugs that reduce joint destruction and slow disease progression; benefits develop slowly.

   a. Disease-modifying antirheumatic drugs (DMARDs)
   b. Glucocorticoids
   c. Nonsteroidal anti-inflammatory drugs (NSAIDs)

CRITICAL THINKING, PRIORITIZATION, AND DELEGATION QUESTIONS

4. Which medication use for rheumatoid arthritis (RA) follows current guidelines? (Select all that apply.)
   a. Do not discontinue glucocorticoid therapy once started because this will cause "flares."
   b. If symptoms cannot be controlled by an NSAID, add a DMARD.
   c. Start with a DMARD within 3 months of diagnosis.
   d. Start with an NSAID and use glucocorticoids for "flares."
   e. Take an NSAID along with a DMARD during the first few months of drug therapy for RA.

5. What is an advantage of COX-2 inhibitors such as celecoxib (Celebrex) over prescription-strength COX-1 and -2 inhibitors such as naproxen?
   a. They decrease production of stomach acid.
   b. They do not decrease gastric mucus production.
   c. They do not irritate the stomach as much.
   d. They are more effective in reducing pain and inflammation.

6. Which teaching is of greatest priority if a patient has taken prednisone 10 mg twice a day for 6 weeks for an RA flare and the flare has subsided?
   a. Avoid people who have infections.
   b. Be sure to get enough rest.
   c. Follow instructions for tapering off of the drug.
   d. Take steps to manage stress.

7. A patient has been prescribed methotrexate (DMARD) immediately after being diagnosed with RA. The patient has heard that these drugs can be dangerous and asks the nurse why the prescriber has not ordered a prescription-strength NSAID. What is the best response by the nurse?
   a. "Methotrexate delays joint degeneration."
   b. "Methotrexate has fewer adverse effects than prescription-strength NSAIDs."
   c. "Methotrexate works faster than NSAIDs."
   d. "Prescription-strength NSAIDs can cause peptic ulcers; methotrexate does not."

8. A patient who is unwilling to take other drugs for his RA has been prescribed aspirin 975 mg (3 tablets) every 6 hours. Which symptom, if experienced by this patient, suggests aspirin toxicity?
   a. Bruising
   b. Epigastric pain
   c. Jaundice
   d. Ringing in the ears

9. A patient with RA is being treated with oral prednisolone for a flare of RA. Which statement by the patient would suggest to the nurse that this patient needs more teaching?
   a. "If I stop taking this drug suddenly, my body may not be able to deal with infection, healing, and stress."
   b. "It is important to keep active if I need to take this drug because it can make my bones weak."
   c. "I should not stop taking this drug without guidance from my doctor."
   d. "Taking this drug with food will prevent me from having any bad effects."

10. A 16-year-old female patient takes methotrexate once a week for juvenile RA. Which laboratory test result for this patient would be of greatest concern for the nurse?
    a. Blood urea nitrogen (BUN) 20 mg/dL
    b. Erythrocyte sedimentation rate (ESR) 30 mm/hr
    c. Urine hCG positive
    d. White blood cell count 11,000/mm^3

11. Which laboratory test result should be monitored when a patient is receiving sulfasalazine (Azulfidine)?
    a. CBC
    b. Electrolytes
    c. Fasting blood glucose
    d. Urine specific gravity

12. When performing a nursing assessment on a patient receiving leflunomide (Arava), which observations would be a reason for the nurse to hold the medication and contact the prescriber?
    a. Abdominal pain and dark urine
    b. Alopecia and skin rash
    c. Nausea and diarrhea
    d. Rhinorrhea and sneezing

✳13. When a female patient is prescribed hydroxychloroquine (Plaquenil) for RA, it is of greatest priority for the nurse to assess if the patient has adhered to recommended follow-up care with which specialist?
    a. Endocrinologist
    b. Gastroenterologist
    c. Gynecologist
    d. Ophthalmologist

14. Which assessment finding, if identified in a patient who is receiving a biologic DMARD, should the nurse report to the prescriber immediately?
    a. Dizziness
    b. Fever
    c. Headache
    d. Injection-site erythema

15. Which symptom suggests that a patient who is prescribed etanercept (Enbrel) may be experiencing the adverse effect of Stevens-Johnson syndrome?
    a. Diminished breath sounds and wheezing
    b. Nausea, vomiting, and diarrhea
    c. Painful, red rash and blisters
    d. Perioral edema and tingling

16. The pediatric office nurse is preparing a referral to a rheumatologist for a child who has juvenile RA that has been unresponsive to methotrexate. It would be most important for the nurse to identify whether the child has received or is scheduled to receive which immunization before the child sees the specialist?
    a. DTaP
    b. IPV
    c. Influenza IM
    d. Varicella

17. It would be of greatest priority to report which test result to the prescriber of infliximab (Remicade)?
    a. ANC 3500/mm³
    b. AST 45 IU/L
    c. BNP 2875 picograms/mL
    d. Troponin T 0.1 ng/mL

18. A patient has returned to the office for reading of the PPD tuberculin test administered 50 hours ago before initiation of treatment for RA with adalimumab (Humira). The nurse would document the test results as positive and consult the prescriber if the skin reaction was greater than
    a. 5 mm of erythema.
    b. 5 mm of induration.
    c. 5 cm of erythema.
    d. 5 cm of induration.

19. A male patient who has been taking a DMARD is planning to try to conceive a child with his wife. The nurse must counsel him about the need for a specific procedure to clear his body of the drug if the patient has been taking which DMARD?
    a. Adalimumab (Humira)
    b. Anakinra (Kineret)
    c. Infliximab (Remicade)
    d. Leflunomide (Arava)

*20. What is the priority nursing concern when administering intravenous rituximab (Rituxan)?
    a. Airway
    b. Hydration
    c. Infection
    d. Infiltration

21. What should be reported STAT to the prescriber when a patient has been receiving tocilizumab (Actemra) once a month for the past 2 years? (Select all that apply.)
    a. ALT 32 IU/L
    b. ANC 1750/mm³
    c. BP 120/72 mm Hg sitting; 110/68 standing
    d. Sudden LLQ pain
    e. Total cholesterol 185 mg/dL

DOSE CALCULATION QUESTIONS

22. Etanercept (Enbrel) 25 mg is prescribed for a 55-lb 10-year-old with JRA. Is the dose safe?

23. Etanercept (Enbrel) 15 mg is prescribed subcutaneous for a child. Available is 25 mg/mL. What amount should the nurse administer?

CASE STUDY

A 34-year-old woman who works as a grocery store clerk has been diagnosed with RA after seeking care for carpal tunnel syndrome.

1. The patient asks how the disease developed from carpal tunnel syndrome. How should the nurse respond?

2. The patient's physician has recommended that the patient see a vocational rehabilitation counselor. The patient asks the nurse, "What type of job should I be thinking about?" What guidance can the nurse provide?

3. When developing a long-range plan of care for this patient, what interventions might the nurse include to address the four goals of RA therapy?

   a. Relieving symptoms

   b. Maintaining joint function

   c. Minimizing systemic joint involvement

   d. Delaying disease progression

4. The rheumatologist has recommended that the patient start a drug regimen that includes NSAIDs and methotrexate (Rheumatrex). Based on the developmental stage of this patient, what teaching would be especially important for the nurse to provide to this patient?

5. What symptoms of methotrexate toxicity to these organs should the nurse teach the patient to report to her prescriber?

   a. Liver

   b. Kidney

   c. Bone marrow

   d. GI

74

Drug Therapy of Gout

STUDY QUESTIONS

True or False

For each of the following statements, enter T *for true or* F *for false.*

1. ___ Colchicine is the most common drug used to prevent gout attacks.
2. ___ Chemotherapy for cancer can cause gout.
3. ___ Gout can be acute or chronic.
4. ___ Gout is usually a systemic disease.
5. ___ In patients with gout, enzymes released when white blood cells break down damage the joints.
6. ___ Urate crystals can damage kidneys.

CRITICAL THINKING, PRIORITIZATION, AND DELEGATION QUESTIONS

7. A patient who experiences an attack of gout once every 1 or 2 years has been self-treating with over-the-counter (OTC) drugs. Which drug would the nurse expect to provide the least relief of gout pain?
   a. Acetaminophen (Tylenol)
   b. Acetylsalicylic acid (Bayer aspirin)
   c. Ibuprofen (Advil, Motrin)
   d. Naproxen (Aleve)

8. A male patient develops an acute gouty attack of the left first toe. He is prescribed colchicine (Colcrys) and is able to return to work in 48 hours. The patient calls the prescriber stating that he is experiencing nausea and abdominal pain. He wants to know what he should do. The telephone triage nurse should advise the patient to
   a. stop taking the medication.
   b. take the medication before going to bed.
   c. take the medication with food.
   d. take the medication with milk.

✳ 9. A patient has been prescribed allopurinol (Zyloprim) for chronic tophaceous gout. Which laboratory test result would be a priority to report to the prescriber?
   a. BUN 22 mg/dL
   b. Creatinine 3.8 mg/dL
   c. ESR 28 mm/hr
   d. Uric acid 9 mg/dL

10. The nurse teaches the patient to stop taking allopurinol (Zyloprim) and contact the prescriber if he experiences which effect?
    a. Diarrhea
    b. Drowsiness
    c. Fever
    d. Headache

11. The nurse is administering allopurinol (Zyloprim) to a patient who also receives warfarin (Coumadin). Which laboratory test result would be a priority to report to the prescriber of the Coumadin?
    a. BUN 15 mg/dL
    b. eGFR 90 mL/min
    c. INR 4.6
    d. WBC 9200/mm^3

12. What is an important nursing action to prevent complications when initiating therapy with probenecid for gouty arthritis?
    a. Avoid taking BP or drawing blood from the affected extremity.
    b. Increase fluid intake to 2500-3000 mL/day.
    c. Elevate the affected extremity.
    d. Measure intake and output.

13. It is of greatest priority to assess for which possible adverse reaction to pegloticase?
    a. Dyspnea
    b. Erythema at injection site
    c. Itching
    d. Flare of pain

DOSE CALCULATION QUESTIONS

14. A patient is prescribed allopurinol 150 mg once a day. Available are 100-mg tablets. How many tablets should be administered per dose?

15. Pegloticase 8 mg is available mixed in a 250-mL bag of normal saline solution. The drug is to be administered over 120 minutes. What is the rate of infusion in mL/hr?

CASE STUDY

A 5-year-old boy who is scheduled to start chemotherapy in 2 weeks for acute leukemia is prescribed allopurinol 150 mg once a day. His father researches the drug on the Internet and asks the nurse why it is being prescribed when his son does not have gout.

1. How should the nurse respond?

2. The patient's father does not like to give drugs to his children. What protective effects of allopurinol would be most important for the nurse to include in an explanation of why this drug is prescribed?

75

Drugs Affecting Calcium Levels and Bone Mineralization

STUDY QUESTIONS

Completion

1. The three factors that regulate serum calcium levels are _____, _____, and _____.

2. Because free calcium is the active form of calcium, a patient with low protein levels can exhibit symptoms of _____.

3. An inadequate level of free, ionized calcium may result in blood taking longer to _____.

4. Central nervous system symptoms of hypercalcemia include _____ and _____.

5. Hypocalcemia increases neuromuscular excitability, which can cause symptoms such as _____, _____, _____, and _____.

6. Parathyroid hormone secretion _____ calcium absorption in the small intestine.

7. Patients should not take calcium supplements with _____ or _____ because they interfere with calcium absorption.

8. Patients should take calcium supplements that also contain _____ because this would increase absorption of the calcium.

9. Calcium supplements decrease the absorption of _____, _____, _____, and _____.

CRITICAL THINKING, PRIORITIZATION, AND DELEGATION QUESTIONS

*10. The priority goal of the body's regulation of calcium levels is maintaining normal calcium levels in which body system?
   a. Cardiovascular
   b. Muscular
   c. Nervous
   d. Skeletal

11. A 55-year-old female consumes 6 oz of plain, low-fat yogurt and 16 oz of skim milk each day. How much daily calcium supplementation (with vitamin D) is recommended for this patient?
   a. 300 mg once a day
   b. 300 mg twice a day
   c. 600 mg once a day
   d. 600 mg twice a day

12. What is a known adverse effect of excessive calcium supplementation?
   a. Bleeding
   b. Diarrhea
   c. Dysrhythmias
   d. Euphoria

*13. The nurse is caring for a patient whose lab results include calcium 12 mg/dL. What is the nursing priority?
   a. Administering medications on time
   b. Ensuring adequate hydration
   c. Preventing falls
   d. Supporting respirations

*14. The nurse is caring for a patient whose lab results include calcium 6.8 mg/dL. What is the nursing priority?
   a. Administering medications on time
   b. Ensuring adequate hydration
   c. Preventing falls
   d. Supporting respirations

15. A 62-year-old woman is receiving chemotherapy for metastatic breast cancer. Which laboratory result suggests the patient is at increased the risk for hypercalcemia?
    a. Creatinine 3.2 mg/dL
    b. H/H 11 g/dL/33%
    c. HDL 35 mg/dL
    d. FBS 145 mg/dL

16. The plan of nursing care for a patient with bone cancer who is at risk for hypercalcemia should include teaching to avoid which food in the diet?
    a. Bran
    b. Canned sardines
    c. Spinach
    d. Whole-grain cereal

17. Which question would provide the most useful information when taking the history of a child diagnosed with rickets?
    a. "Does your child have any difficulties in school?"
    b. "Has your child ever had a kidney infection?"
    c. "Have you noticed a change in your child's energy level?"
    d. "How many hours a day does your child watch television?"

18. The nurse is assessing a postoperative thyroidectomy patient. Which assessments suggest that the parathyroid glands may have been damaged or removed during the surgery? (Select all that apply.)
    a. Dorsiflexion of the first toe and fanning of the other toes when the sole of the foot is stroked with a blunt object from lateral heel to medial toes
    b. Inflation of a BP cuff for 3 minutes producing involuntary spasms of the wrist
    c. Loss of balance when standing with the eyes closed, arms at sides, and legs together
    d. Sharp calf pain with dorsiflexion of the foot
    e. Twitching of facial muscles when the facial nerve is tapped

19. A 58-year-old woman is at risk for osteoporosis caused by a history of hypothyroidism treated with levothyroxine (Synthroid) 0.15 mg every morning. She has been instructed to take supplemental calcium. She is considering taking calcium carbonate (TUMS) with 400 mg of elemental calcium. Which statement, if made by the patient, would indicate a need for further teaching?
    a. "I can take TUMS with food, but it will not be as well absorbed if I take it when eating bran cereal."
    b. "I should take the TUMS with a large glass of water."
    c. "The calcium will be better absorbed if I take each tablet at separate times throughout the day."
    d. "TUMS are not as good a source of calcium as oyster-shell calcium, but they are less expensive."

20. It is of greatest priority for the nurse to monitor for which symptom when administering parental calcium to a patient who is prescribed digoxin (Lanoxin)?
    a. Hypertension
    b. Decreased urine output
    c. Dehydration
    d. Bradycardia

21. The pediatric nurse is explaining why vitamins should be kept out of the reach of children. Which are possible effects of vitamin D toxicity? (Select all that apply.)
    a. Diarrhea
    b. Constipation
    c. Bone pain
    d. Tetany
    e. Vomiting

22. Patients with which chronic disorders are less able to activate vitamin D from sunlight? (Select all that apply.)
    a. Chronic renal failure
    b. Chronic obstructive pulmonary disease (COPD)
    c. Cirrhosis
    d. Osteoarthritis
    e. Type 2 DM

23. A 3-year-old child is admitted after ingesting an unknown number of chewable multiple vitamins including vitamin D. Which assessment finding, if present, would be of most concern to the nurse?
    a. BP 80/50 mm Hg
    b. One watery stool in past 4 hours
    c. Pulse 102 beats/min
    d. Confusion and ataxia

24. Which statements are true regarding calcitonin (Miacalcin)? (Select all that apply.)
    a. It is usually administered once a week.
    b. It is the safest effective drug for osteoporosis in men.
    c. Nasal pumps must be primed before each use.
    d. The drug promotes bone formation.
    e. The drug should be administered using hand opposite of nostril.

✱25. Which assessment finding, if identified in a patient who is receiving a biphosphonate such as alendronate (Fosamax), would be of greatest priority for the nurse to report to the prescriber?
    a. Dysphagia
    b. Dysphasia
    c. Headache
    d. Muscular pain

26. Monitoring of estimated glomerular filtration, serum creatinine, urine output, weight, and intake and output is especially important for the nurse to monitor when a patient is receiving which biphosphonate?
    a. Alendronate (Fosamax)
    b. Etidronate (Didronel)
    c. Tiludronate (Skelid)
    d. Zoledronic acid (Zometa)

27. Taking calcium supplements at the same time as a dose of a biphosphonate for osteoporosis does what?
    a. Increases bone-building
    b. Interferes with absorption of the biphosphonate
    c. Potentiates the action of the biphosphonate
    d. Prevents adverse effects

28. A patient who has just started taking tiludronate (Skelid) for Paget's disease calls the prescriber's office and reports that she is experiencing nausea since starting the drug. What is the first thing the nurse should do?
    a. Advise the patient to stop taking the drug.
    b. Determine if the patient is taking the drug with a full glass of water.
    c. Instruct the patient to take the drug with an antacid.
    d. Instruct the patient to take the drug with food.

29. A patient with hypercalcemia of malignancy (HCM) receives zoledronate (Zometa). Which symptom, if present, suggests that the patient may be experiencing drug-induced hypomagnesemia? (Select all that apply.)
    a. Anorexia
    b. Dry, sticky mucous membranes
    c. Muscle weakness
    d. Muscle spasms

30. When a patient is prescribed a biphosphonate, which nursing measure would be most effective to prevent the possible adverse effect of osteonecrosis?
    a. Emphasizing the importance of excellent oral hygiene
    b. Taking calcium supplementation with the drug
    c. Teaching the importance of weight-bearing exercise
    d. Teaching the importance of avoiding alcohol and tobacco

31. What causes osteonecrosis when a patient is prescribed biphosphonates?
    a. Decreased bone breakdown
    b. Increased bone deposition
    c. Impaired perfusion to bone
    d. Reduction in blood calcium

32. Which is true of raloxifene (Evista), a selective estrogen receptor modulator?
    a. It may damage the eyes so the nurse should teach to report blurring of vision.
    b. It may stimulate the occurrence of hot flushes (hot flashes).
    c. It reduces the risk of hip, forearm, and vertebral fractures.
    d. It should be avoided in women with a history of breast cancer.

✱33. Which information, if elicited from a patient who is receiving raloxifene (Evista), would be of greatest priority for the nurse to communicate to the prescriber?
    a. Has an aunt who has been diagnosed with estrogen receptor–positive breast cancer
    b. Has had a hysterectomy
    c. Is experiencing hot flashes
    d. Does work that requires frequent, long airplane trips

∗34. Which laboratory test result, if found in a woman who has just been prescribed raloxifene, would be the priority concern to the nurse?
  a. Calcium 11.1 mg/dL
  b. Hemoglobin (Hb) 11.6 g/dL
  c. Hemoglobin A1c 6.8%
  d. Human chorionic gonadotropin (hCG) 330 mIU/mL

35. To increase bone mineral density, teriparatide (Forteo) should be administered how?
  a. Continually
  b. Injection
  c. Intravenously
  d. Orally

36. Which action should the nurse perform when scheduled to administer teriparatide (Forteo) to a patient with osteoporosis?
  a. Administer in the deltoid or vastus lateralis muscle with a 1-inch needle.
  b. Administer subcutaneously in the upper arm, alternating arms daily.
  c. Date the injection pen for disposal 28 days after first use.
  d. Remove the pen from refrigeration 20 minutes before administration to allow the solution to warm.

37. Which symptoms would be a priority to report to the prescriber if a patient who is receiving chemotherapy is scheduled to receive denosumab (Xgeva)?
  a. Fatigue and anorexia
  b. Flank pain and fever
  c. Nausea and vomiting
  d. Redness at injection site after previous injection

38. Which action should the nurse perform when scheduled to administer denosumab (Prolia) to a patient with osteoporosis? (Select all that apply.)
  a. Administer into the posterior gluteal muscle.
  b. Assess current dental needs.
  c. Inspect solution for clarity and color.
  d. Discard if particles present in solution.
  e. Warm to room temperature for 15-30 minutes.

39. The nurse would withhold cinacalcet (Sensipar) and consult with the prescriber if which new finding was discovered during patient assessment?
  a. Anorexia
  b. Diarrhea
  c. Headache
  d. Numbness

40. Intravenous furosemide has been prescribed for a patient in a hypercalcemic emergency. The nurse knows that which imbalance would be least likely to occur as a result of this therapy?
  a. Hypocalcemia
  b. Hypoglycemia
  c. Hypokalemia
  d. Hyponatremia

DOSE CALCULATION QUESTIONS

41. The nurse's drug book recommends that calcium gluconate be infused at a rate of 0.5 to 2 mL/min. If the nurse infuses 5 mL of 10% calcium gluconate, how long will it take to infuse the entire amount?

42. Denosumab (Xgeva) 120 mg subcutaneous injection is prescribed every 4 weeks. Available is 120 mg/1.7 mL. What amount should be administered?

CASE STUDY

A 50-year-old patient who states that she is going through menopause is undergoing a thyroidectomy today. The literature states that the nurse should be sure IV calcium is available postoperatively. The patient has just been admitted to the nursing unit from the postanesthesia care unit (PACU).

1. Knowing the anatomy of the thyroid gland, why would the nurse anticipate a potential need for IV calcium?

2. What is the average normal value for total serum calcium?

3. The patient's calcium level drops to 6.8 mg/dL. Intravenous 10% calcium gluconate 5 mL via IV (push) infusion is prescribed. The patient is sitting in a chair when the nurse prepares to administer the calcium gluconate. Why is it important for the nurse to assist the patient back to bed before the drug is administered?

4. What should be monitored while the nurse is administering the calcium gluconate?

5. The patient's spouse has assumed that calcium is in the bone. The spouse asks how surgery on the neck can cause an imbalance in the calcium in the body. What could the nurse include in the discussion of the functions of calcium and the mechanism for calcium regulation?

76

Drugs for Asthma and Chronic Obstructive Pulmonary Disease

STUDY QUESTIONS

Matching

Match the term with its definition.

1. ____ Adventitious breath sound that occurs with bronchoconstriction of asthma
2. ____ Drug that may increase the number of bronchial beta$_2$ receptors as well as their responsiveness to beta$_2$ agonists
3. ____ Devices which attach directly to the MDI to increase delivery of drug to the lungs and decrease deposition of drug on the oropharyngeal mucosa
4. ____ Hoarseness, speaking difficulty
5. ____ Measures taken to maintain health and prevent illness
6. ____ Most effective drugs available for relieving acute bronchospasm and preventing exercise-induced bronchospasm
7. ____ Persisting for a long period of time
8. ____ A small machine used to convert a drug solution into a mist
9. ____ Used to deliver drugs in the form of a dry, micronized powder directly to the lungs
10. ____ Handheld, pressurized devices that deliver a measured dose of drug with each actuation
11. ____ Spasm of bronchial smooth muscle that narrows airways
12. ____ Underlying cause of asthma

   a. Beta$_2$ agonist
   b. Bronchoconstriction
   c. Chronic

   d. Dry-powder inhaler (DPI)
   e. Dysphonia
   f. Glucocorticoid
   g. Inflammation
   h. Metered-dose inhaler (MDI)
   i. Nebulizer
   j. Prophylaxis
   k. Spacer
   l. Wheezing

CRITICAL THINKING, PRIORITIZATION, AND DELEGATION QUESTIONS

*13. Which outcome would be of greatest priority for most asthma patients?
   a. Avoiding pollution
   b. Increasing exercise tolerance
   c. Preventing airway inflammation
   d. Stimulating release of eosinophils

14. A patient has received instructions from the nurse to administer two puffs of a beta$_2$-agonist drug via a metered-dose inhaler (MDI). Which statement by the patient would indicate a need for further teaching?
   a. "I need to inhale slowly and deeply so the drug goes deep into my lungs."
   b. "I need to count the MDI doses that I use so that I know when it is empty."
   c. "I should start to inhale after activating the inhaler."
   d. "It is best to wait 1 full minute before I take the second puff."

15. What are current recommendations for use of inhaled glucocorticoids for persistent asthma?
    a. Administer daily even on days where there are no symptoms.
    b. Administer first when giving with a bronchodilator.
    c. Only use as a rescue drug for acute flares of wheezing.
    d. Only use on a regular basis if acute attacks occur every day because of adverse effects.

16. Which symptom suggests that a child with asthma is not rinsing his or her mouth after using a glucocorticoid inhaler?
    a. Enlarged tonsils
    b. Gray membrane in the throat
    c. Persistent cough
    d. White patches in mouth

17. The nurse would question the prescriber if which drug regimen is ordered for an asthmatic patient? (Select all that apply.)
    a. Albuterol inhaler, two puffs before exercise, not exceeding eight puffs in 24 hours for a 14-year-old patient
    b. Albuterol (AccuNeb) followed by budesonide suspension (Pulmicort Respules) via ultrasonic nebulizer for a 6-year-old patient
    c. Budesonide suspension (Pulmicort Respules) followed by albuterol (AccuNeb) via jet nebulizer with a mask for a 4-year-old patient
    d. Salmeterol (Serevent Diskus), two inhalations every 12 hours for a 20-year-old patient
    e. Salmeterol (Serevent Diskus), one inhalation and budesonide (Pulmicort Flexhaler) every 12 hours for a 40-year-old patient

18. It is of greatest priority to teach strategies to maintain adequate bone mass if an asthmatic patient is prescribed which drug?
    a. Flunisolide (AeroBid) MDI
    b. Fluticasone-salmeterol (Advair) DPI
    c. Nebulized levalbuterol (Xopenex)
    d. Prednisolone oral tablets

▶19. A hospitalized patient has orders for budesonide (Pulmicort Flexhaler) and salmeterol (Serevent Diskus), one inhalation every 12 hours and albuterol (Proventil) MDI, two puffs every 4 hours as needed. The patient has not required albuterol for the last 24 hours. When preparing to administer the budesonide and salmeterol, the nurse notes audible wheezing and dyspnea. Which action by the nurse is correct?
    a. Administer albuterol only.
    b. Administer albuterol, wait 5 minutes, and then administer the salmeterol and then budesonide.
    c. Administer salmeterol and then budesonide, and reassess in 15 minutes for the need for albuterol.
    d. Administer budesonide, wait 5 minutes, administer the salmeterol, and reassess in 15 minutes for the need for albuterol.

✳20. The nurse is caring for several patients who receive beta-agonist inhalation treatments for asthma. After treatments are administered, it is of greatest priority to reassess the patient who also has a history of which condition?
    a. Heart failure (HF)
    b. Deep vein thrombosis (DVT)
    c. Gastroesophageal reflux (GERD)
    d. Rheumatoid arthritis (RA)

21. A 42-year-old patient with asthma is admitted for a surgery. Which information would be of greatest priority for the nurse to share with the anesthesiologist?
    a. This patient experiences an asthma attack whenever exposed to tobacco smoke.
    b. The patient has degenerative joint disease (osteoarthritis) of the knees.
    c. The patient uses albuterol (Proventil) MDI, two puffs every 4 hours as needed.
    d. The patient was recently changed from long-term oral methylprednisolone to inhaled beclomethasone.

22. The nurse administers albuterol via nebulizer when a patient with asthma experiences severe wheezing while trying to eat lunch. Several minutes after the treatment, the patient is resting quietly with his eyes closed. What should the nurse do?
    a. Allow the patient to rest.
    b. Assess the patient's breathing and lung sounds.
    c. Inform the dietary department that another lunch will be needed later.
    d. Wake the patient and encourage him to try to finish his lunch.

23. Which assessment finding in a patient who is prescribed a beta$_2$-adrenergic agonist would be a reason for the nurse to consult the prescriber?
    a. BP 140/90 mm Hg
    b. SMBG 165 mg/dL
    c. Unexplained fainting
    d. Unexplained tremor

24. If flunisolide (AeroBid) and pirbuterol (Maxair) are both ordered to be administered at 0900, how should they be administered?
    a. Flunisolide first, then pirbuterol 1 minute later, using a spacer for both drugs
    b. Flunisolide first, using a spacer, then pirbuterol 3 minutes later
    c. Pirbuterol first, using a spacer, then flunisolide 5 minutes later
    d. Pirbuterol first, then flunisolide 10 minutes later, using a spacer for both drugs

25. Why does the FDA recommend that patients with asthma who use an inhaled long-acting beta-adrenergic agonist (LABA) bronchodilator only be prescribed a combination product with a glucocorticoid rather than the two drugs as separate inhalers?
    a. It decreases the risk that the patient will take the LABA and not the glucocorticoid.
    b. The two drugs given together as one inhalation produces faster bronchodilation.
    c. The combination drug is a DPI and therefore is less harmful to the environment.
    d. The combination drug is less expensive than the two drugs given separately.

26. The nurse is caring for a patient who is prescribed zafirlukast (Accolate) for asthma and warfarin for atrial fibrillation. Which is a possible result of the interaction of these two drugs?
    a. Bradycardia
    b. Hemorrhage
    c. Pulmonary emboli
    d. Myocardial infarction

27. The nurse would be most concerned about drug interactions if a patient who has asthma is prescribed both zileuton and
    a. albuterol.
    b. prednisolone.
    c. terbutaline.
    d. theophylline.

28. Zafirlukast (Accolate) is listed on the MAR to be administered at 7:00 AM (0700). Breakfast is served at 8:30 AM (0830). What should the nurse do?
    a. Administer the drug as ordered.
    b. Change the timing of the drug to 8:30 AM (0830).
    c. Change the timing of the drug to 10:00 AM (1000).
    d. Consult the prescriber.

29. The nurse is explaining therapy with cromolyn to a patient who has asthma. Which statement should not be included in the teaching?
    a. Cromolyn must be taken on a regular basis to control inflammation.
    b. Rinse the mouth immediately after administration to remove the unpleasant taste.
    c. Timing doses 15 minutes before activities involving exertion or exposure to known allergens may prevent bronchospasm.
    d. The drug is not effective in stopping an episode once it has begun.

*30. The nurse is caring for a patient who has asthma who takes omalizumab (Xolair) in an emergency department. Which symptom would warrant immediate, priority care?
    a. Fever
    b. Headache
    c. Perioral edema
    d. Severe pharyngitis

*31. An adolescent patient with asthma has controlled her asthma using a drug regimen that includes theophylline. Which new behavior would be of greatest priority to report to the prescriber?
    a. Joining the soccer team
    b. Occasionally skipping school when not ill
    c. Becoming sexually active
    d. Smoking a pack of cigarettes per day

32. Which finding, if identified in a patient who has been prescribed ipratropium-albuterol (Combivent), would be of greatest priority to report to the prescriber?
    a. Allergy to peanuts
    b. Complaint of sore throat
    c. Drinking 4-6 cups of coffee per day
    d. Smoking two packs of cigarettes per day

33. Which adverse effect would the patient be most likely to experience when prescribed the anticholinergic bronchodilator drug tiotropium (Spiriva)?
    a. Blurred vision
    b. Constipation
    c. Dry mouth
    d. Urinary retention

34. A patient who has asthma has had peak expiratory flow rates at approximately 70% of his personal best despite regular and as-needed use of drugs. What are current treatment recommendations for this patient?
    a. Continue the regularly prescribed treatment.
    b. Use a rescue inhaler and continue regularly prescribed treatment.
    c. Use a rescue inhaler and consult the prescriber for possible treatment changes.
    d. Seek immediate emergency medical attention.

▶35. A child with moderate asthma is distressed because she has just learned that she is allergic to the family dog. Which intervention would most effectively address the physical and psychosocial needs of the child?
    a. Advise the family that there are no interventions that will help.
    b. Advise the family to increase the dose of the child's asthma drugs when the dog is around.
    c. Advise the family to take the dog to the local shelter.
    d. Advise the family to train the dog to stay out of bedrooms and off of furniture.

DOSE CALCULATION QUESTIONS

36. Budesonide (Pulmicort Respules) 0.2 mg is prescribed via nebulizer. Budesonide is available as 250 mcg/2 mL. How much budesonide should be administered via nebulizer at each dose?

37. Omalizumab (Xolair), once reconstituted, is available as a solution of 150 mg/1.2 mL. 300 mg subcutaneous is prescribed once every 4 weeks. How much drug should be administered?

CASE STUDY

A 7-year-old boy, who was first diagnosed with asthma at age 4 years, has been admitted to a medical unit from intensive care after experiencing a severe acute exacerbation. Based on the frequency, characteristics, and severity of his symptoms, he is currently classified as having severe persistent asthma. The pediatrician has ordered oral prednisolone 10 mg every 8 hours, budesonide (Pulmicort Respules) 0.2 mg, and albuterol 1.25 mg via nebulizer every 6 hours as needed.

1. What is the difference between administering budesonide and albuterol via nebulizer?

2. The boy's parents tells the nurse that they have heard negative things about steroids and are concerned about their son receiving them. What does the nurse need to teach regarding the importance of steroid therapy for this child?

3. The parents have heard that steroids prevent growth. What information can the nurse provide about the effects of steroids on growth?

4. What teaching does the nurse need to provide about the inhaled steroid therapy to prevent adverse effects?

5. The nebulizer is more time-consuming to use than dry-powder inhalers (DPI) and metered-dose inhalers (MDI). What are possible reasons why this route was prescribed for this child?

6. Allergy workup identified that the child is allergic to house dust mites. What teaching should be provided regarding exposure to allergens?

7. In addition to allergens, what other things should be avoided because they are common triggers of acute asthma episodes?

8. After 2 years of standard allergy treatment, the child is still experiencing asthma attacks two to three times a week, and he is missing many days of school. The allergist has prescribed omalizumab (Xolair) 200 mg to be administered subcutaneously every 4 weeks. What is the procedure for administering this drug?

77
Drugs for Allergic Rhinitis, Cough, and Colds

STUDY QUESTIONS

Matching

Match the term with its description.

1. ____ Conjunctivitis
2. ____ Erythema
3. ____ Immunoglobulins
4. ____ Perennial
5. ____ Pruritus
6. ____ Rhinitis
7. ____ Rhinorrhea
8. ____ Seasonal

   a. Antibodies
   b. Inflammation of the upper airway
   c. Inflammation of mucous membrane lining the eyelids and eye surface
   d. Itching
   e. Occurs during spring and fall in reaction to outdoor allergens
   f. Nonseasonal, triggered by indoor allergens
   g. Redness as a result of injury or irritation
   h. Runny nose

Match the drug with its descriptor.

9. ____ Renders cough more productive by stimulating the flow of respiratory tract secretions
10. ____ Decreases sensitivity of respiratory tract stretch receptors
11. ____ Antibody directed against IgE
12. ____ Blocks cholinergic receptors, thereby decreasing rhinorrhea

13. ____ The most effective OTC nonopioid cough medicine, and the most widely used of all cough medicines
14. ____ Smells like rotten eggs
15. ____ Cough suppression is achieved only at doses that produce prominent sedation
16. ____ Somewhat more potent than codeine and carries a greater liability for abuse

   a. Acetylcysteine
   b. Benzonatate
   c. Dextromethorphan
   d. Diphenhydramine
   e. Guaifenesin
   f. Hydrocodone
   g. Ipratropium
   h. Omalizumab

CRITICAL THINKING, PRIORITIZATION, AND DELEGATION QUESTIONS

17. A patient exhibits watery nasal discharge and sneezing every winter when the house is closed and the forced-air furnace is running. How is this classified?
   a. Perennial rhinitis
   b. Seasonal rhinitis

18. Allergic rhinitis involves the release of (Select all that apply.)
   a. glucocorticoids.
   b. histamine.
   c. leukocytes.
   d. leukotrienes.
   e. prostaglandins.

19. What are the most effective drugs for prevention and treatment of symptoms of seasonal and perennial rhinitis?
    a. First-generation oral antihistamines
    b. Intranasal glucocorticoids
    c. Oral glucocorticoids
    d. Second-generation oral antihistamines

▶20. The school nurse notes that a child is receiving long-term therapy with intranasal glucocorticoids for seasonal rhinitis. The nurse must monitor the child's
    a. blood sugar.
    b. hearing.
    c. height.
    d. weight.

21. A patient was prescribed fluticasone (Flonase) 2 sprays in each nostril 2 weeks ago. She calls the nurse to report that the drug has not helped. Which question should the nurse ask to identify a common cause of early treatment failures?
    a. "Do you have nasal burning after administration?"
    b. "Do you have nasal congestion?"
    c. "How often are you administering the sprays?"
    d. "What is the expiration date on the bottle?"

22. The nurse teaches a patient with allergic rhinitis that antihistamines are not effective in reducing which symptom?
    a. Nasal itching
    b. "Runny nose"
    c. "Stuffy nose"
    d. Sneezing

23. A patient has received instructions regarding administration of a second-generation oral antihistamine for seasonal allergic rhinitis. Which of these statements made by the patient would indicate that the patient needs further teaching?
    a. "I should only use the medication when I am experiencing symptoms."
    b. "I should take the medication as prescribed throughout the season when I have allergy symptoms."
    c. "This drug can still cause sedation, so I need to be careful when driving."
    d. "This drug is not any more effective than over-the-counter antihistamines."

24. What is an advantage of intranasal cromolyn (Nasalcrom) in allergic rhinitis?
    a. It can be used prophylactically.
    b. It has once-a-day dosing.
    c. It is more effective than other drugs.
    d. It is safe.

▶25. Which of these assessment findings, if identified in a patient who is taking an oral decongestant, would be a priority to report to the prescriber?
    a. Agitation
    b. Chest pain
    c. Epistaxis
    d. Sore throat

▶26. In which situation would it be most beneficial for the nurse to administer a prescribed as-needed dose of an antitussive medication?
    a. Barking cough of croup
    b. Cough that interferes with work because the patient cannot carry tissues at work in which to expectorate the mucus
    c. Cough associated with upper respiratory infection that keeps the patient awake at night
    d. Severe episodes of coughing with sputum production that only occur on arising

27. A patient who recently saw a commercial for montelukast (Singulair) asks the office nurse why the prescriber will not order this for her allergic symptoms. The nurse knows that prescribers may not readily prescribe this drug for allergic rhinitis for what reason?
    a. It frequently causes irritation inside the nose.
    b. It has many adverse effects.
    c. It is limited in effectiveness as a decongestant.
    d. It treats only sneezing and itching.

28. A patient is prescribed omalizumab (Xolair) for allergic rhinitis. Which statement, if made by the patient, suggests a need for further teaching about this drug therapy?
    a. "I can finally go to a Labor Day picnic and not sneeze all day."
    b. "I need to continue taking this drug during the winter to control my allergy to house dust."
    c. "The doctor has prescribed this drug to control my allergy symptoms because allergies trigger my asthma."
    d. "This drug will be injected into the fat under my skin."

29. Research suggests that codeine, dextromethorphan, and diphenhydramine are not effective in suppressing coughs induced by
    a. chemical irritation.
    b. common cold.
    c. mechanical irritation.
    d. smoking.

30. A patient has received instructions regarding administration of benzonatate (Tessalon Perles). Which statement made by the patient would indicate that the patient needs further teaching?
    a. "The drug should not be given to infants."
    b. "I can take the drug three times a day."
    c. "I need to be careful because the drug may make me drowsy."
    d. "I should crush the beads and mix them in a soft food such as applesauce."

*31. Despite instruction by the nurse to swallow the benzonatate (Tessalon Perles) whole, the patient proceeds to chew the capsule. What is a priority nursing concern until the effect of this drug has diminished?
    a. Aspiration
    b. Bronchospasms
    c. Respiratory depression
    d. Severe constipation

32. Which statements are true about the common cold? (Select all that apply.)
    a. Antibiotics are not effective.
    b. Antihistamines do not help.
    c. It is best treated with multiple symptom medications.
    d. Fever usually means there is a bacterial infection.
    e. Vitamin C prevents colds.

DOSE CALCULATION QUESTIONS

Diphenhydramine 50 mg orally every 6 hours is prescribed. The patient has purchased 25-mg capsules.

33. How many capsules should the patient take for each dose?

34. The nurse would teach the patient not to take more than how many capsules in 24 hours?

CASE STUDIES

Case Study 1

A 19-year-old college student presents to the student health clinic during spring semester with complaints of runny and itchy nose, sneezing, and nasal congestion. He is diagnosed with allergic rhinitis. The student states that he has been using an over-the-counter nasal spray for 2 weeks. It really helps but the congestion comes back and seems to be getting worse.

1. Explain what is happening and how he can discontinue use of this drug.

2. The nurse practitioner prescribes loratadine (Claritin) 10 mg daily and triamcinolone (Nasacort) 2 sprays twice a day. What teaching can the nurse provide?

3. If he develops a common cold, how should he change his medications?

Case Study 2

A patient asks the nurse why she doesn't need a prescription but can't buy Sudafed off the shelf. She says that she had to go to the pharmacy counter and sign a paper to get her Sudafed, but they wouldn't let her buy enough to take on her Peace Corps assignment.

4. What should the nurse include in the response?

5. The patient asks why she can buy Sudafed PE off the shelf if Sudafed can be made into an abused substance. What should the nurse include in the explanation?

Case Study 3

Parents of a 17-month-old girl ask the pediatric on-call nurse why their doctor did not give them samples of PediaCare cold medication like she did with their older children. The parents came to the office 2 days ago and their daughter is still coughing.

6.   How should the nurse respond?

7.   The parents ask what they can do to help their child feel better. What current nonpharmacologic recommendations can the nurse provide?

8.   The parents ask the nurse what they should do if their 4-year-old catches the cold from his younger sister. What instructions should the nurse provide if the parents choose to use cold remedies for this child?

78

Drugs for Peptic Ulcer Disease

STUDY QUESTIONS

Matching

Match the drug with its mechanism of action.

1.   ___   Can cause a disulfiram-like reaction, and hence must not be combined with alcohol
2.   ___   Works quickly to neutralize acid in the stomach
3.   ___   Serves as a replacement for endogenous prostaglandins
4.   ___   Creates protective barrier in stomach against acid and pepsin
5.   ___   Disrupts the cell wall of *H. pylori*, thereby causing lysis and death
6.   ___   Causes irreversible inhibition of H^+, K^+-ATPase, the enzyme that generates gastric acid
7.   ___   Suppresses growth of *H. pylori* by inhibiting protein synthesis
8.   ___   Blocks H_2 receptors thereby reducing both the volume of gastric juice and its hydrogen ion concentration

   a.   Aluminum hydroxide
   b.   Bismuth
   c.   Clarithromycin (Biaxin)
   d.   Cimetidine (Tagamet)
   e.   Misoprostol (Cytotec)
   f.   Omeprazole (Prilosec)
   g.   Sucralfate (Carafate)
   h.   Tinidazole (Tindamax)

True or False

For each of the following statements, enter T for true or F for false.

9.   ___   Aluminum hydroxide antacids bind phosphate, warfarin, and digoxin, decreasing absorption.
10.   ___   Aluminum hydroxide antacids frequently cause diarrhea.
11.   ___   Calcium carbonate antacids can constipate.
12.   ___   Calcium carbonate antacids do not cause belching and flatus.
13.   ___   Use of calcium carbonate has declined because of acid rebound.
14.   ___   Magnesium hydroxide antacids are used to help diagnose abdominal pain.
15.   ___   Magnesium hydroxide antacids should not be used in severe renal impairment.
16.   ___   Sodium bicarbonate antacids can be absorbed into systemic circulation.
17.   ___   Sodium bicarbonate decreases blood pH.

CRITICAL THINKING, PRIORITIZATION, AND DELEGATION QUESTIONS

18. It is a priority to teach patients who have PUD the importance of
    a. avoiding use of alcohol.
    b. consuming more dairy products.
    c. not using tobacco products.
    d. using ibuprofen, not acetaminophen, for headaches.

19. Hypersecretion of gastric acid is the etiology of what?
    a. Duodenal ulcers
    b. Gastric ulcers
    c. Peptic ulcers
    d. Zollinger-Ellison syndrome ulcers

20. Drug therapy that prevents recurrence of peptic ulcers associated with *H. pylori* must include
    a. antacids.
    b. antibiotics.
    c. antisecretory agents.
    d. mucosal protectants.

21. Which dietary alteration may facilitate recovery from ulcers?
    a. Avoiding caffeine intake
    b. Eating only bland foods
    c. Six small meals a day
    d. Frequent intake of milk

22. A 36-year-old woman who is taking bismuth subsalicylate, tetracycline, and metronidazole experiences black-colored stool. What is the priority nursing action at this time?
    a. Completing an abdominal assessment
    b. Consulting the prescriber
    c. Continuing nursing care; this is a harmless effect of bismuth
    d. Teaching that tetracycline can discolor fetal teeth if the patient gets pregnant

∗23. A patient is prescribed drug therapy including bismuth subsalicylate, metronidazole, and tetracycline. The patient reveals to the nurse that she does not like taking medications all at once. The nurse should explain that it is important for the patient to take the therapy as prescribed, because taking the drugs alone may cause what to occur?
    a. Increasing the risk of developing resistance.
    b. Increasing the incidence of adverse effects.
    c. Need for increased dose of the individual drugs.
    d. Experience of nausea and diarrhea.

24. A patient with gastroesophageal reflux disease (GERD) who has difficulty following drug regimens with multiple doses has been prescribed cimetidine (Tagamet) 800 mg once a day at bedtime. The patient complains that the medication effects wear off before taking the next dose. To prolong the beneficial effects of the drug, the nurse instructs the patient to take the medication
    a. twice a day.
    b. with food.
    c. on an empty stomach.
    d. with an antacid.

▶25. Cimetidine (Tagamet) inhibits the CYP2D6 and CYP3A4 hepatic enzymes. The nurse must be particularly cautious for toxic effects of which drugs that are metabolized by these enzymes when they are administered with cimetidine, because of their narrow margin of safety? (Select all that apply.)
    a. Nateglinide (Starlix)—diabetes
    b. Phenytoin (Dilantin)—seizures
    c. Prednisone (Deltasone)—anti-inflammatory
    d. Theophylline—asthma
    e. Warfarin (Coumadin)—anticoagulant

26. The generic names of histamine$_2$ receptor antagonists (H$_2$RAs) share which common suffix?
    a. -azole
    b. -lol
    c. -dine
    d. -sartan

27. A patient with Zollinger-Ellison syndrome asks why he was prescribed ranitidine (Zantac) since his spouse takes cimetidine (Tagamet) for GERD. The nurse will base the response which fact?
    a. Ranitidine only needs to be taken once a day.
    b. Ranitidine has fewer adverse effects than cimetidine.
    c. Ranitidine is less expensive than cimetidine.
    d. Ranitidine is less potent than cimetidine.

28. The generic names of proton pump inhibitors (PPIs) share which common suffix?
    a. -azole
    b. -lol
    c. -dine
    d. -sartan

29. Which action by the nurse would be of greatest priority when a patient experiences five watery stools in 24 hours when prescribed a PPI?
    a. Consult the prescriber for an order for stool for ova and parasite.
    b. Encourage oral intake of 2000 mL of fluids in 24 hours.
    c. Place the patient in isolation.
    d. Wash hands with soap and water after caring for the patient.

▶ 30. A patient had been prescribed omeprazole (Prilosec) for GERD. The patient recently had a percutaneous endoscopic gastrostomy (PEG) tube inserted, and the pharmacy substituted omeprazole (Zegerid) immediate-release oral suspension because Prilosec capsules cannot be crushed. Because of differences between Prilosec and Zegerid, which concurrent diagnoses would be a reason for the nurse to consult the prescriber? (Select all that apply.)
    a. Chronic obstructive pulmonary disease (COPD)
    b. Heart failure (HF)
    c. Diabetes mellitus (DM)
    d. Hyperthyroidism
    e. Uncontrolled hypertension

31. The nurse is preparing to administer lansoprazole (Prevacid) IV. Administration directives include which of the following? (Select all that apply.)
    a. It may be diluted in normal saline.
    b. It may be diluted in lactated Ringer's solution.
    c. It may be diluted in 5% dextrose in water.
    d. It may be infused over 15 minutes.
    e. It must be used with an inline filter.

▶ 32. Which laboratory result would be a reason for the nurse to consult the prescriber regarding administration of rabeprazole (AcipHex)?
    a. Digoxin 2.5 ng/mL
    d. INR 1
    c. LDL 138 mg/dL
    d. WBC 10,000/mm³

33. A patient who has recently been prescribed omeprazole (Prilosec) asks why he has been told to stop taking sucralfate (Carafate). The nurse's response is based on what knowledge?
    a. The two drugs are not necessary.
    b. The sucralfate prevents the absorption of the omeprazole.
    c. The adherent coating of sucralfate requires a gastric pH of less than 4.
    d. Both drugs are metabolized by the CYP450 cytochrome system.

▶ 34. A 47-year-old woman who has been taking an NSAID for rheumatoid arthritis and an oral contraceptive is prescribed misoprostol (Cytotec) to treat GI distress relating to NSAID use. She informs the nurse that she has stopped taking her oral contraceptives because she has not had a period for 2 months and thinks she could be in menopause. What should the nurse do?
    a. Administer all the medications as ordered and consult the prescriber regarding tests for menopause.
    b. Administer the NSAID and misoprostol (Cytotec), hold the oral contraceptive, and inform the prescriber.
    c. Administer all the medications as ordered and inform the prescriber that the patient has not been taking the oral contraceptives.
    d. Hold the medications and consult the prescriber regarding a pregnancy test.

35. Antacids for PUD should be administered
    a. half an hour before meals and bedtime.
    b. 1 and 3 hours after meals and at bedtime.
    c. as soon as symptoms occur.
    d. as infrequently as possible.

DOSE CALCULATION QUESTIONS

36. Sucralfate is available in a suspension (1 g/10 mL) for oral dosing. The patient is prescribed 2 g a day in two divided doses. How many mL should be administered at each dose?

37. Cimetidine IV infusion is diluted in 100 mL of normal saline solution and is to be administered over 15 minutes. The IV tubing has a drip factor of 10 drops/mL. What is the drip rate per 15 seconds?

CASE STUDIES

Case Study 1

A 47-year-old woman with a history of type 2 diabetes mellitus (T2DM) and hypertension is seen by her primary care practitioner (PCP) with the complaint of midepigastric pain, especially at night. The pain radiates to the back and is relieved by antacids, but returns within an hour. The pain is worse when bending forward and better after eating. The PCP wants to rule out PUD. A urea breath test and gastroesophageal-duodenoscopy are ordered. The patient asks the nurse how breathing into a bag can test for the presence of bacteria in the stomach.

1. Describe how the nurse explains this test.

2. The urea breath test results indicate the presence of *H. pylori*; the and gastroesophageal-duodenoscopy results reveal a duodenal ulcer. What are the goals of drug therapy for PUD?

3. Initial therapy includes cimetidine intravenous (IV) infusion. The nurse is preparing to administer an IV bolus of 300 mg of cimetidine. What assessments, actions, and teaching should the nurse perform when administering this medication?

4. The drug handbook states that cimetidine is the drug of choice to prevent aspiration pneumonia. Why is it important to do a careful respiratory assessment of this patient?

5. Assessment findings of the patient on the second day include severe pain and a rigid abdomen. What should the nurse do and why?

6. At discharge, the patient is prescribed drug therapy including bismuth subsalicylate, metronidazole, and tetracycline for PUD associated with *H. pylori*. What teaching should the nurse provide relating to therapy with metronidazole?

7. The patient asks why she is not on a special diet. She has heard that ulcer patients should eat bland foods and drink a lot of milk. How should the nurse respond?

Case Study 2

A 47-year-old man with a history of T2DM and osteoarthritis has recently been experiencing GI distress attributed to use of NSAIDs for joint pain. Eating small, frequent meals has helped, but not relieved, the GI distress. The patient asks how his arthritis medication can cause stomach distress.

8. Describe the nurse's response.

9. Ranitidine (Zantac), an H_2RA, is prescribed. Based on the patient's need to take medications for his chronic conditions and his developmental level, describe why ranitidine is a better choice than cimetidine (Tagamet) for this patient.

10. Why is this patient at risk for accumulation of ranitidine, and what laboratory tests should be monitored?

79
Laxatives

STUDY QUESTIONS

Matching

Match the type of laxative to its mechanism of action.

1. ___ Increase secretion of water and ions into the intestine, and reduce water and electrolyte absorption.
2. ___ Lower surface tension, which facilitates penetration of water into the feces.
3. ___ Swell in water to form a viscous solution or gel, thereby softening the fecal mass.
4. ___ Draw water into the intestinal lumen causing the fecal mass to soften and swell, thereby stretching the intestinal wall, which stimulates peristalsis.

    a. Bulk-forming
    b. Osmotic
    c. Stimulant
    d. Surfactant

CRITICAL THINKING, PRIORITIZATION, AND DELEGATION QUESTIONS

5. What is a reason to use castor oil?
   a. Avoid straining with defecation
   b. Compensate for lack of fiber in diet
   c. Prevent constipation due to chronic opioid use
   d. Prepare for a colonoscopy

✳ 6. When clarifying a patient's complaint of constipation, what priority information does the nurse need to obtain?
   a. Amount of stool
   b. Color of stool
   c. Consistency of stool
   d. Frequency of stool

7. The nurse is teaching a patient about measures to prevent and treat constipation, which is a common adverse effect of a newly prescribed drug. Which statement made by the patient indicates a need for additional instruction?
   a. "Drinking 6-8 glasses of water each day will keep my bowels regular."
   b. "Eating fruits and vegetables or whole grains every day will help prevent constipation."
   c. "I should eat more whole grains and drink more water if my stool is hard, even if I go a couple of times a day."
   d. "Laxatives do not normally work overnight."

8. The nurse teaches a patient that which is the best source of fiber to promote proper colon function?
   a. Dietary bran
   b. Methylcellulose
   c. Psyllium
   d. Vegetable fiber

9. A nursing student is sharing research on laxatives. Which statement by the student would indicate a need for further study?
   a. "Bulk-forming agents can form a mass in the esophagus if the patient does not drink enough water when taking the drug."
   b. "Cathartics are useful as bowel preparations for colon procedures."
   c. "Patients should be warned that stimulant laxatives can cause electrolyte imbalances."
   d. "Stimulant laxatives are a good choice to prevent constipation associated with pregnancy."

✳10. The nurse is caring for a 45-year-old woman who is receiving antibiotic therapy. The patient takes a fiber laxative twice a day. It would be a priority to report which assessment finding to the prescriber?
   a. Bubbling sounds throughout the abdomen and dull sound with percussion of the left lower quadrant (LLQ)
   b. Gurgling bowel sounds throughout abdomen and one soft, liquid stool this morning
   c. High-pitched tinkling bowel sounds in the right lower quadrant (RLQ) and absent bowel sounds in other quadrants
   d. Soft bowel sounds throughout the abdomen occurring every 1-2 minutes in all quadrants on awakening

▶11. What is the most important teaching the nurse should provide regarding bulk-forming laxatives?
   a. They should never be taken more than once a day.
   b. They should be taken with 8 oz of water or juice.
   c. The fiber increases bulk but has no effect on peristalsis.
   d. They are contraindicated if the patient has irritable bowel syndrome.

12. Which directive should be included in instructions for administration of bisacodyl tablets?
   a. "You will have the best response if you take the laxative with a meal."
   b. "You should chew the bisacodyl tablets to achieve the maximum effect."
   c. "You should not take antacids within 1 hour of taking the laxative."
   d. "You should take the laxative with a full glass of milk."

▶13. It is important for the nurse to assess a patient who regularly uses Milk of Magnesia as a laxative for signs of hypermagnesemia. What is a sign of hypermagnesemia?
   a. Hypertension and rapid, bounding pulse
   b. Paresthesias around mouth, fingers, and toes
   c. Tremors, twitching, and hyperactive deep tendon reflex (DTR)
   d. Weakness, diminished bowel sounds, and bradycardia

✳14. The nurse is administering lactulose 30 mL to a patient who has hepatic encephalopathy. Which of these outcomes is a priority as the nurse plans care with this patient?
   a. Ammonia 110 mcg/dL
   b. ALT 35 international units/L
   c. One soft, formed stool within 24 hours
   d. Relief of constipation

▶15. Which result would be a reason to not administer Milk of Magnesia, prescribed as needed for constipation, and to consult with the prescriber?
   a. BUN 10 mg/dL
   b. eGFR 30 mL/min
   c. FBS (FBG) 135 mg/dL
   d. Na^+146 mEq/L

16. A patient who has a history of type 2 diabetes mellitus (T2DM) and hypertension who takes insulin, hydrochlorothiazide, and valsartan is having bowel preparation for a colonoscopy. The patient asks why the prescriber has ordered polyethylene glycol-electrolyte solutions (GoLYTELY) instead of the Fleet Phospho-Soda (sodium phosphate) that she took in past. Which statement would not be included in the nurse's response?
   a. "GoLYTELY does not cause electrolyte imbalances."
   b. "Sodium phosphate can harm the kidneys."
   c. "You are at greater risk for kidney damage due to your medical history and drug therapy."
   d. "This preparation (GoLYTELY) is better because you do not have to drink as much liquid."

▶17. A healthy pregnant patient complains of chronic constipation. Which would be the best initial intervention?
   a. Bulk-forming laxative daily and increase fiber and fluid in diet
   b. Moderate exercise after meals and increase fiber and fluid in diet
   c. Stool softener and increase fiber and fluid in diet
   d. Stool softener and moderate exercise after meals

18. Which would be a reason to withhold administration of lubiprostone (Amitiza) and consult the prescriber?
   a. The patient takes multiple drugs that are metabolized by the P450 metabolizing enzymes.
   b. The patient experiences mild nausea after taking the drug.
   c. The patient is older than 60 years.
   d. The patient is taking the drug for constipation associated with chronic opiate use.

✳19. A patient has been using mineral oil daily as a laxative. Because excessive use can interfere with vitamin K absorption, it would be a priority to report which symptom?
   a. Bruising
   b. Fatigue
   c. Pallor
   d. Sore tongue

20. Which laxative is best for reestablishing normal bowel functioning when discontinuing chronic stimulant laxative use?
    a. Castor oil
    b. Glycerin suppository
    c. Lactulose
    d. Mineral oil

DOSE CALCULATION QUESTIONS

21. Milk of Magnesia, 1 oz, is prescribed. How many mL will the nurse administer?

22. Lubiprostone, 0.008 mg twice a day, is prescribed for irritable bowel syndrome with constipation. Available are 8-mcg soft gelatin capsules. How many capsules should the nurse administer at each dose?

CASE STUDY

During a routine physical examination, the nurse discovers that a 78-year-old woman who lives alone uses several over-the-counter (OTC) laxatives every day to have a daily bowel movement. She has a history of hypertension and heart failure.

1. What additional information does the nurse need to know about this patient before she can address the problem of laxative overuse?

Further data collection reveals that this patient describes her daily bowel movement as light brown, mushy, and with some watery discharge.

2. What lifestyle changes are appropriate to help establish an acceptable bowel pattern for this patient?

3. What problems does this patient's medical history present when trying to address normalizing bowel patterns and laxative use for this patient?

4. What laxatives are contraindicated for this patient?

80

Other Gastrointestinal Drugs

STUDY QUESTIONS

Completion

1. The vomiting center is a group of neurons located in the _____ _____.

2. Vomiting is a(n) _____ action.

3. Chemotherapy drugs cause vomiting by directly stimulating the _____ _____ _____.

4. Signals that stimulate nausea and vomiting travel via the _____ nerve.

5. Drugs for chemotherapy-induced nausea and vomiting (CINV) are most effective if administered _____ _____.

6. Ondansetron (Zofran) exerts its antiemetic action by blocking _____ receptors.

7. The effectiveness of ondansetron (Zofran) is increased by also administering _____.

8. First-line therapy for nausea and vomiting of pregnancy is _____ plus _____.

9. Slowing down intestinal motility with drugs in uncomplicated diarrhea can _____ traveler's diarrhea.

10. _____ _____ _____ is the most common disorder of the GI tract.

CRITICAL THINKING, PRIORITIZATION, AND DELEGATION QUESTIONS

✱11. It would be of greatest priority to monitor which laboratory test results when a patient is experiencing the adverse effect of diarrhea when prescribed ondansetron (Zofran) for prolonged vomiting?
   a. ALT and creatinine
   b. BUN and electrolytes
   c. CBC and differential
   d. INR and PT

12. What is the primary reason why aprepitant (Emend) is often used with other antiemetics for CINV?
   a. It is only moderately effective.
   b. It has fewer adverse effects when given with other drugs.
   c. It is more effective than drugs that block serotonin receptors.
   d. It is effective only for acute nausea and vomiting.

13. A postoperative patient is prescribed IV prochlorperazine as needed for nausea and vomiting. After being transferred from the bed to a chair with the assistance of three people, the patient vomits and requests the medication. What should the nurse do? (Select all that apply.)
   a. Administer the medication while the patient is sitting in the chair.
   b. Assess vital signs before and after administration.
   c. Hold the medication if the patient is hypertensive.
   d. Incorporate safety precautions after medication administration.
   e. Transfer the patient back to the bed before administering the medication.

✱14. What action would be of greatest priority if a patient with postoperative vomiting reports burning at the IV promethazine (Phenergan) infusion site?
   a. Apply ice.
   b. Contact the prescriber.
   c. Page the IV team.
   d. Stop the IV infusion.

15. What is an appropriate nursing focus when a patient is prescribed haloperidol (Haldol) for nausea and vomiting after knee replacement surgery?
   a. Anxiety
   b. Body image
   c. Safety
   d. Swallowing

✱16. It would be of greatest priority to report to the prescriber which new finding when a patient is prescribed dronabinol (Marinol) for CINV?
   a. Need to take two naps per day
   b. Blood pressure of 110/72 mm Hg
   c. Pulse increase from 82 to 122 beats/min
   d. Two-pound weight gain in past month

17. Why is it recommended that a patient with nausea and vomiting of pregnancy take doxylamine at bedtime?
   a. It is more effective with this dosing.
   b. Sedation is a common effect.
   c. Severity of nausea is usually the worst at night.
   d. There is a longer time between doses.

18. Which planned activity would be of most concern if a patient has been prescribed scopolamine (Transderm-Scōp)?
   a. Taking a charter fishing trip
   b. Taking a cross-country rail trip
   c. Driving a delivery truck
   d. Taking a jet airliner trip to Europe

19. Which symptoms would be of greatest concern when a patient is experiencing prolonged diarrhea?
   a. BUN 22 mg/dL
   b. Hct 35%
   c. K 3.3 mEq/L
   d. Na 135 mEq/L

20. What is the primary reason why Lomotil, an antidiarrheal drug, contains atropine in addition to diphenoxylate?
   a. Its adverse effects limit abuse of the drug.
   b. It antagonizes the opiate effects.
   c. It inhibits gastric acid secretion.
   d. It relieves pylorospasm.

▶21. Which is the best intervention for a healthy child who has had two loose stools in the past 12 hours?
a. Difenoxin
b. Loperamide
c. Paregoric
d. Watchful waiting

▶22. Which symptom would warrant directing a parent to immediate medical care when his or her 10-year-old child had flulike symptoms that were treated with acetaminophen and bismuth subsalicylate (Pepto-Bismol)?
a. Two loose stools in the last 24 hours
b. Black tongue and black stool
c. Fatigue and poor appetite
d. Vomiting and confusion

23. A patient is prescribed alosetron (Lotronex) 1 mg once a day. How long after administration of the drug should the patient expect relief from symptoms?
a. 30-40 minutes
b. 1-2 hours
c. 3-4 days
d. 1-4 weeks

24. It is important for the nurse to teach a female patient who is taking alosetron (Lotronex) to stop taking the medication and immediately report symptoms if she experiences
a. abdominal pain and dyspepsia.
b. abdominal pain relieved by defecation.
c. constipation or bloody diarrhea.
d. fever or headache.

✳25. It is of greatest priority to specifically document the presence or absence of chest pain and dyspnea before administering which drug?
a. Alosetron (Lotronex)
b. Lubiprostone (Amitiza)
c. Sulfasalazine (Azulfidine)
d. Tegaserod (Zelnorm)

26. A patient is prescribed sulfasalazine (Azulfidine) for moderate ulcerative colitis. The nurse would consult the prescriber if which allergy was listed on the patient's chart? (Select all that apply.)
a. Cefazolin (Ancef)
b. Glipizide (Glucotrol)
c. Meperidine (Morphine)
d. Nafcillin (Unipen)
e. Quinapril (Accupril)
f. Trimethoprim-sulfamethoxazole (Bactrim)

▶27. Which laboratory result for a 37-year-old female patient suggests possible adverse effects of sulfasalazine (Azulfidine)?
a. Hemoglobin 10 g/dL
b. MCV 90/mm^3
c. Neutrophils 75%
d. WBC 10,500/mm^3

✳28. A 43-year-old female patient who has been taking
▶ hydrochlorothiazide (HydroDIURIL) for hypertension and olsalazine (Dipentum) for ulcerative colitis is admitted to the hospital. What would be the greatest nursing priority if nursing assessment findings include severe muscle weakness and paresthesias?
a. Anxiety
b. Breathing pattern
c. Fluid volume deficit
d. Knowledge deficit

29. A patient has received acute relief from dexamethasone for an exacerbation of Crohn's disease at the ascending colon. He is concerned because the prescriber is discontinuing this drug and prescribing budesonide (Entocort EC). How should the nurse respond? (Select all that apply.)
a. "Systemic effects are lower than with dexamethasone."
b. "Budesonide is released in the area of the colon where it needs to work."
c. "The drugs are the same, but budesonide is less expensive."
d. "Tolerance develops to long-term use of dexamethasone."

▶30. Which laboratory test result would be of most concern to the nurse when caring for a patient who is receiving cyclosporine for severe Crohn's disease?
a. BUN 22 mg/dL
b. Creatinine 3.6 mg/dL
c. ESR 22 mm/hr
d. FBG 122 mg/dL

✳31. It would be of greatest priority for a patient who is prescribed infliximab (Remicade) for Crohn's disease to report which symptom for over 6 weeks?
a. Abdominal pain
b. Blood in the stool
c. Fatigue
d. Productive cough

► 32. Which would be a reason for the nurse to withhold certolizumab (Cimzia) prescribed for severe ulcerative colitis and consult the prescriber?
   a. Butterfly rash on the face and joint pain
   b. Headache and photophobia
   c. Pruritic eruption on the ankles
   d. Serous rhinitis and optic tearing

33. The nurse would consult the prescriber if a patient with Crohn's disease reported new paresthesias after prolonged use of which drug?
   a. Budesonide (Entocort EC)
   b. Ciprofloxacin (Cipro)
   c. Infliximab (Remicade)
   d. Metronidazole (Flagyl)

∗ 34. A patient with diabetes has been experiencing episodes of abdominal pain, nausea, and vomiting of undigested food, especially at night. Metoclopramide (Reglan) 10 mg orally four times a day is prescribed. Because the drug promotes gastric motility, the nurse would expect to administer the doses within which time frame?
   a. After meals and at bedtime
   b. Before meals and at bedtime
   c. Every 6 hours
   d. With meals and at bedtime.

► 35. Which outcome would be appropriate for a patient who is taking palifermin (Kepivance)?
   a. Absence of nausea and vomiting after chemotherapy
   b. ALT/AST within normal limits
   c. Comfortable consumption average of 70% of meals and snacks each day
   d. Weight gain of 1 lb each week

► 36. The school nurse cares for a student with cystic fibrosis. When should the child receive her pancrelipase?
   a. With lunch
   b. One half-hour before lunch
   c. One hour before lunch
   d. Two hours after breakfast and lunch

DOSE CALCULATION QUESTIONS

37. Dronabinol (Marinol) 5 mg is prescribed 2 hours before the start of chemotherapy for a patient who is 4' 2" tall and weighs 70 lb. Based on BSA, is the dose safe and effective?

38. What is a safe and effective maintenance dose of infliximab (Remicade) for a 166-lb man with ulcerative colitis?

CASE STUDIES

Case Study 1

A patient who has a history of motion sickness receives a prescription for a scopolamine patch for use when flying cross-country and embarking on a 7-day cruise. The patient has many questions, so the prescriber asks the office nurse to explain the use of this medication.

1. How should the nurse describe the medication's action and administration?

2. Research the drug in a drug handbook and list precautions that the nurse should teach the patient to take.

3. What interventions can the nurse suggest to prevent adverse effects?

Case Study 2

A first-year college student is diagnosed with diarrhea-dependent irritable bowel syndrome (IBS) at the college health center.

4. What nonpharmacologic measures can the nurse teach to assist this patient with controlling his IBS?

5. Alosetron (Lotronex) is prescribed. The patient should stop taking the medication and return to the health center if he experiences what symptoms?

81
Vitamins

STUDY QUESTIONS

Matching

Match the term with its definition.

1. ____ Average daily dietary intake sufficient to meet the nutrient requirements of nearly all healthy individuals
2. ____ An estimate of the average daily intake required to meet nutritional needs
3. ____ Five reference values on dietary vitamin intake
4. ____ The highest average daily intake that can be consumed by nearly everyone without a significant risk of adverse effects
5. ____ The level of intake that will meet nutrition requirements for 50% of the healthy individuals in any life-stage or gender group

   a. Adequate intake (AI)
   b. Dietary reference intakes (DRIs)
   c. Estimated average requirement (EAR)
   d. Recommended dietary allowance (RDA)
   e. Tolerable upper intake (UI)

CRITICAL THINKING, PRIORITIZATION, AND DELEGATION QUESTIONS

6. The nurse knows that which statements are true about vitamins?
   a. They are inorganic compounds.
   b. They are needed for energy transformation and regulation of metabolic processes.
   c. They are required in megadoses for growth and maintenance of health.
   d. They are sources of energy.

7. The nurse knows that which statement is true about published RDAs?
   a. They do not consider increased needs during illness.
   b. They include values for older adults.
   c. They may be excessive for a chronically ill person.
   d. They need to be ingested every day.

8. Routine vitamin supplementation is recommended with which vitamin(s)? (Select all that apply.)
   a. Alpha-tocopherol (vitamin E) to protect against heart disease and cancer
   b. Ascorbic acid (vitamin C) to prevent colds
   c. Beta carotene (vitamin A) for smokers to protect from lung cancer
   d. Cyanocobalamin (vitamin B_{12}) to prevent anemia in people older than 50 years
   e. Folic acid for women before and during pregnancy

✳ 9. It would be a priority for the nurse to report which laboratory test result when a patient is taking high doses of vitamin A for acne?
   a. ALT 250 IU/L
   b. BUN 20 mg/dL
   c. hCG 0.6 mIU/mL
   d. INR 1

10. A patient with rough, scaling skin and a sore tongue may be experiencing niacin deficiency. The nurse teaches that which foods are high in niacin?
    a. Enriched grain products, green leafy vegetables, and legumes
    b. Chicken, peanuts, and cereal bran
    c. Dairy products and fortified cereal and bread
    d. Pork and enriched breads and cereals

11. The preoperative patient's medication history includes hydrochlorothiazide 25 mg once a day, calcium 400 mg 4 times a day, a senior multivitamin once a day, cholestyramine (Questran) 4 g 4 times a day, and vitamin E 1000 mg twice a day. The nurse should document the findings and notify the surgeon of the medication history because the patient is at risk for what issue?
    a. Excessive bleeding during surgery
    b. Hypotension during surgery
    c. Poor wound healing
    d. Vomiting during surgery

12. The nurse would teach a patient who follows a vegan diet the importance of supplementation with which vitamin?
    a. Alpha-tocopherol
    b. Ascorbic acid
    c. Cyanocobalamin
    d. Folic acid

∗13. It would be a priority to educate which patient on the possible adverse effects of self-prescribing megadoses of vitamin A for healthy skin?
    a. Adolescent female
    b. Adolescent male
    c. Older adult female
    d. Middle-aged male

14. The nurse should be aware that which disorder puts the patient at greatest risk for bleeding and bruising because of vitamin K deficiency?
    a. Addison's disease
    b. Celiac disease
    c. Gastroesophageal reflux disease (GERD)
    d. Peptic ulcer disease (PUD)

∗15. A patient tells the nurse that he takes a multivitamin containing vitamin K. The nurse reports this information to the patient's prescriber because the patient has been prescribed which drug?
    a. Digoxin
    b. Furosemide
    c. Heparin
    d. Warfarin

16. The nurse includes in her health promotion teaching that vitamin C supplementation has been approved for which use?
    a. Decreased bronchoconstriction of asthma
    b. Prevention of colds
    c. Promotion of wound healing
    d. Treatment of scurvy

17. An oncology nurse is providing health teaching to a patient who is starting chemotherapy. The patient has heard that chemotherapy can cause painful mouth ulcers. The patient would like to know if there is anything that she can do to help prevent these ulcers. The nurse could teach about adequate consumption of which foods that are rich in vitamin A ?
    a. Citrus fruits, strawberries, and red peppers
    b. Deep yellow, orange, and green vegetables and fruits
    c. Nuts, nut oils, and vegetable oils
    d. Pork and enriched breads and cereals

∗18. The nurse is providing nutritional teaching to a patient with advanced esophageal cancer. It is most important for the nurse to assess if the patient is self-medicating with which vitamin that has been falsely promoted as a treatment for cancer and can cause upper GI irritation?
    a. Vitamin A
    b. Vitamin B
    c. Vitamin C
    d. Vitamin E

19. Which characteristic of the older adult could cause a vitamin D deficiency?
    a. Older adults buy less fresh fruit because it is expensive.
    b. Older adults consume fewer dairy products.
    c. Older adults do not eat fresh vegetables because they cause indigestion.
    d. Older adults have difficulty chewing meat.

20. A teacher sends a Hispanic migrant worker's child to the school nurse's office because he is concerned that the child has a smooth, swollen tongue and cracks in the corners of her mouth and lips. The nurse knows that this may be a vitamin deficiency, possibly caused by a diet whose main component is
    a. home-ground corn.
    b. commercial cereals.
    c. dairy products.
    d. freshly picked vegetables.

DOSE CALCULATION QUESTIONS

21. Niacinamide is available in 100-mg tablets. The medication administration record indicates the dose is 150 mg. How many tablets should the nurse administer?

22. Vitamin K_1 0.5 mg IM is ordered for a neonate. Available is vitamin K_1 2 mg/mL. Calculate the dose.

CASE STUDIES

Case Study 1

A 46-year-old man has been admitted to a medical unit after 4 days in an alcohol detoxification center. He was admitted because of complaints of extreme weakness and an unsteady gait. His wife provided a history that his alcohol intake has steadily increased since he lost his job 3 years ago. During the past 6 months, he has been living on the street and drinking 1-2 quarts of wine daily. He is a poor historian and does not recall being admitted to the hospital. His response when asked about his diet is, "Whatever I can get." Physical assessment reveals ataxia, edema of the lower extremities, nystagmus, dry skin with cracks in the corners of his mouth, and multiple bruises. He states that the bruises are caused by any slight pressure. He is anorexic, taking sips of fluid and eating only a few bites of his lunch. He complains that his mouth is "too sore" to eat many foods. Endoscopy reveals severe gastritis with no obvious bleeding. The patient is diagnosed with vitamin deficiency and started on an IV drip with one ampule of vitamins C and B complex per liter.

1. Describe the symptoms exhibited that suggest deficiency of the following vitamins.

    a. Thiamine

    b. Niacin and pyridoxine

    c. Riboflavin

    d. Ascorbic acid

    e. Cyanocobalamin and folic acid

2. Why is the patient less likely to be showing symptoms of fat-soluble vitamin deficiencies?

3. Blood studies include hemoglobin 8.4 g and hematocrit 25%. Which vitamins are essential in red blood cell production?

4. The patient's wife has agreed that he may come home with her after his discharge from the hospital as long as he continues to stay in an outpatient rehabilitation program and does not drink. She asks the nurse to tell her some of the foods she should prepare to be certain that he gets the necessary vitamins. What foods or food groups would you suggest to her to ensure intake of vitamin A, vitamin C, niacin, pyridoxine, riboflavin, thiamine, and folate?

5. The patient's wife asks the nurse whether it would be a good idea to go to the health-food store and buy him some high-dose vitamin pills that include all vitamins. What is the best response?

Case Study 2

A high-school nurse has developed a rapport with a female student who has acne. The student states that she has been seeing a dermatologist without success. At the last appointment, the doctor stated that she would be considering isotretinoin, a megadose form of vitamin A, as the next step in therapy.

6. What precautions and instruction should the nurse provide?

82

Drugs for Weight Loss

STUDY QUESTIONS

Matching

Match the drug with its characteristics.

1. ___ Suppresses appetite by increasing the availability of norepinephrine at receptors in the brain
2. ___ Suppresses appetite and creates a sense of satiety
3. ___ Acts in the GI tract to reduce absorption of fat

   a. Orlistat
   b. Lorcaserin
   c. Phentermine

CRITICAL THINKING, PRIORITIZATION, AND DELEGATION QUESTIONS

4. The nurse is teaching health promotion to adolescent girls. Developmentally, which health risk would most likely be a motivator for change to healthier eating and exercise habits?
   a. Cardiovascular disease
   b. Decreased fertility
   c. Diabetes mellitus
   d. Hypertension

5. Research suggests that which change has not been shown to occur when patients lose weight?
   a. Decrease in high-density lipoproteins
   b. Decrease in low-density lipoproteins
   c. Decrease in level of hypertension
   d. Decrease in hemoglobin A1c in patients with type 2 diabetes mellitus

6. What is the most important factor when the nurse is devising a weight management plan for a patient?
   a. Developing strategies to help the patient minimize stress
   b. Including aerobic exercise, as possible, in the patient's plan
   c. Advising the patient to limit overly processed foods in the diet
   d. Seeking the patient's input in creating and revising the plan

7. Which statement, if made by a patient who has been prescribed a drug for weight loss, suggests that the patient needs additional teaching?
   a. "If I follow the directions regarding drug therapy, exercise, and diet, I should be able to lose a pound each week during the first month."
   b. "If Xenical works for me, I may need to take it long-term to maintain my weight loss."
   c. "My doctor is starting drug therapy because I have followed the recommended diet and exercise prescribed for the past 7 months and lost only 4% of my starting body weight."
   d. "My doctor is starting drug therapy for me because I am too heavy to exercise."

✳ 8. Which laboratory test result would be a priority to report to the prescriber of warfarin if a patient has self-prescribed orlistat (Alli)?
   a. ALT 30 IU/L
   b. BUN 22 mg/dL
   c. INR 5.2
   d. Potassium 5.2 mEq/L

9. Research on drugs for weight loss suggests that some patients will lose weight even when receiving a placebo.
   a. True
   b. False

10. Which result would be of most concern if a patient is prescribed phentermine?
    a. BP 180/98 mm Hg
    b. P 52 beats/min
    c. R 24/minute
    d. T 102.2° F (39° C)

11. A patient who is prescribed levothyroxine (Synthroid) for hypothyroidism has self-prescribed orlistat (Alli) for weight loss. Which teachings would be of greatest priority for this patient? (Select all that apply.)
    a. It is important to decrease dietary fat consumption.
    b. It is important to take supplements of vitamins B and C.
    c. Take the orlistat (Alli) before breakfast, lunch, and dinner.
    d. Take the prescribed Synthroid 30 minutes before breakfast.
    e. Taking fiber supplements such as psyllium can reduce GI effects.

DOSE CALCULATION QUESTIONS

12. Prescription orlistat (Xenical) dose is equal to how many capsules of OTC orlistat (Alli)?

13. Phentermine 18.75 mg is prescribed twice a day. Available are 37.5-mg tablets. How many tablets should be administered at each dose?

CASE STUDY

A 48-year-old man with a history of sleep apnea, hypertension, and type 2 diabetes weighs 285 lb and is 5' 8" tall. His waist circumference is 44". His total cholesterol is 330 mg.

1. The patient asks the nurse what is considered a realistic goal for weight loss, and how much he needs to cut back in his eating. How should the nurse respond?

2. The patient is prescribed orlistat 120 mg three times a day with meals. What strategies can the nurse suggest to minimize these adverse effects, which can be serious?
   a. GI effects

   b. Liver damage

   c. Reduced absorption of vitamin D

   d. Reduced absorption of vitamin K

3. The patient is concerned about the adverse effects of orlistat and asks if there are ways to improve his health without taking diet drugs. How should the nurse respond?

83

Basic Principles of Antimicrobial Therapy

STUDY QUESTIONS

True or False

For each of the following statements, enter T *for true or* F *for false.*

1. ___ Mammalian cells do not have a rigid cell wall.
2. ___ Patients should not take folic acid supplements when prescribed sulfonamide drugs.
3. ___ Cephalosporins kill bacteria by weakening the cell wall and promoting bacterial lysis.
4. ___ Aminoglycosides inhibit folic acid production by the microbe.
5. ___ Metronidazole inhibits DNA synthesis in certain microbes.
6. ___ Many drugs that are prescribed for HIV infection inhibit enzymes needed for viral reproduction.
7. ___ MRSA, VRE, and *C. difficile* are a problem because infection with these microbes is usually fatal.
8. ___ When patients take antibiotics as prescribed, resistance to antibiotics does not occur.
9. ___ Bacteria can become resistant to antibiotics by producing enzymes that inactivate the antibiotic.
10. ___ If a bacterium changes its receptors, an antibiotic may not be able to bind to the microbe and exert effects.
11. ___ The human body can make compounds that prevent an antibiotic from exerting the desired effect.
12. ___ Some microbes can change so that they stop taking antibiotics into the cell.
13. ___ The New Delhi Metallo-Beta-Lactamase 1 (NDM-1) gene is common in people of Indian or Pakistani decent.
14. ___ Broad-spectrum antibiotics kill more competing organisms than do narrow-spectrum drugs and do the most to facilitate emergence of resistance.
15. ___ Narrow-spectrum antibiotics tend to promote overgrowth of normal flora that possess mechanisms for resistance.
16. ___ Infants do not have a well-developed blood-brain barrier and drugs can enter the CNS more readily than in a child or adult.
17. ___ Antibiotics have difficulty penetrating an abscess.
18. ___ The American Heart Association has recently stressed that prophylactic use of antibiotics is more important than previously thought.
19. ___ Antibiotics that are added to animal feed can cause humans to develop a resistance to those antibiotics.

CRITICAL THINKING, PRIORITIZATION, AND DELEGATION QUESTIONS

▶20. A patient is admitted to a medical unit and prescribed intravenous (IV) ampicillin/sulbactam (Unasyn) after a specimen was sent for culture and sensitivity (C&S) from the emergency department (ED). The nurse knows the priority reason for notifying the prescriber of culture results as soon as they are available is that ampicillin/sulbactam (Unasyn)
   a. has many more adverse effects than most other antibiotics.
   b. is a broad-spectrum antibiotic, and there may be an effective narrow-spectrum antibiotic.
   c. is a very expensive antibiotic.
   d. is a narrow-spectrum antibiotic and may not be effective for the cultured organism.

21. Which patient would most likely have an infection that is resistant to antibiotic therapy?
   a. A child with asthma who develops pneumonia
   b. An adult construction worker who drinks from a worksite water supply and develops giardiasis
   c. An adult who developed a wound infection while in the hospital after surgery
   d. An older adult who got an infected paper cut

22. Which infection would be classified as a suprainfection?
    a. Monilial vaginal infection that develops during antibiotic therapy
    b. Peritonitis that develops after surgery for a ruptured appendix
    c. Pneumonia in a patient with chronic bronchitis
    d. Varicella outbreak after injection with varicella vaccine

23. Microscopic examination of gram-stained preparations has the advantage(s) of (Select all that apply.)
    a. detecting microbes when only a minute amount are present.
    b. Being more sensitive and specific than polymerase chain reaction (PCR).
    c. Providing rapid results.
    d. Being a more simple test.

24. The nurse has consulted the prescriber because a patient reports an allergy to the prescribed penicillin antibiotic. The prescriber is aware of the allergy, but the patient is experiencing a life-threatening infection and no other suitable antibiotic is available. What is the priority nursing action?
    a. Administer the antibiotic.
    b. Ask the patient if he or she is willing to take the antibiotic.
    c. Obtain orders for treatment of a possible allergic reaction.
    d. Refuse to administer the antibiotic.

✳25. It would be a priority to report which test result if a patient is prescribed tetracycline?
    a. G6PD 8.2 U/g of hemoglobin
    b. hCG 5325 mIU/mL
    c. INR 1.1
    d. Sodium 132 mEq/L

26. What test results should the nurse monitor when caring for a patient who is at risk for a glucose-6-phosphate dehydrogenase deficiency who is prescribed a sulfonamide antibiotic?
    a. AST and ALT
    b. BUN and creatinine
    c. Glucose and A1c
    d. Hemoglobin and hematocrit

27. In most infections, the level of antibiotic at the site of infection needs to be
    a. at the minimum inhibitory concentration (MIC).
    b. 2-3 times the MIC.
    c. 4-8 times the MIC.
    d. 10-20 times the MIC.

28. Which are valid reasons for prescribing two different antibiotics? (Select all that apply.)
    a. Cases of infection with *Mycobacterium tuberculosis*
    b. Results of the C&S indicate multiple drugs are effective
    c. Results of C&S indicate multiple organisms sensitive to different drugs are present
    d. Severe infection in the immunocompromised patient
    e. Foreign material is present on the sample specimen

29. Which is an acceptable reason for giving antibiotic prophylaxis?
    a. Before cardiac surgery
    b. Before examination of the eyes where dilating drops are instilled
    c. When patient experiences yellowish or yellow-green nasal discharge
    d. Whenever the patient has a fever

CASE STUDIES

Case Study 1

A 78-year-old nursing home patient with a history of hypertension, type 2 diabetes mellitus, and chronic obstructive pulmonary disease (COPD) is brought into the ED with a history of fever for 72 hours and moist cough. The extended care nursing report states that he was very irritable last night, and then was difficult to awaken this morning. Assessment findings include temperature 103° F (39.4° C), pulse 112 beats/min, BP 100/56 mm Hg, respirations 26 and labored, fine late inspiratory crackles (rales) throughout the lung fields, Glasgow coma scale 12. Chest x-ray demonstrates lung consolidation. Intravenous fluids are infusing. Other orders include admit and sputum (C&S).

1. What are nursing responsibilities regarding these orders?

2. What type of antibiotic would the nurse expect to be ordered and why?

3. The IV antibiotic that was ordered is cefotetan (Cefotan) 1 g every 12 hours. The unit nurse reviews the following (C&S) results. What action should the nurse take?

Organism: *Moraxella catarrhalis*	
Antibiotic	*Sensitivity*
Amikacin	R
Amoxicillin	R
Azithromycin	S
Cefepime	R
Cefotetan	R
Clarithromycin	R
Gatifloxacin	S
Levofloxacin	S
Piperacillin	R
Tobramycin	R

S = sensitive; R = resistant.

4. The cultured organism is sensitive to more than one drug. In this case, what other factors are considered when choosing among the effective antibiotics?

5. What assessment should be monitored by the nurse to determine clinical response to the antibiotic?

Case Study 2

A neighbor asks a student nurse why her doctor will not phone in prescriptions when she has a "sinus infection" anymore.

6. How can the nurse explain these changes in antibiotic prescription practices?

7. The neighbor states that she has antibiotics left over from the last infection. "I always save some in case I need them," she says. She asks the nurse if it is okay to take the leftover drug since it was prescribed for her. How should the student nurse respond?

8. The neighbor asks what she can do to prevent resistance to antibiotics. What suggestions should the student nurse make?

9. Where can the student nurse direct people for more information on preventing antibiotic resistance?

84

Drugs That Weaken the Bacterial Cell Wall I: Penicillins

STUDY QUESTIONS

True or False

For each of the following statements, enter T *for true or* F *for false.*

1. ___ All penicillins are able to penetrate the gram-negative cell membrane.
2. ___ Penicillins are able to destroy many bacteria when taken as prescribed.
3. ___ Penicillins are in the same antibiotic family as macrolide antibiotics.
4. ___ Penicillins are only active against bacteria that are undergoing growth and division.
5. ___ Penicillins are more effective against gram-negative than gram-positive bacteria.
6. ___ Penicillins are toxic to human tissue when prescribed in high doses.
7. ___ Penicillins can cause diarrhea by altering the normal GI flora.
8. ___ Penicillins must bind to special proteins on the outer surface of cytoplasmic membrane to be effective.
9. ___ People can drastically reduce their chance of catching methicillin-resistant *Staphylococcus aureus* (MRSA) by simple hygiene measures.
10. ___ MRSA can be treated by penicillinase-resistant penicillin such as nafcillin.
11. ___ Many people have MRSA in their nose and do not know it.
12. ___ Most infections with MRSA come from sports equipment.
13. ___ The germ that causes MRSA is commonly found on the skin.

CRITICAL THINKING, PRIORITIZATION, AND DELEGATION QUESTIONS

✳14. Which assessment is of greatest priority for the nurse to complete before administering a penicillin antibiotic?
   a. Allergy history
   b. BUN
   c. Temperature
   d. Wound drainage

15. Parents ask why their son has been prescribed amoxicillin and calcium clavulanate (Augmentin) if amoxicillin (Amoxil) has been ineffective in the past. The nurse's response is based on the fact that the addition of calcium clavulanate
   a. aids the penicillin in attaching to microbial penicillin-binding proteins.
   b. affects a wider spectrum of bacteria.
   c. prevents penicillinase from inactivating the amoxicillin.
   d. provides additional activity to disrupt the bacterial cell wall.

16. Which organism was previously susceptible to penicillin but has developed resistance to penicillin G?
   a. Gas gangrene caused by *Clostridium perfringens*
   b. Gonorrhea caused by *Neisseria gonorrhoeae*
   c. Meningitis caused by *Streptococcus pneumoniae*
   d. Syphilis caused by *Treponema pallidum*

17. A child is prescribed amoxicillin. When asked if their son is allergic to penicillin, the child's parents state that the child has never received any medication except immunizations. Why is it important to assess for an allergic response despite this history?
   a. Most people who experience a penicillin allergy experience the first incident in childhood.
   b. Most people who are allergic to penicillin do not know of the allergy.
   c. Parents often are poor historians.
   d. People can have an initial exposure to penicillin present in foods.

✳18. Which assessment finding would be a priority to report to the prescriber if it occurred after administration of a large IV dose of penicillin?
   a. Discomfort at IV site
   b. Fever higher than 100.4° F (38° C)
   c. Wheezing
   d. Shivering

▶19. The nurse is preparing to administer 8 AM (0800) medications to a patient who is to receive nafcillin 2 g via secondary intravenous (IV) infusion. The drug is dissolved in 100 mL of normal saline solution. The drug handbook states that the drug should be infused over 30-90 minutes. Just before the nurse hangs the nafcillin, the nurse is informed the patient is to be placed on a cart to go off the unit for a diagnostic test in 30-45 minutes. The patient is expected to be off the floor for 30 minutes. What should the nurse do?
   a. Hold the drug infusion until the patient returns from the test.
   b. Infuse the drug in 30 minutes before placing the patient on the cart.
   c. Infuse the drug in 45 minutes while loading the patient on the cart.
   d. Set the infusion to run over 90 minutes.

20. What does the nurse do when assisting with skin testing for penicillin allergy with the minor determinant mixture (MDM)?
   a. Instruct the patient how to assess for a local reaction during the following week.
   b. Be aware that the test carries little risk of a systemic reaction.
   c. Make respiratory support and epinephrine available.
   d. Be aware that the test involves injection of a small amount of penicillin under the skin.

21. The nurse would be concerned about the increased possibility of an allergic reaction when administering which antibiotic(s) if the patient's allergy record includes penicillin allergy? (Select all that apply.)
   a. Ampicillin/sulbactam (Unasyn)
   b. Azithromycin (Zithromax)
   c. Clindamycin (Cleocin)
   d. Gatifloxacin (Tequin)
   e. Piperacillin/tazobactam (Zosyn)
   f. Vancomycin (Vancocin)

22. What is the drug of choice for MRSA?
   a. Dicloxacillin
   b. Nafcillin
   c. Oxacillin
   d. Vancomycin

23. Which of these findings, if identified in a patient who is receiving ticarcillin/clavulanate (Timentin), should the nurse report to the prescriber immediately?
   a. Capillary refill 2 seconds
   b. Respirations 16 per minute
   c. Temperature 101° F
   d. Weight gain of 2 lb in 24 hours

✶24. The nurse reviews current laboratory test results before administering ticarcillin/clavulanate (Timentin). It would be a priority to report which laboratory result to the prescriber?
   a. BNP 65 picograms/dL
   b. BUN 22 mg/dL
   c. Hgb 8 g/dL
   d. WBC 15,000/mm^3

25. The nurse would be concerned about toxicity if a patient receiving penicillin had which laboratory result?
   a. ALT 52 international units/L
   b. BUN 20 mg/dL
   c. Creatinine 2.6 mg/dL
   d. Potassium 3.3 mEq/L

DOSE CALCULATION QUESTIONS

26. Amoxicillin 125 mg every 6 hours for 10 days is prescribed for a child with acute otitis media who weighs 16.5 lb. The recommended dose is 20-40 mg/kg/day. Is the prescribed dose safe?

27. Ampicillin 1 g/sulbactam 0.5 g (Unasyn) is supplied in 50 mL of solution to be infused over 15 minutes. The nurse should program the IV pump to deliver how many mL per hour?

CASE STUDIES

Case Study 1

An 8-year-old is diagnosed with streptococcal pharyngitis. She is prescribed amoxicillin 250 mg 3 times a day for 10 days.

1. What important information should the nurse obtain before the penicillin is administered?

2. What information about the possible side effects and adverse reactions of penicillin does the nurse need to provide to the patient's parents?

3. Describe the types of allergic reactions that might develop with the administration of penicillin and the interventions that should be included in nursing care to prevent complications from an allergic reaction.

4. The patient's parents ask how and when amoxicillin should be given. How should the nurse respond?

5. Why is it critical that the nurse teach the patient's parents not to stop the medication even if the child's throat stops hurting in 4-5 days?

6. What outcome would indicate that the antimicrobial effects were successful?

Case Study 2

The nurse is working in a public health clinic. A 15-year-old with no known allergies is diagnosed with syphilis and prescribed 1 dose of 2 million units of procaine penicillin G2 intramuscularly (IM).

7. Developmentally, why is this drug a good choice for this patient?

8. The patient asks why he cannot get this medication in a pill. How should the nurse respond?

9. Describe the technique the nurse should use to administer this IM injection, including precautions to prevent administration complications.

10. The patient has denied an allergy to penicillin. Why does the nurse need to be cautious about possible allergy?

11. What actions/policies should the clinic have in place to prevent death from an anaphylactic reaction?

85

Drugs that Weaken the Bacterial Cell Wall II: Cephalosporins, Carbapenems, Vancomycin, Telavancin, Aztreonam, Teicoplanin, and Fosfomycin

STUDY QUESTIONS

Completion

1. Cephalosporins are often resistant to _____.

2. First-generation cephalosporins are highly active against gram-_____ bacteria.

3. First-generation cephalosporins are not effective against _____.

4. Second-generation cephalosporins have _____ resistance to beta-lactamases produced by gram-negative organisms.

5. Third-generation cephalosporins are considerably more active against gram-_____ aerobes.

6. _____ is the only cephalosporin with activity against methicillin-resistant *Staphylococcus aureus* (MRSA).

7. Penetration of cerebrospinal fluid (CSF) by fourth-generation cephalosporins is

_____.

CRITICAL THINKING, PRIORITIZATION, AND DELEGATION QUESTIONS

8. Which result would be of greatest priority to report to the prescriber of cefotaxime?
   a. Albumin 3.4 g/dL
   b. ALT 158 international units/L
   c. eGFR 48 mL/min
   d. INR 1

9. Which result would be of greatest priority to report to the prescriber of ceftriaxone?
   a. Albumin 3.4 g/dL
   b. eGFR 88 mL/min
   c. H/H 9.2 g/dL/27%
   d. INR 1

10. When performing shift assessment, the nurse notes a maculopapular rash over the trunk of a patient who has been taking a ceftriaxone for 4 days. What is the priority nursing action?
   a. Administer PRN epinephrine.
   b. Complete the assessment.
   c. Consult the prescriber.
   d. Withhold the ceftriaxone.

11. Nursing interventions when administering cephalosporins include (Select all that apply.)
   a. always administer on an empty stomach.
   b. assess for severe allergy to carbapenems due to cross-allergy.
   c. instruct the patient to immediately report pain or warmth at IV site.
   d. store oral suspensions in the refrigerator.

12. A patient who is receiving ceftazidime has three loose, brown bowel movements in 24 hours. What should the nurse do?
   a. Administer the drug and continue nursing care.
   b. Continue to administer the drug and notify the prescriber of the change in bowel movements.
   c. Discontinue administering the drug and notify the prescriber.
   d. Page the prescriber STAT.

13. A patient with hospital-acquired pneumonia has just been prescribed cefotaxime and probenecid. The patient has no history or evidence of gout. What should the nurse do?
   a. Administer both medications as ordered.
   b. Administer the cefotaxime as ordered and ask the patient if he or she was taking probenecid at home.
   c. Administer the cefotaxime, but contact the prescriber before administering the probenecid.
   d. Contact the prescriber before administering either of the medications.

✴14. An alert and oriented patient with a history of penicillin allergy is prescribed cephalexin. What is the priority action by the nurse?
   a. Administer the cephalexin.
   b. Administer the cephalexin and carefully assess for allergic reaction.
   c. Assess the type of reaction that the patient had to the penicillin.
   d. Notify the prescriber of the allergy and ask for a different antibiotic order.

15. The nurse is reviewing new laboratory results, including creatinine clearance (eGFR) 82 mL/min for a patient receiving cefotetan 2 g every 12 hours. What should the nurse do?
   a. Administer the medication.
   b. Withhold the medication and notify the prescriber of the laboratory results.

16. Cefazolin has been prescribed at discharge for a patient with pelvic inflammatory disease. Due to the possibility of a disulfiram-like reaction, during discharge teaching it is important for the nurse to teach the patient to avoid consuming what?
   a. Alcohol
   b. Antacids
   c. Aspirin
   d. Ibuprofen

17. The nurse is preparing to administer an IV minibag of ceftriaxone in 50 mL of 5% dextrose to an infant. The infant has an IV of lactated Ringer's solution infusing at 35 mL/hr. What should the nurse do?
   a. Start a second IV for concurrent administration of the minibag and IV fluids.
   b. Run the minibag as a piggyback at a Y site.
   c. Consult with the prescriber.
   d. Stop the running IV, infuse the minibag, then restart the running IV.

▶18. Which laboratory result, if present, would be a reason to withhold administering cefotetan to an adult male and to notify the prescriber?
   a. ALT 254 international units/L
   b. BUN 34 mg/dL
   c. Creatinine 2.1 mg/dL
   d. FBS 230 mg/dL

19. Cefditoren is prescribed on discharge for a patient diagnosed with bronchitis caused by *Moraxella catarrhalis,* type 2 DM, GERD, and end-stage renal failure. Why is this antibiotic a good choice for this patient?
   a. Its absorption is not affected by antacids.
   b. Cefditoren is effective for beta-lactamase producing *M. catarrhalis.*
   c. Cefditoren is inexpensive.
   d. Cefditoren has once-a-day dosing.

▶20. Ceftriaxone 1 gram intramuscular is ordered for a 130-lb woman. The drug is reconstituted to a solution of 250 mg/mL. How should the nurse administer it?
   a. 1 mL each in the right and left vastus lateralis and deltoid muscles
   b. 2 mL each in the right and left ventrogluteal muscles
   c. 2 mL each in the right and left deltoid muscle
   d. 4 mL in the right or left gluteus maximus muscle

21. When imipenem (Primaxin) and valproate are prescribed for a patient, what is the priority nursing concern?
   a. Hydration
   b. Nutrition
   c. Safety
   d. Skin integrity

22. The carbapenem antibiotic imipenem (Primaxin) is a combination of the antibiotic and cilastatin. What is the purpose of the additive cilastatin?
   a. To decrease adverse effects of nausea and vomiting
   b. To improve absorption in the GI tract
   c. To prevent destruction of the antibiotic by beta-lactamase
   d. To prevent inactivation by an enzyme present in the kidney

23. The nurse is preparing to administer an intermittent infusion of ertapenem (Invanz). This drug can be administered concurrently with which intravenous (IV) solution?
   a. 5% dextrose in water
   b. 0.9% sodium chloride
   c. 0.45% sodium chloride
   d. 0.45% sodium chloride/5% dextrose solution

▶24. Vancomycin is being administered by mouth for pseudomembranous colitis caused by *Clostridium difficile*. The nurse receives laboratory results on the patient that include creatinine 2.2 mg/dL. What should the nurse do?
   a. Administer the medication.
   b. Hold the medication and notify the prescriber.

25. Which pre-drug administration assessment finding would be of most concern when a patient is prescribed telavancin?
   a. Facial flushing
   b. Foamy urine
   c. Maculopapular rash on cheeks and nose
   d. Bibasilar crackles

DOSE CALCULATION QUESTIONS

26. Telavancin 0.75 grams is prescribed for a patient who weighs 72 kg and whose eGFR (CrCl) is 34 mL/min. Is the dose safe?

27. Meropenem (Merrem) 250 mg is prescribed every 8 hours for a 14-lb child. The recommended safe pediatric dose of meropenem (Merrem) for meningitis is 40 mg/kg every 8 hours. Is this a safe dose?

CASE STUDIES

Case Study 1

A 45-year-old, gravida 4, para 4 woman is admitted to the nursing unit with the diagnosis of acute diverticulitis. She complaints of abdominal pain, nausea, and vomiting. She has a fever of 101°F and a white count of 18,000/mm³. A nasogastric tube is placed, an IV is started, and 1 g of ceftriaxone is ordered every 12 hours. Pain management is provided by IV morphine.

1. The nurse should assess the patient for which possible adverse reactions to the antibiotic?

2. How can the possibility of thrombophlebitis be minimized?

3. Why would a broader spectrum antibiotic not be prescribed for this patient?

4. What should the nurse do if the nurse discovers the patient has had an anaphylactic reaction to penicillin?

Case Study 2

The nurse is caring for a patient who is prescribed IV cefotaxime 2 g every 12 hours and Amikacin (Amikin) 300 mg 3 times a day after surgery for a ruptured appendix.

5. What assessments and laboratory results should be monitored while this patient is on this drug therapy?

6. What precautions does the nurse need to take when administering these two antibiotics through the same IV site?

7. The nurse notes that the patient's INR is 3.5. What should the nurse do?

8. Three days postoperatively, the patient has progressed to a soft diet and develops severe watery diarrhea. What are possible causes of the diarrhea?

9. What are possible electrolyte imbalances that could occur and what are their symptoms?

Case Study 3

A patient is prescribed vancomycin (Vancocin) 1 g every 12 hours scheduled at 0900 (9 AM) and 2100 (9 PM). The pharmacy provides a solution of 1 g in 200 mL.

10. Why is it critical to use an IV pump when administering this drug rather than hanging this drug by gravity?

11. If the drug is administered at 0900, at what time should blood be drawn to assess trough levels of the drug?

12. The drug will reach its therapeutic level after how many doses of the drug?

13. Describe red man syndrome and the nursing measures that can be taken to prevent this reaction.

14. Does experiencing red man syndrome create a contraindication for further administration of vancomycin?

15. Describe how the nurse will assess for the possible adverse effects of
    a. ototoxicity.

    b. immune-mediated thrombocytopenia.

86

Bacteriostatic Inhibitors of Protein Synthesis: Tetracyclines, Macrolides, and Others

STUDY QUESTIONS

True or False

For each of the following statements, enter T *for true or* F *for false.*

1. ___ Tetracyclines should be taken on an empty stomach.
2. ___ Low doses of doxycycline can be used to prevent destruction of gingival connective tissue.
3. ___ Resistance to tetracycline is increasing.
4. ___ Tetracyclines are the first drug of choice for most nonseptic infections.
5. ___ Tetracycline easily crosses mammalian cell membranes.
6. ___ Tetracycline is active against the bacilli that cause anthrax.
7. ___ Tetracycline is a narrow-spectrum antibiotic.
8. ___ Tetracyclines are bactericidal.
9. ___ Minocycline reduces symptoms of rheumatoid arthritis.
10. ___ Tetracycline should be used for mild acne.

CRITICAL THINKING, PRIORITIZATION, AND DELEGATION QUESTIONS

11. The nurse teaches a patient who has been prescribed oral tetracycline that the medication should not be taken with which over-the-counter medication(s)? (Select all that apply.)
    a. Ascorbic acid
    b. Centrum silver
    c. Ferrous sulfate
    d. Folic acid
    e. TUMS

12. A patient who was admitted with severe abdominal pain has been diagnosed with *H. pylori*–associated peptic ulcer. Tetracycline 500 mg, metronidazole 250 mg, and bismuth subsalicylate 525 mg have been prescribed 4 times a day. The nurse notes that the patient's 24-hour fluid intake has been approximately 2500 mL and urine output has been 600-800 mL for each of the past 2 days. What should the nurse do?
    a. Administer the medications and continue nursing care.
    b. Administer the medications and report the changes.
    c. Withhold the medication and continue nursing care.
    d. Withhold the medication and notify the prescriber of the changes.

13. Tetracycline can cause esophageal ulceration. What can the nurse teach to minimize the risk of this adverse effect?
    a. Stay upright for at least 30 minutes after taking the medication.
    b. Take the medication at bedtime.
    c. Take the medication with an antacid.
    d. Take the medication with milk.

14. A patient is prescribed a tetracycline antibiotic. Which patient information is a reason for the medication to be withheld by the nurse and the prescriber consulted?
    a. Patient has an allergy to penicillin.
    b. Patient is a 12-year-old child.
    c. Pregnancy status of patient is unknown.
    d. Theophylline for asthma is also prescribed.

15. The nurse should assess for adverse effects of lightheadedness and dizziness when a patient is receiving which medication?
    a. Demeclocycline
    b. Doxycycline
    c. Minocycline
    d. Oxytetracycline

＊16. A patient is prescribed tetracycline for *Chlamydia trachomatis*. Which change in assessment findings would be a priority to report to the prescriber?
    a. Burning on urination
    b. Perineal itching
    c. Vaginal discharge
    d. Watery stool

17. A patient with a penicillin allergy is prescribed erythromycin ethylsuccinate 250 mg every 6 hours for pneumonia caused by *Haemophilus influenzae*. The medication administration record (MAR) has the medication scheduled at 0600, 1200, 1800, and 2400. On the second day of therapy, the patient complains that he does not like taking the drug because it causes heartburn. What would be an appropriate intervention by the nurse?
    a. Administer the drug with food.
    b. Change the timing of the drug so that most doses are administered with meals.
    c. Explain that taking the drug with food or antacids will prevent absorption of the drug.
    d. Withhold the drug and notify the prescriber.

18. How should an enteric-coated erythromycin base be administered? (Select all that apply.)
    a. On an empty stomach
    b. Once a day
    c. Whole, not chewed
    d. With a full glass of water
    e. With food

19. Because of the risk of prolonged QT interval and torsades de pointes, the nurse would consult the prescriber before administering erythromycin to a patient who has experienced
    a. frequent headaches.
    b. nausea.
    c. unexplained fainting.
    d. wheezing.

20. A patient is prescribed erythromycin. What is one reason why careful review of all drugs this patient is prescribed is important?
    a. Erythromycin's action is prevented by clindamycin.
    b. Erythromycin becomes ineffective because metabolism is increased by nondihydropyridine CCB.
    c. Erythromycin can increase levels of warfarin and cause bleeding.
    d. Erythromycin prevents the absorption of -azole antifungals.

21. The nurse teaches that to be well-absorbed, which form of clarithromycin (Biaxin) must be administered with food?
    a. Standard tablets
    b. Extended-release tablets
    c. Granules
    d. Suspension

22. What teaching can the nurse provide regarding administration of antibiotics that helps decrease the development of resistance?
    a. Always take antibiotics with food.
    b. Only take antibiotics when symptoms are present.
    c. Go to the doctor and ask for antibiotics as soon as you think you have an infection.
    d. When prescribed, take the full course as directed even if symptoms are gone.

23. It is important for the nurse to monitor which laboratory test when a patient is prescribed azithromycin or erythromycin and warfarin?
    a. BUN
    b. CK-MM
    c. INR
    d. RBC

24. The MAR has azithromycin (Zithromax) listed to be administered at 0800. Breakfast arrives on the nursing unit around 0800, lunch at 1230, and dinner at 1730. The patient does not receive any antacids. What should the nurse do?
    a. Administer the drug at 0730, within the acceptable time frame.
    b. Administer the drug at 0800 and hold the patient's breakfast until 0900.
    c. Consult the prescriber.
    d. Reschedule the drug for 1030.

25. A diabetic patient is receiving clindamycin (Cleocin) for gas gangrene. Which drug, if also taken by this patient, could decrease bowel motility and prevent the body's attempt to rid the colon of overgrowth of *C. difficile*?
    a. Bethanechol (Urecholine)
    b. Digoxin (Lanoxin)
    c. Tolterodine (Detrol)
    d. Warfarin (Coumadin)

26. The nurse would consult the prescriber regarding oral administration of linezolid (Zyvox) if the nurse discovered the patient has a history of which disorder?
    a. Asthma
    b. Celiac disease
    c. Gout
    d. Phenylketonuria

27. It would be a priority to monitor which laboratory test when a patient is prescribed linezolid (Zyvox)?
    a. AST and ALT
    b. BUN
    c. CBC and differential
    d. Fasting blood glucose

28. A patient with a history of hypertension controlled by an angiotensin-converting enzyme inhibitor is prescribed linezolid (Zyvox) for a vancomycin-resistant enterococcal (VRE) infection. The patient should be instructed to avoid consuming what substance while on this antibiotic?
    a. Aged cheese
    b. Milk
    c. Red meat
    d. Seafood

29. The nurse should include in teaching to a patient who has been receiving linezolid (Zyvox) to immediately report which symptom of a *rare* adverse effect that has been associated with prolonged therapy?
    a. Dizziness when changing positions
    b. Headache
    c. Numbness or tingling in any extremity
    d. Vomiting

*30. A patient was receiving telithromycin (Ketek) for community-acquired pneumonia (CAP) caused by *Chlamydia pneumoniae*. The patient developed nausea, vomiting, dark urine, and fatigue. The prescriber discontinued the drug after evaluating ALT levels at 287 international units/L. What is a priority teaching for this patient?
    a. "If you ever take this drug again, you should take it with food to minimize adverse effects on the GI tract."
    b. "If you ever take this drug again, you need to drink 80-100 oz of fluids each day."
    c. "If you ever take this drug again, you should look at your stool and contact the prescriber if it turns black or bloody."
    d. "You should never take this drug again."

*31. Which laboratory result, if identified in a patient who is receiving dalfopristin/quinupristin (Synercid), should the nurse report to the prescriber immediately?
    a. ALT 250 international units/L
    b. BUN 20 mg/dL
    c. CK-MM 50 units/mL
    d. FBG 250 mg/dL

*32. The nurse is caring for a patient whose peak chloramphenicol level is 28 mcg/mL. Which assessment finding would be a priority to report to the prescriber relating to administration of this drug?
    a. BP 135/80 mm Hg
    b. Facial flushing with activity
    c. Pallor
    d. Vomiting

33. What is a major advantage of tigecycline (Tygacil) in treating VRE?
    a. No change to the metabolism of any drugs including warfarin
    b. Decreased development of antibiotic resistance
    c. Oral administration
    d. Safe for use in pregnant patients and pediatric patients

34. When used to treat colonized MRSA, mupirocin (Bactroban) is administered in which way?
    a. Intranasally
    b. Intravenously
    c. Orally
    d. Topically

DOSE CALCULATION QUESTIONS

35. Erythromycin oral suspension, 200 mg 4 times a day, has been prescribed for a child. The pharmacy provided erythromycin 250 mg/5 mL. How much erythromycin should the nurse teach the parent to administer per dose?

36. Chloramphenicol sodium succinate 1 g every 6 hours is prescribed IV for a 67-kg patient. The recommended dose is 12.5 mg/kg every 6 hours due to slightly elevated liver enzymes. Is the prescribed dose safe?

CASE STUDIES

Case Study 1

A 30-year-old attorney reports to the health care facility with a fever of 101° F and a nonproductive cough that has lasted 10 days. Her medical history reveals that she has asthma, takes theophylline (Theo-Dur), and is allergic to penicillin. On physical examination, her respiratory rate is 24/min and nonlabored, and bibasilar rhonchi are heard. The patient is given a prescription for erythromycin, 250 mg 4 times a day for 10 days, to treat what is suspected to be mycoplasma pneumonia. She is advised to take Tylenol 325 mg every 4 hours for fever, increase her fluids to 6-8 glasses of water per day, and stay home from work for 2-3 days.

1. What serious adverse effect is this patient at risk for based on drug interactions, and what symptoms would suggest this syndrome?

2. What should the nurse do regarding the possibility of this syndrome?

Case Study 2

A 15-year-old patient is readmitted after being discharged following an appendectomy with shaking chills, fever of 103° F, and purulent drainage from the incision site. Culture and sensitivity results of the wound drainage reveal *Enterococcus faecium* that is resistant to vancomycin. Dalfopristin/quinupristin (Synercid), 500 mg intravenous every 12 hours, is prescribed.

3. What laboratory tests and symptoms should the nurse monitor to assess for hepatotoxicity?

4. What nursing assessments and interventions should the nurse include in the plan of care relating to the significant risk of infusion-related thrombophlebitis?

5. Dalfopristin/quinupristin (Synercid) inhibits CYP3A4 hepatic drug-metabolizing enzyme. What are the ramifications for nursing care?

87

Aminoglycosides: Bactericidal Inhibitors of Protein Synthesis

STUDY QUESTIONS

Completion

1. Aminoglycosides kill bacteria so their action is
   _____.

2. Aminoglycosides are highly polar polycations and therefore cannot enter the _____
   _____.

3. Aminoglycosides are rapidly excreted by the
   _____.

4. Aminoglycosides are _____
   -spectrum antibiotics.

5. Aminoglycosides are primarily used to treat serious infections with aerobic gram-
   _____ bacilli.

6. Aminoglycosides can be toxic to the _____ and _____ _____.

7. Aminoglycosides can kill bacteria for several _____ after serum levels drop below the minimal bactericidal concentration.

8. Cell kill by aminoglycosides is _____ _____.

9. The principal cause of bacterial resistance is production of _____ that can inactivate _____.

10. Aminoglycosides cannot kill _____.

CRITICAL THINKING, PRIORITIZATION, AND DELEGATION QUESTIONS

11. Major adverse effects of aminoglycoside antibiotics include damage to (Select all that apply.)
    a. cochlea.
    b. heart.
    c. kidneys.
    d. lungs.
    e. stomach.
    f. vestibular apparatus.

12. Facultative bacteria survive in what condition?
    a. anaerobic
    b. both anaerobic and aerobic
    c. aerobic

＊13. A patient who is prescribed tobramycin (Nebcin) complains of a headache. What is the priority nursing action?
    a. Assess the onset, characteristics, and associated symptoms of the headache.
    b. Medicate with acetaminophen and reassess in 1 hour.
    c. Withhold the tobramycin and notify the prescriber when making rounds.
    d. Withhold the tobramycin and notify the prescriber STAT.

14. The nurse is assessing a patient who is scheduled to receive a dose of gentamicin (Garamycin). In the last 12 hours, fluid intake has been 900 mL, urine output has been 300 mL, and the patient's bladder is not distended. What should the nurse do?
    a. Administer the drug.
    b. Administer the drug and notify the prescriber of the output.
    c. Instruct the patient to drink a full glass of water each time the medication is administered.
    d. Withhold the drug and notify the prescriber of the output.

15. The nurse is taking a history from the spouse of a patient who was admitted in a septic state and prescribed an aminoglycoside antibiotic. Which question is most important to ask the patient's spouse about the patient's history?
    a. "Has your spouse ever had any surgery performed?"
    b. "Has your spouse been told to follow any specific diet?"
    c. "Has your spouse received a flu vaccine this year?"
    d. "What medications is your spouse currently taking?"

16. The nurse is assessing for adverse effects of IV tobramycin. Which change would be a priority to report to the prescriber?
    a. Dilute urine
    b. Headache
    c. Limp, weak muscles
    d. Ringing in the ears

17. The nurse is aware that the risk of ototoxicity is significantly increased if a hypertensive patient is also receiving which medication?
    a. Bumetanide
    b. Ethacrynic acid
    c. Furosemide
    d. Hydrochlorothiazide

＊18. What is the priority nursing action before administering an aminoglycoside to a patient with an eGFR of 50 mL/min?
    a. Ask the patient if he or she has had a headache.
    b. Assess peak levels of the drug.
    c. Assess liver function tests.
    d. Compare prescribed dose to recommended dose.

▶19. When aminoglycosides are prescribed IV as a once-daily dose, it is important to monitor trough levels
a. 30 minutes before the next dose.
b. 1 hour after completing the infusion.
c. 1 hour before the next dose.
d. 30 minutes after completing the infusion.

▶20. The nurse is caring for a patient who is receiving gentamicin twice a day. Peak and trough levels were drawn after the fourth dose. Results were peak 3 mcg/mL and trough 0.6 mcg/mL. What should the nurse do?
a. Administer an additional dose.
b. Continue nursing care.
c. Consult with the prescriber.
d. Withhold future doses until the prescriber can be consulted.

✳21. Which of these laboratory tests would be a priority for the nurse to assess when a patient is receiving an aminoglycoside?
a. Creatinine
b. Fasting blood glucose
c. Hemoglobin and hematocrit
d. INR

▶22. A patient received a neuromuscular blocking agent during surgery. In the postanesthesia care unit, the prescriber orders gentamicin 40 mg IV STAT. What is the most appropriate nursing action?
a. Administer the drug as quickly as possible.
b. Assess the patient's vital signs.
c. Clarify the order.
d. Refuse to administer the drug.

DOSE CALCULATION QUESTIONS

23. Based on the recommended dose of gentamicin, what is the recommended dose range for a patient with a gram-negative infection, who weighs 220 lb, if the gentamicin is to be administered every 8 hours?

24. A patient weighs 65 kg and has been prescribed amikacin 175 mg every 8 hours. Is the prescribed dose appropriate for this patient?

CASE STUDIES

Case Study 1

A 72-year-old male patient with a history of type 2 diabetes mellitus (T2DM) treated with metformin, and rheumatoid arthritis treated for many years by nonsteroidal anti-inflammatory drugs, had a prostatectomy 14 days earlier. He is readmitted to a medical-surgical unit for a surgical site infection. Assessment findings include BP 100/70 mm Hg, pulse 98 beats/min, respirations 24/min, and temperature 104° F (40° C). He is difficult to arouse and his skin is hot and dry. *Escherichia coli* cultured from the wound drainage is sensitive to amikacin (Amikin). His dose of amikacin is less than the normal recommended dose.

1. What are possible reasons for the prescribed dose not being equivalent to the recommended dose?

2. The drug is to be administered at 0600 (6 AM), 1400 (2 PM), and 2200 (10 PM). Peak and trough levels of the amikacin are ordered. When will the nurse schedule the collection of the blood sample for this testing?

3. Why are serum trough levels more significant than serum peak levels?

4. The trough level of the amikacin (Amikin) is 15 mcg/mL. What should the nurse do?

Case Study 2

A 40-year-old male patient is recovering in the trauma unit from a major accident. He is on a ventilator and has a central line for IVs and antibiotics, a Swan-Ganz catheter to measure cardiac status, an arterial line to measure continuous blood pressure, a small-bore feeding tube, two chest tubes, and a Foley catheter. After 3 days, he develops gram-negative septicemia and pneumonia and is started on gentamicin sulfate (Garamycin) and ampicillin (Unasyn) IV.

5. Describe the assessments the nurse should perform to detect nephrotoxicity and neurotoxicity.

6. How does nephrotoxicity increase the risk of developing ototoxicity?

7. Which toxicity is most likely to be permanent?

8. How can the nurse prevent drug interactions?

9. What type of urine collection bag should the nurse use with this patient?

10. What changes in the dosages of medications would be necessary if the patient were 80 years old instead of 40?

88
Sulfonamides and Trimethoprim

STUDY QUESTIONS

True or False

For each of the following statements, enter T *for true or* F *for false.*

1. ____ Sulfonamide antibiotics are chemically related to glipizide, glyburide, furosemide, and hydrochlorothiazide.
2. ____ Sulfonamides are narrow-spectrum antibiotics.
3. ____ Sulfonamides are no longer active against many microbes for which they initially were effective.
4. ____ Sulfonamides are currently used to treat urinary tract infections (UTIs).
5. ____ Sulfonamides are usually administered intramuscularly or intravenously.
6. ____ Sulfonamides are widely used because of low toxicity.
7. ____ Sulfonamides are effective in treating an organism common in pneumonia occurring in patients with AIDS.
8. ____ Sulfonamides cause folic acid deficiency in the patient.
9. ____ Sulfonamides cross the placenta.
10. ____ Sulfonamides do not cause toxicity when applied topically.
11. ____ Sulfonamides inhibit microbial synthesis of folic acid.
12. ____ Sulfonamides were the first systemic antibiotics developed.

CRITICAL THINKING, PRIORITIZATION, AND DELEGATION QUESTIONS

✱13. Which type of rash would most likely indicate the start of Stevens-Johnson syndrome when a patient is receiving sulfonamides?
   a. Amber-colored, crusty rash on the cheeks
   b. Papular rash on the shoulders
   c. Pruritic rash on lower arms
   d. Vesicular rash in the mouth

✱14. What is the priority reason why the nurse teaches a patient who is prescribed sulfamethoxazole to take this medication with a full glass of water?
   a. Decrease the risk of esophageal irritation
   b. Minimize crystal formation in the urine
   c. Prevent nausea
   d. Stimulate frequent voiding

✱15. Which laboratory test result would be a priority to report to the prescriber of a sulfonamide?
a. Neutrophils 65%
b. Platelets 200,000/mm³
c. RDW 18.4%
d. WBC 11,800/mm³

16. Sulfonamides can cause the adverse effect of kernicterus. How does this present?
a. Damage to the brain in neonates caused by deposition of bilirubin in the brain
b. Damage to the kidney tubules by crystals in the urine
c. Inability of the bone marrow to produce blood cells
d. Unusual sensitivity to sunlight

17. A patient who takes glyburide for type 2 diabetes mellitus (T2DM) is prescribed sulfamethoxazole-trimethoprim (TMP/SMZ) for a UTI. Because of the possibility of intensifying the effect of glyburide, the nurse should assess for
a. bleeding and bruising.
b. fever and photophobia.
c. hot, dry skin and thirst.
d. paresthesias and abdominal cramps.

18. The patient has been receiving mafenide application to a second-degree burn for over 2 weeks. Which laboratory results suggest that the drug might be causing acidosis?
a. pH 7.32, HCO_3 18 mEq/L, pco_2 31 mm Hg
b. pH 7.35, HCO_3 22 mEq/L, pco_2 37 mm Hg
c. pH 7.41, HCO_3 24 mEq/L, pco_2 40 mm Hg
d. pH 7.45, HCO_3 21 mEq/L, pco_2 47 mm Hg

✱19. The nurse is preparing to apply topical mafenide to second-degree burns on the anterior of a 7-year-old patient's arms, upper legs, and trunk. What is the priority nursing action, aimed at preventing the common adverse effect relating to application of this drug?
a. Employ aseptic technique.
b. Explain the importance of therapy.
c. Prevent pain.
d. Shield so the patient cannot see the wounds.

20. The nurse is administering trimethoprim to a patient who has a history of alcohol use disorder. Because folate deficiency is associated with alcohol use disorder, the nurse should assess for symptoms of possible adverse effects of trimethoprim, which include
a. nausea and vomiting.
b. rash and malaise.
c. pallor and sore throat.
d. photosensitivity and drug fever.

21. Trimethoprim (Primsol) is classified as pregnancy category C. What does this mean? (Select all that apply.)
a. Animal studies have shown a risk for fetal problems, but human studies have not shown any problems.
b. Controlled studies have shown no risk to a developing fetus.
c. This drug must not be used while the patient is pregnant.
d. Risks are possible during pregnancy but the potential benefits may justify the risk.
e. There is definite evidence of risk to a developing fetus.

✱22. Because of the risk of hyperkalemia when prescribed trimethoprim, it is a priority for the nurse to teach the patient to report what symptom?
a. Bruising
b. Weakness
c. Pallor
d. Sore throat

23. The nurse is preparing to administer trimethoprim 50 mg prescribed orally every 12 hours. Laboratory test results include eGFR 30 mL/min. What should the nurse do?
a. Administer the drug.
b. Check the patient's intake and output.
c. Consult the prescriber.
d. Withhold the drug.

24. What is a benefit of trimethoprim-sulfamethoxazole (TMP/SMZ) over the components used alone?
a. Lack of interaction with drugs that have a narrow therapeutic range
b. Fewer adverse effects
c. Less resistance has developed
d. Lower incidence of toxicity

25. A physician who is on call for another physician gives a verbal order for sulfamethoxazole-trimethoprim (TMP/SMZ) for a patient. The nurse would consult the prescriber about this order if the patient had a history of which condition?
a. Megaloblastic anemia
b. Chronic obstructive lung disease
c. Diabetes mellitus
d. Hypertension

26. Which INR result would be a reason to contact the prescriber in a patient with atrial fibrillation taking warfarin who has also been prescribed a sulfonamide?
    a. INR 2
    b. INR 2.5
    c. INR 3
    d. INR 3.5

DOSE CALCULATION QUESTION

27. The child is prescribed 72 mg TMP/360 mg SMZ. Available is an oral suspension of 8 mg TMP and 40 mg SMZ per mL. How many mL should the nurse administer?

CASE STUDIES

Case Study 1

A 30-year-old IV drug addict who is HIV-positive has been treated with AZT for more than 1 year. She presents to the clinic with a low-grade fever, nonproductive cough, and shortness of breath. A chest x-ray shows diffuse infiltrates. A diagnosis of pneumocystis pneumonia (PCP) caused by *Pneumocystis jiroveci* is made.

1. The patient states that she knows about getting pneumonia from *Pneumocystis carinii*. Now she has something new and she is sure that she is going to die. How should the nurse respond?

2. The patient is started on trimethoprim-sulfamethoxazole (TMP/SMZ). Why is TMP/SMZ a good choice for this patient?

3. Why is it important to wait for the results of hCG levels before this patient starts taking TMP/SMZ?

4. What adverse effects should the nurse teach the patient to report, should they occur?

5. What can the nurse teach to decrease the incidence and severity of these possible adverse effects to TMP/SMZ?
    a. Photosensitivity

    b. Stevens-Johnson syndrome

    c. Renal damage

6. What forms of sulfonamide drugs have less risk of Stevens-Johnson syndrome?

Case Study 2

The nurse has volunteered to make a trip to provide health care to Rwandan refugees in Uganda. A clinic has been set up, and doctors and nurse practitioners are diagnosing cases and providing donated samples of medications. The RN is providing teaching via an interpreter. Sulfonamides are being provided to patients with urinary tract infections.

7. What adverse effect would these patients be at greater risk for than the general population?

8. What type of sulfonamides would be more likely to cause hemolytic anemia?

9. The nurse should assess for what symptoms that suggest possible development of hemolytic anemia?

10. An HIV-positive patient comes to the clinic with a 2-week-old infant who appears toxic. The only antibiotic the team has in a liquid form is a sulfonamide. Why is this dangerous to give to this infant?

89

Drug Therapy of Urinary Tract Infections

STUDY QUESTIONS

Matching

Match the term with its definition.

1. ___ Inflammation of the kidney and its pelvis
2. ___ Inflammation of the tube that takes urine from the bladder to the urinary meatus
3. ___ Inflammation of the gland surrounding the bladder neck in men
4. ___ Inflammation of the urinary bladder
5. ___ Recolonization with the same organism
6. ___ Colonization with a new organism

    a. Cystitis
    b. Prostatitis
    c. Pyelonephritis
    d. Reinfection
    e. Relapse
    f. Urethritis

CRITICAL THINKING, PRIORITIZATION, AND DELEGATION QUESTIONS

7. What is an example of a complicated urinary tract infection (UTI)?
   a. UTI acquired in the hospital
   b. UTI caused by an enlarged prostate
   c. UTI caused by multiple organisms
   d. UTI of the kidney pelvis

＊ 8. The nurse is caring for an incontinent patient who has repeated episodes of UTIs (*E. coli*) treated with TMP/SMZ. What is the priority action to prevent recurrence of infection?
   a. Assessing for sore throat and fever
   b. Carefully wiping from front to back during perineal care
   c. Encouraging ingestion of at least 2000 mL of fluids each day
   d. Offering cranberry juice each day

9. A female patient has been prescribed an antibiotic for 3 days. What are some advantages of shorter-course therapy? (Select all that apply.)
   a. Fewer adverse effects
   b. Less potential for antibiotic resistance
   c. Lower cost
   d. Greater likelihood of patients completing therapy as prescribed
   e. Treatment of upper urinary tract involvement

＊10. A prescriber's orders for a new admission include urine culture and sensitivity and ciprofloxacin 400 mg intravenously (IV) every 12 hours. What is a priority nursing responsibility?
   a. Calculate the drip rate for the IV infusion.
   b. Flush the IV cap.
   c. Mix the antibiotic in the correct IV solution.
   d. Obtain the urine culture specimen before administering the antibiotic.

11. What is true about nitrofurantoin and methenamine?
   a. They are first-line agents for prostatitis.
   b. They are not absorbed from the GI tract.
   c. Therapeutic levels are achieved only in urine.
   d. They have few adverse effects.

＊12. Which of these assessment findings, if identified in a patient who is receiving nitrofurantoin (Macrodantin), should the nurse report to the prescriber immediately?
   a. Brown-colored urine
   b. Dyspnea
   c. Nausea
   d. Headache

13. A patient is receiving 50 mg of nitrofurantoin (Macrodantin) at bedtime for prophylaxis of recurrent cystitis. This means that the patient
   a. is taking low doses of the drug to prevent reinfection.
   b. is taking low doses of the drug to prevent relapse.
   c. is taking very high doses of the drug because he or she cannot get rid of the infection.
   d. has a UTI caused by a resistant microorganism.

14. A patient has been prescribed nitrofurantoin (Furadantin) for recurrent UTIs. The nurse should teach the patient to do what? (Select all that apply.)
    a. Not to take the drug if there is any chance that she might be pregnant.
    b. Report any shortness of breath and coughing.
    c. Report the onset of numbness or tingling.
    d. Take the medication on an empty stomach.
    e. Use caution when driving because the drug can cause drowsiness.

＊15. Which laboratory test result is of greatest priority to review before the nurse administers nitrofurantoin (Furadantin)?
    a. ALT
    b. Bilirubin
    c. eGFR
    d. Sodium

16. The nurse is reviewing the other over-the-counter products taken by a patient who has been prescribed methenamine (Mandelamine). Which of these home treatments might reduce the urinary antiseptic action of methenamine?
    a. Baking soda in water for heartburn
    b. Drinking 10 glasses of water each day for general health
    c. Taking ibuprofen twice a day for joint pain
    d. Taking megadoses of vitamin C to prevent colds

DOSE CALCULATION QUESTIONS

17. Nitrofurantoin macrocrystals (Macrodantin) 50 mg twice a day is prescribed. Available are 25-mg capsules. How many should be administered per dose?

18. Methenamine hippurate (Hiprex) 500 mg twice a day is prescribed for a 10-year-old child. The pharmacy dispenses methenamine hippurate (Hiprex) 1-g tablets. How many tablets should be administered at each dose?

CASE STUDIES

Case Study 1

A 75-year-old male patient with known benign prostatic hyperplasia (BPH) has had numerous episodes of cystitis.

1. If the patient develops flank pain, chills, fever, or other signs of infection higher in the urinary tract suggesting pyelonephritis, what actions should be taken?

2. The patient has been successfully treated with TMP/SMZ and has been prescribed nitrofurantoin (Macrodantin) to prevent recurrence of UTIs until he can be evaluated for surgery for his enlarged prostate. The nurse should teach the patient to be alert for what possible adverse effects from Macrodantin?

3. What nursing assessments and teaching can the nurse employ to prevent complications from nitrofurantoin (Macrodantin) therapy?

4. The patient calls to tell the office nurse that his urine has changed to a brown color. What should the nurse tell him?

5. Why is it important to monitor creatinine levels in this patient?

Case Study 2

A female patient is seen at the college health center. She constantly feels that she needs to urinate, but she does not want to because it hurts, and the urge to urinate persists after she voids. She denies fever and flank pain and has not looked at her urine.

6. What additional questions should the nurse ask the patient to assist the practitioner with diagnosing?

7. Why is it important to determine how frequently the patient has had UTIs in the past?

8. The college health nurse knows that most UTIs treated with sulfonamides are due to *Escherichia coli* infection. Why are female patients more prone to get this infection?

9. What instruction should the nurse provide the patient to prevent future infections?

90

Antimycobacterial Agents: Drugs for Tuberculosis, Leprosy, and *Mycobacterium avium* Complex Infection

STUDY QUESTIONS

True or False

For each of the following statements, enter T *for true or* F *for false.*

1. ____ The principal cause underlying the emergence of resistance is inadequate drug therapy.
2. ____ Microscopic examination of sputum is the best way to diagnose TB.
3. ____ Culture and sensitivity for *Mycobacterium tuberculosis* takes 24-48 hours.
4. ____ Individuals infected with TB, but symptom-free, cannot infect other people.
5. ____ Individuals infected with TB have a risk of developing active TB without additional exposure to the bacteria even if the infection has been dormant for many years.
6. ____ Infection with TB is best treated in the hospital.
7. ____ TB is an infection limited to the lungs.
8. ____ TB is more prevalent in jails and homeless populations than the general population.
9. ____ Primary infection with TB usually is evident on chest x-ray.
10. ____ Resistance to drugs for TB is increasing.
11. ____ Treatment of active infection with TB should always include at least two drugs.

CRITICAL THINKING, PRIORITIZATION, AND DELEGATION QUESTIONS

12. A male patient who has been diagnosed with active TB has been prescribed isoniazid, rifampin, ethambutol, and pyrazinamide. The patient asks the nurse why he has to take so many drugs. The basis of the nurse's response should include that this multidrug therapy has which effect(s)? (Select all that apply.)
    a. Decreased adverse effects
    b. Decreased risk of relapse
    c. No increased risk of suprainfection
    d. Elimination of actively dividing and resting tuberculosis mycobacteria
    e. Prevention of mycobacteria from developing resistance to a drug

13. A male patient asks the nurse why he has to continue to take medication after completion of the initial induction phase if his sputum is "clean." What does the nurse say?
    a. Dormant bacteria are still present inside cells and can become active at a later time.
    b. Sputum cultures are not sensitive enough to ensure that the active bacteria are eliminated.
    c. Sputum cultures are not specific for mycobacterium.
    d. This therapy is in case the patient comes into contact with the person who originally infected him.

14. An HIV-infected patient who is receiving drug therapy, including delavirdine (Rescriptor) and saquinavir, is diagnosed with an active TB infection. Because of the drug interaction that decreases the effect of these drugs for HIV infection, this patient should not be prescribed which drug?
    a. Ethambutol
    b. Isoniazid
    c. Pyrazinamide
    d. Rifampin

15. A 19-year-old nursing student with no history of medical problems, no symptoms of disease, and no risk factors for contracting TB is being screened for TB before starting a clinical nursing course. He has a 20-mm area of erythema surrounding an 11-mm area of induration 48 hours after receiving a PPD tuberculin test. Chest x-ray and sputum culture are negative. The nurse would expect prophylactic treatment to involve
    a. multidrug therapy.
    b. watchful waiting.
    c. isoniazid.
    d. rifampin.

*16. A nurse is receiving isoniazid therapy for latent TB. It would be of greatest priority to contact the prescriber if the nurse experiences
    a. frontal headache.
    b. dry mouth.
    c. heartburn at night.
    d. persistent nausea.

17. The public health nurse would withhold administration of TB drug therapy with rifampin and pyrazinamide and contact the prescriber if the patient's laboratory test results include
    a. AST 75 international units/L.
    b. bilirubin, total 3 mg/dL.
    c. BUN 22 mg/dL.
    d. creatinine 1 mg/dL.

18. The nurse should be particularly vigilant when monitoring intake and output and creatinine levels when a patient is receiving which antitubercular drugs? (Select all that apply.)
    a. Amikacin
    b. Gatifloxacin
    c. Kanamycin
    d. Isoniazid
    e. Streptomycin

19. A patient with a history of peripheral vascular disease, type 2 diabetes mellitus, and latent TB is prescribed isoniazid and pyridoxine. What is the purpose of the pyridoxine?
    a. Improve arterial blood flow
    b. Prevent hypoglycemia
    c. Prevent peripheral neuropathy
    d. Treat resting mycobacteria within cells

20. Why is the interaction of isoniazid and phenytoin especially important?
    a. Isoniazid levels can become subtherapeutic.
    b. Phenytoin has a narrow therapeutic range.
    c. Phenytoin levels can become subtherapeutic.
    d. The risk of hepatotoxicity increases.

21. A patient who is paranoid schizophrenic who has been involuntarily committed to a psychiatric institution has been diagnosed with latent TB and is refusing drug therapy with isoniazid. What would be an appropriate nursing response?
    a. Consult the prescriber and psychiatrist regarding possible intramuscular administration of isoniazid.
    b. Explain the importance of drug therapy.
    c. Withhold the drug and isolate the patient until he agrees to take the drug.
    d. Withhold the drug; the patient cannot infect others.

22. The nurse knows that oral rifampin may not reach therapeutic levels if it is administered
    a. on an empty stomach.
    b. with food.
    c. with other drugs that are metabolized by the hepatic cytochrome P450 enzymes.
    d. with protease inhibitors and nonnucleoside reverse transcriptase inhibitors (NNRTIs) for HIV infection.

23. A patient takes prophylactic warfarin because of a history of atrial fibrillation. The patient has recently been diagnosed with TB and is prescribed antimicrobial drugs, including rifampin. Because of the interaction between warfarin and rifampin, it is important for the nurse to assess the patient for which symptom?
    a. Abdominal pain
    b. Bleeding
    c. Change in mental status
    d. Oliguria

24. A patient has received instructions regarding TB therapy with rifampin. Which of these statements made by the patient would indicate the patient needs further teaching?
    a. "I should contact my ophthalmologist regarding use of my contact lenses."
    b. "I should contact my prescriber if I experience reddish-colored urine."
    c. "My oral contraceptive birth control may not work."
    d. "This drug can stain my contact lenses."

25. Several second-line agents for TB have the potential to damage the eighth cranial nerve. The nurse would assess for this damage by noting changes in what? (Select all that apply.)
    a. Balance
    b. Extraocular movements
    c. Facial movements
    d. Hearing
    e. Sense of smell

✳26. It is of greatest priority to teach a patient who is prescribed ethambutol to
    a. call the prescriber if experiencing nausea.
    b. contact the prescriber if experiencing any visual changes.
    c. take the drug on an empty stomach with or without food.
    d. take the drug with food if it causes upset stomach.

27. Multidrug therapy for Hansen's disease (leprosy)
    a. is curative.
    b. is prophylactic.
    c. is futile.
    d. is unnecessary.

28. The current recommendation for use of rifampin for Hansen's disease (leprosy) is to administer the drug how often?
    a. Once a day
    b. Once a week
    c. Once a month
    d. Once a year

29. A patient with G-6-PD deficiency, who is receiving dapsone for leprosy, is at increased risk for
    a. destruction of red blood cells.
    b. fluid retention.
    c. infection.
    d. liver damage.

✳30. Which of these assessment findings, if identified in a patient who is receiving clofazimine, is of greatest priority to report to the prescriber?
    a. Darkening of the skin
    b. Diarrhea, nausea, and vomiting
    c. Hyperactive bowel sounds in right upper quadrant and absent bowel sounds in left lower quadrant
    d. Red-tinged sputum and urine

DOSE CALCULATION QUESTIONS

31. The nurse is preparing to administer rifampin 420 mg intravenously. The solution was prepared by dissolving 600 mg of powdered rifampin in 10 mL of sterile water. Seven milliliters of the prepared solution was added to a 500-mL intravenous (IV) bag of 5% dextrose. The infusion is to run over 3 hours. What is the hourly rate of infusion that the nurse should program into the IV infusion pump?

32. The safe dose of cycloserine (Seromycin Pulvules) is 10-20 mg/kg per day. An 88-lb child is prescribed a 250-mg capsule twice a day. Is the dose safe?

CASE STUDIES

Case Study 1

A 36-year-old woman who works as a social worker and has sole custody of her two children is prescribed rifampin, isoniazid, ethambutol, and pyrazinamide after being diagnosed with active TB.

1. Why is therapy for active infection always initiated with at least two drugs?

2. What information should the nurse provide to ensure that these medications are taken exactly as prescribed?

3. What obstacles might this patient face regarding compliance with drug therapy?

4. What will be necessary to determine the effectiveness of drug therapy?

5. The public health nurse is consulted regarding the need to identify all of the people who share facilities with the patient to screen them for TB and prophylactically treat the individuals without active infection with isoniazid. Why is it essential to treat TB contacts prophylactically for TB?

6. When evaluating the contacts associated with an active TB patient, what considerations are made to determine whether they are candidates for isoniazid prophylactic therapy?

7. What is the drug of choice as the primary agent for treatment and prophylaxis of TB, and why is this true?

8. Two months into therapy, the nurse is reviewing laboratory results for the original patient, which include ALT 65 international units/L, AST 80 units/L, total bilirubin 0.3 mg/dL, creatinine 0.8 mg/dL, and uric acid 12 mg/dL. What questions should the nurse ask this patient?

9. What organ function is the nurse most concerned about when a patient is taking this combination of drugs? What symptoms would suggest this adverse effect?

10. What are the benefits of directly observed therapy (DOT) for this patient?

11. What interventions could the public nurse implement to improve compliance with drug therapy with this patient?

12. If this patient were found to be HIV-positive, what drug-drug interactions may occur between the TB drug regimen and his HIV drug therapy?

13. The nurse is evaluating the patient when he comes in for DOT. The patient reports vision changes in which he feels like he is looking through a tunnel. What could possibly be causing this visual change? What should the nurse do?

14. The nurse is writing a letter to a legislator because of proposed cuts to funding for health care that would affect patients with TB. What could the nurse include in the letter to justify the expense of the government providing assistance for people who cannot afford to pay for therapy for TB?

Case Study 2

A 45-year-old man who is homeless comes to the emergency department with weight loss, lethargy, a low-grade fever, and a productive cough streaked with blood. His chest x-ray indicates a suspicious area in the middle right lobe. He is hospitalized, and sputum cultures are ordered. The sputum cultures reveal *M. tuberculosis*. His active TB is to be treated with a combination of drugs based on the sputum culture drug sensitivity. The patient is started on isoniazid, ethambutol, and pyrazinamide in the initial phase of therapy.

91

Miscellaneous Antibacterial Drugs: Fluoroquinolones, Metronidazole, Daptomycin, Rifampin, Rifaximin, Bacitracin, and Polymyxins

STUDY QUESTIONS

Completion

1. An unusual adverse effect of fluoroquinolones is _____ rupture.

2. Resistance has become common in _____; therefore, these drugs are no longer recommended for this infection.

3. Ciprofloxacin (Cipro) is not useful against infections caused by _____.

4. Fluoroquinolones pose a risk of _____.

5. The most common site of tendonitis from a fluoroquinolone is the _____.

CRITICAL THINKING, PRIORITIZATION, AND DELEGATION QUESTIONS

✳ 6. The nurse is preparing to administer IV ciprofloxacin to a patient with septic arthritis after arthroscopic surgery. It would be a priority to review which ordered diagnostic test result as soon as it is available?
   a. Culture and sensitivity (C&S)
   b. MRI
   c. Urinalysis
   d. X-ray

✳ 7. The nurse assesses a 6-year-old child who is receiving ciprofloxacin (Cipro) for a complicated UTI. What is a priority concern?
   a. Abdominal pain
   b. Fluid and electrolyte balance
   c. Nutrition
   d. Skin integrity

8. All patients are at risk for developing tendon rupture when prescribed a fluoroquinolone. Which patients have an increased risk? (Select all that apply.)
   a. Older adult patients
   b. Patients who frequently take antacids for heartburn
   c. Patients who are prescribed calcium supplements for osteopenia
   d. Patients who are prescribed glucocorticoids
   e. Patients who are post-solid organ transplantation

9. Which situation would warrant assessing for candida infection when the nurse is caring for a 6-month-old, breast-fed infant who is prescribed ciprofloxacin for pyelonephritis?
   a. Parents supplement breast milk with rice cereal.
   b. Infant has stool after every feeding.
   c. Infant's stool is mushy and seedy.
   d. Infant's suckling is interrupted by crying.

▶10. A consulting urologist orders ciprofloxacin 250 mg twice a day for a 72-year-old woman with a UTI. The patient is also receiving ferrous sulfate 300 mg for anemia and calcium carbonate 400 mg 4 times a day for osteopenia. What should the nurse do?
   a. Administer the ciprofloxacin 1 hour before the other medications.
   b. Administer the ciprofloxacin 2 hours after the other medications.
   c. Consult with the prescriber for directions.
   d. Hold the ferrous sulfate and calcium during ciprofloxacin therapy.

▶11. The nurse is administering ciprofloxacin (Cipro) to a patient who receives theophylline for asthma. Because of potential drug interactions, the nurse should monitor theophylline levels and assess for
   a. constipation.
   b. drowsiness.
   c. tachycardia.
   d. weakness.

12. A common symptom of suprainfection that can occur with extended ciprofloxacin therapy is
    a. circumoral cyanosis.
    b. high fever.
    c. pinpoint maculopapular rash.
    d. white patches in the mouth.

►13. Which assessment finding suggests hypokalemia and should be reported to the prescriber of moxifloxacin (Avelox)?
    a. Confusion and irritability
    b. Constipation and weakness
    c. Diarrhea and vomiting
    d. Tremor and numbness

14. When a patient is prescribed a fluoroquinolone that is known to cause prolongation of the QT interval on ECG, the nurse should monitor the electrolytes for which result that is most likely to increase the risk of this adverse effect? (Select all that apply.)
    a. Chloride less than 98 mEq/L
    b. Magnesium less than 1.3 mEq/L
    c. Potassium less than 3.5 mEq/L
    d. Sodium less than 135 mEq/L

15. Which goal is most appropriate when a patient is prescribed metronidazole (Flagyl) for *C. difficile* (CDAD)?
    a. Clear lung sounds
    b. No burning on urination
    c. Soft, formed stool
    d. Temperature within normal limits

16. The nurse finds the pharmacy-prepared minibag of metronidazole in the patient's medication drawer and notes that it has been mixed to a concentration of 5 mg/mL. What should the nurse do?
    a. Administer the drug.
    b. Discard the solution and get a new bag from the pharmacy.
    c. Dilute the solution to a 2.5 mg/mL solution.
    d. Return the bag to the pharmacy and request a refrigerated preparation.

17. The nurse is preparing to administer daptomycin. When should the nurse withhold the medication and contact the prescriber?
    a. If the patient is diagnosed with MRSA of the skin.
    b. If the patient's INR is 1.8.
    c. If the patient reports sudden severe muscle pain.
    d. If peak and trough plasma levels have not been ordered.

18. A nursing measure to prevent the most common adverse effect of daptomycin (Cubicin) is to
    a. include increased fiber and fluids in the patient's diet.
    b. dim the lights in the patient's room.
    c. elevate the patient's IV site.
    d. limit noise in the halls during the night.

19. Which isoenzyme of CPK would be most helpful when monitoring for the most common serious adverse effect if a patient is prescribed daptomycin (Cubicin) and simvastatin (Zocor)?
    a. CPK
    b. CPK-BB
    c. CPK-MB
    d. CPK-MM

20. The prescriber has asked the nurse to provide teaching for a 34-year-old female patient who has requested a prescription for rifaximin (Xifaxan) before a trip to Central America. Teaching should include not administering the drug if the patient experiences what issue? (Select all that apply.)
    a. Amenorrhea
    b. Bloody stool
    c. Fever
    d. Flatulence
    e. Nausea

DOSE CALCULATION QUESTIONS

21. The drug handbook states that the therapeutic dose of metronidazole is 7.5 mg/kg every 6 hours. A child is prescribed IV metronidazole (Flagyl) 500 mg in 100 mL D₅W every 6 hours. The child is 5'6" and weighs 145 lb. Is the dose safe and effective?

22. A prophylactic dose of 1 g of metronidazole (Flagyl) IV is ordered for a patient who weighs 176 lb. The recommended dose is 15 mg/kg. Is the dose safe?

CASE STUDIES

Case Study 1

A 68-year-old female patient returns to her prescriber after taking 10 days of ampicillin for her upper respiratory infection. She continues with a low-grade fever and does not seem to have improved. She has a productive cough and thick secretions. Her x-ray does not indicate pneumonia. The patient has a history of atrial fibrillation, for which she takes an anticoagulant. She is given ciprofloxacin 250 mg, orally, 2 times a day for 7 more days. The patient's nurse wants to be sure she understands this medication.

1. What in the patient's history may contribute to potential drug-drug interactions?

2. What foods should the patient avoid when taking oral ciprofloxacin?

3. The patient calls the prescriber's office in 2 days to report that she is much better. She asks whether she can stop taking the medication since it is so expensive and she is improving so much. How should the nurse respond?

4. What new problem might the patient develop while taking this antibiotic?

Case Study 2

A 15-year-old male patient is admitted to the nursing unit after emergency surgery for a ruptured appendix. He is prescribed IV metronidazole (Flagyl) 500 mg in 100 mL D_5W every 6 hours and ampicillin/sulbactam (Unasyn) 1.5 g (in 50 mL NSS) every 8 hours. Both are to run at a rate of 100 mL per hour.

5. Metronidazole is scheduled at 0000-0600-1200-1800 at a rate of 100 mL/hr. Ampicillin/sulbactam is scheduled at 0600-1400-2200. Which would the nurse administer first at 0600, and when would the nurse start each drug?

6. What procedures need to be followed when administering these drugs?

7. Because the family delayed seeking treatment for their child's abdominal pain and GI bacteria were expelled into the peritoneum, the nurse would monitor for what symptoms that suggest the bacteria have invaded the retroperitoneal region?

92
Antifungal Agents

STUDY QUESTIONS

Completion

1. The term for fungal disease is
   _____.

2. *Superficial* means _____.

3. *Systemic* means _____
   _____ _____.

True or False

For each of the following statements, enter T *for true or* F *for false.*

4. ____ Amphotericin B can bind to cholesterol in human cell membranes causing toxicity.

5. ____ Amphotericin B damages the kidneys.

6. ____ Amphotericin B doses must be decreased if initial creatinine clearance is less than 40 mL/min.

7. ____ Amphotericin B is rarely associated with fungal resistance.

8. ___ Amphotericin B has broad-spectrum bacteri-cidal activity.

9. ___ Amphotericin B is only used for systemic fungal infections.

10. ___ Amphotericin B is the best drug for systemic fungal infections despite the potential for toxicity.

11. ___ Amphotericin B readily penetrates the central nervous system (CNS).

12. ___ Amphotericin B remains in human tissue more than a year after treatment is discontinued.

Matching

Match the fungal infection to its site of occurrence.

13. ___ Body
14. ___ Foot
15. ___ Groin
16. ___ Scalp

a. Tinea capitis
b. Tinea corporis
c. Tinea cruris
d. Tinea pedis

CRITICAL THINKING, PRIORITIZATION, AND DELEGATION QUESTIONS

17. When administering drugs that are potentially nephrotoxic, the nurse should consult the prescriber before administering which over-the-counter (OTC) drug(s)?
    a. Antacids
    b. Acetaminophen
    c. NSAIDs
    d. Laxatives

18. At what point is the patient most likely to experience fever, chills, rigors, nausea, and headache when receiving amphotericin B?
    a. Immediately after the infusion begins
    b. 20-30 minutes after the infusion begins
    c. 1-3 hours after the infusion begins
    d. 3-6 hours after the infusion begins

19. A patient experiences sudden episodes of shaking chills after receiving a dose of amphotericin B. Which drug, ordered as-needed for this patient, should the nurse administer at this time?
    a. Acetaminophen (Tylenol)
    b. Dantrolene (Dantrium)
    c. Diphenhydramine (Benadryl)
    d. Lorazepam (Ativan)

20. How does dantrolene relieve rigors and fever associated with amphotericin B infusion?
    a. Blocking the action of amphotericin B
    b. Counteracting an allergic reaction
    c. Decreasing the set point of temperature in the hypothalamus
    d. Relaxing muscles and preventing shivering

✱21. The nurse is reviewing laboratory tests before preparing to administer a dose of amphotericin B. Before administering the drug, it is a priority to review which lab result?
    a. Creatinine levels
    b. ECG
    c. Liver function tests
    d. WBC count

22. Which laboratory results of an adult male patient suggest bone marrow suppression caused by amphotericin B?
    a. Hemoglobin 10 g/dL; hematocrit 30%; MCV 110 mcg³; MCH 28 pg/cell
    b. Hemoglobin 10 g/dL; hematocrit 30%; MCV 67 mcg³; MCH 30 pg/cell
    c. Hemoglobin 10 g/dL; hematocrit 30%; MCV 89 mcg³; MCH 28 pg/cell
    d. Hemoglobin 10 g/dL; hematocrit 30%; MCV 105 mcg³; MCH 20 pg/cell

23. A patient with a systemic fungal infection is prescribed amphotericin B and flucytosine. The nurse expects what drug interaction?
    a. Decreased risk of amphotericin toxicity
    b. Increased risk of renal damage
    c. Increased risk of rigor
    d. Needing a higher dose of amphotericin B

24. What is true of itraconazole (Sporanox)?
    a. It is always administered intravenously (IV).
    b. It is capable of impairing liver metabolism of other drugs.
    c. It is effective against more fungi than amphotericin.
    d. It is nephrotoxic.

25. To achieve maximum absorption of itraconazole (Sporanox) capsules, the nurse administers the drug with which liquid?
    a. Apple juice
    b. Milk
    c. Cola
    d. Water

∗26. The nurse is reviewing test results for a patient who is prescribed itraconazole (Sporanox). Which result would warrant immediate consultation with the prescriber?
   a. AST 35 international units/L
   b. BNP 745 pg/mL
   c. Echocardiogram—ejection fraction 60%
   d. Potassium 3.8 mEq/L

27. The nurse is administering itraconazole (Sporanox) to a patient who also is prescribed simvastatin (Zocor). Because of the effect of itraconazole on hepatic isoenzyme CYP3A4, the combination increases the risk of rhabdomyolysis from the -statin drug. The nurse should monitor the patient for what symptoms?
   a. Bleeding and bruising
   b. Hypoglycemia and tremors
   c. Hypotension and dizziness
   d. Muscle pain and dark urine

28. Which drug may prevent absorption of itraconazole (Sporanox), no matter when it is administered?
   a. Cyclosporin (Sandimmune)
   b. Digoxin (Lanoxin)
   c. Esomeprazole (Nexium)
   d. Ranitidine (Zantac)

∗29. It would be a priority to report which symptoms in a patient who is prescribed the -azole antifungal drug fluconazole (Diflucan)?
   a. Abdominal pain and diarrhea
   b. Fever and blisters in the mouth
   c. Headache and photophobia
   d. Nausea and vomiting

30. The nurse reviews the laboratory results of a female patient who is prescribed voriconazole (Vfend) 200 mg by mouth. Which laboratory result warrants withholding the drug and immediately notifying the prescriber?
   a. AST 37 international units/L
   b. FBG 222 mg/dL
   c. Hgb 11.8 g/dL
   d. hCG 172 international units/mL

31. A patient who has been receiving ketoconazole for 5 days experiences nausea and vomiting. What should be the initial response of the nurse?
   a. Administer the medication with food.
   b. Assess the skin, abdomen, urine, and stool.
   c. Consult the prescriber.
   d. Withhold the medication.

∗32. A patient is prescribed posaconazole (Noxafil) for thrush (oral candidiasis) that occurred after treatment of pneumonia with IV antibiotics. It would be of greatest priority to promptly inform the prescriber if drug reconciliation reveals that the patient takes which drug(s) for cluster headaches?
   a. Aspirin, acetaminophen, caffeine (Excedrin Migraine)
   b. Dihydroergotamine (Migranal)
   c. Ibuprofen (Motrin IB)
   d. Sumatriptan (Imitrex)

33. What is the first thing the nurse should do when preparing to administer caspofungin (Cancidas)?
   a. Assess the IV site.
   b. Check the dose provided with the dose ordered.
   c. Reconstitute the drug in sterile saline.
   d. Prime the IV tubing.

34. The nurse would be concerned that a patient who is receiving micafungin (Mycamine) is experiencing a histamine reaction and might have an anaphylactic reaction if the patient reports a sudden feeling of
   a. bloating.
   b. headache.
   c. itching.
   d. nausea.

35. The nurse reviews the CBC of a patient who is prescribed flucytosine (Ancobon) and notes neutrophils 27%. This patient is especially at risk for which issue?
   a. Fatigue
   b. Fluid volume deficit
   c. Impaired skin integrity
   d. Infection

36. The medication administration record lists a clotrimazole troche to be administered at 0900. The nurse administers this medication by
   a. applying it to the skin.
   b. dissolving it in 8 ounces of water.
   c. instructing the patient to chew it.
   d. instructing the patient to let it dissolve in the mouth.

37. A postoperative patient who had knee replacement surgery is prescribed Lovenox to prevent clot formation related to immobility. The patient develops candidiasis under the breasts and in the groin. The prescriber orders miconazole cream. What should the nurse do?
    a. Administer both the Lovenox and miconazole and monitor INR.
    b. Administer the Lovenox, but consult the prescriber regarding the miconazole.
    c. Administer the miconazole but consult the prescriber regarding the Lovenox.
    d. Withhold both the Lovenox and miconazole and consult the prescriber.

38. What is a potential problem of patients' self-prescribing OTC miconazole for vaginal discharge?
    a. Local irritation
    b. Systemic toxicity
    c. The cause may not be a yeast infection
    d. The treatment is usually not effective

DOSE CALCULATION QUESTIONS

39. The nurse is preparing to administer anidulafungin (Eraxis) 100 mg IV to a patient with esophageal candidiasis. The drug books states a 100-mg vial is reconstituted with 30 mL sterile water yielding a concentration of 3.33 mg/mL, then further diluted in 100 mL of 0.9% normal saline. The infusion is to run over 90 minutes. The IV pump should be set to run at how many mL/hr?

40. The drug book recommends after a successful test dose that the first dose of amphotericin B should be 0.25 mg/kg of drug. The patient weighs 110 lb. The prescriber has ordered 12 mg. Is this a safe dose?

CASE STUDIES

Case Study 1

A 25-year-old female patient was recently diagnosed with acute myelogenous leukemia (AML). She is admitted for the induction phase of chemotherapy. Her platelet count is low, and she has vaginal candidiasis. OTC topical treatments for vaginal candidiasis are available.

1. What problems might this produce?

2. The treatment of choice for this patient's fungal infection is clotrimazole. It is essential that extreme care be taken in providing nursing care to this patient because she is at high risk for additional infections that could now be lethal. The nurse must consider many areas when treatment includes combining the treatment for fungus with the numerous other physical problems a patient with AML faces. What possible adverse effects of intravaginal clotrimazole vaginal suppositories should the nurse instruct this patient to report?

3. The patient asks why she must use the vaginal suppositories when she already has an IV for chemotherapy administration. What should the nurse tell her?

4. The patient's fungal infection has advanced because of her severely immunocompromised state. She now has systemic mycoses requiring amphotericin B for treatment. All of her medications must be carefully evaluated to determine whether they are toxic. What system is almost always damaged in some way by amphotericin B and can increase the risk of toxicity of other drugs?

5. What intervention can the nurse employ to reduce the risk of kidney damage by amphotericin B?

6. Why is it important for the prescriber to first order a 1-mg test dose of amphotericin B (Fungizone) before starting full therapy?

7. Amphotericin B vial is supplied as a powder for reconstitution using sterile water that does not contain a bacteriostatic agent. Why must the drug be mixed in sterile water without a bacteriostatic agent?

8. What nursing measures should the nurse take when infusing amphotericin to prevent infusion-related adverse effects?

9. What teaching does the nurse need to provide this patient regarding drug therapy?

Case Study 2

A 42-year-old male truck driver has been prescribed voriconazole (Vfend) for esophageal candidiasis secondary to immune deficiency caused by HIV.

10. Why is this patient more at risk for hepatotoxicity and drug interactions than the average person?

93

Antiviral Agents I: Drugs for Non-HIV Viral Infections

STUDY QUESTIONS

True or False

For each of the following statements, enter T *for true or* F *for false.*

1. ____ It is hard to develop antiviral drugs that do not harm human tissue.
2. ____ Oral acyclovir will cure active herpes labialis (cold sore).
3. ____ Oral therapy with acyclovir is only effective for varicella (chickenpox) if dosing is begun within 24 hours of rash onset.
4. ____ IV acyclovir should administered slowly, be in a large volume of fluid, and the patient should be well-hydrated.
5. ____ It is possible to spread the infection when applying acyclovir (Zovirax) ointment.
6. ____ Research suggests valacyclovir eliminates the risk of transmitting genital herpes between monogamous heterosexual partners.
7. ____ It is important to teach a patient who is prescribed valacyclovir to report unexpected bruising.
8. ____ Valacyclovir should not be administered to a person who is also prescribed a drug that causes bone marrow suppression.

9. ____ Famciclovir decreases the number of episodes of postherpetic neuralgia associated with herpes zoster (shingles).
10. ____ Penciclovir (Denavir) and docosanol (Abreva) topical preparations decrease the duration of pain of cold sores by 50%.

CRITICAL THINKING, PRIORITIZATION, AND DELEGATION QUESTIONS

11. A college student who has been diagnosed with her first genital herpes infection is discussing the disorder and prescribed topical acyclovir treatment with the college health center nurse. Which statement, if made by the patient, would suggest that the patient needs teaching about this disorder and drug therapy?
    a. "I can get a different infection in the sores if I am not careful about cleaning after having a bowel movement."
    b. "I should use gloves when applying the ointment, immediately dispose of them, then wash my hands because I can spread the infection to other parts of my body."
    c. "I should not have sex when sores are present."
    d. "Using the ointment as soon as I get a sore will stop the outbreak."

12. What should the nurse teach regarding condom use to a patient who is currently in a long-term committed monogamous relationship and who has been prescribed continuous oral acyclovir therapy for recurrent genital herpes?
    a. Condoms prevent the spread of infection, even during active outbreaks.
    b. Use a condom if any symptoms of outbreak are present.
    c. Use a condom with every sexual contact except if conception is desired; conception should be planned when symptoms are absent.
    d. Your partner is already infected, so condom use does not matter.

*13. Which action by the nurse would be a priority for preventing the most common complications of intravenous (IV) acyclovir (Zovirax) therapy?
    a. Assessing the IV site before infusing the drug
    b. Ensuring a fluid intake of 2500 to 3000 mL/24 hr
    c. Reporting vomiting to the prescriber
    d. Teaching perineal hygiene

*14. The nurse is preparing to administer intravenous acyclovir. It would be a priority for the nurse to provide nursing interventions for which assessment finding?
    a. BP 150/85 mm Hg
    b. Creatinine 0.9 mg/dL
    c. Dry, sticky oral mucous membranes
    d. Eight-hour urine output 750 mL

15. It would be a priority to report which laboratory result to the prescriber if a patient is prescribed valacyclovir (Valtrex)?
    a. CD4 less than 100/mm³
    b. Hgb (Hb) 11 g/dL
    c. Platelets 220,000/mm³
    d. WBC 12,800/mm³

16. The nurse is preparing to administer famciclovir (Famvir) 500 mg prescribed orally once a day to a patient admitted with exacerbated chronic obstructive pulmonary disease (COPD) who has developed shingles. The nurse reviews laboratory test results that include eGFR 35 mL/min. What should the nurse do at this time?
    a. Administer the drug as ordered.
    b. Consult the prescriber STAT regarding timing of doses.
    c. Consult the prescriber STAT regarding the need for more laboratory tests.
    d. Withhold the drug and consult the prescriber during her next hospital rounds.

17. The nurse would withhold ganciclovir and notify the prescriber if patient laboratory test results included
    a. BUN 20 mg/dL.
    b. hCG 2775 mIU/mL.
    c. neutrophils 2000/mm³.
    d. platelets 75,000/mm³.

18. The nurse is discussing planned care with the CNA who is assigned to a patient receiving ganciclovir. Because of possible serious adverse effects, which precaution would the nurse include in instructions regarding care?
    a. Do not provide any food 1 hour before or 2 hours after drug administration.
    b. Elevate all four side rails.
    c. Turn and reposition the patient every 2 hours.
    d. Use an electric razor to shave the patient.

19. Which step is most important for a female nurse to follow when administering valganciclovir?
    a. Administer with the patient in an upright position.
    b. Assess vital signs before administering the drug.
    c. Avoid touching the drug.
    d. Dissolve the drug completely in 8 ounces of water or juice.

20. Laboratory results for a patient who is prescribed foscarnet (Foscavir) include FBS 90 mg/dL, AST 87 units/L, potassium 3.6 mEq/L, calcium 8.4 mg/dL, and magnesium 2 mEq/L. The nurse should assess for what symptom of electrolyte imbalance?
    a. Cool, clammy skin
    b. Headache
    c. Muscle spasms
    d. Thirst

21. When explaining prescribed pegylated interferon (peginterferon), the nurse should include which information about the drug that makes it different from conventional interferon?
    a. It can be administered orally.
    b. It prevents relapse when discontinued.
    c. It produces fewer adverse effects.
    d. It produces more consistent therapeutic blood levels.

22. When administering adefovir (Hepsera), which assessment would suggest that therapy could be toxic?
    a. Decreased sperm count
    b. Nausea
    c. Oliguria
    d. Yellow-colored sclera

23. It is important for the nurse to assess for suicidal ideation if a patient is prescribed which drug?
    a. Interferon alfa
    b. Lamivudine
    c. Ribavirin
    d. Valacyclovir

24. Which assessment finding would be of greatest priority to report to the prescriber if identified in a patient who is receiving lamivudine (Epivir HBV), adefovir (Hepsera), or entecavir (Baraclude) for hepatitis B because it suggests possible lactic acidosis?
    a. Deep, rapid breathing
    b. Fever
    c. Poor appetite
    d. Nausea

25. A patient is prescribed adefovir (Hepsera) 10 mg by mouth once a day. Results of recent laboratory tests include CrCl 62 mL/min. What nursing action is warranted?
    a. Administer the medication as prescribed.
    b. Consult the prescriber regarding the need for dose reduction.
    c. Withhold the medication and contact the prescriber immediately.
    d. Request dosing be changed to every other day.

26. The nurse is reviewing the chart of a patient prescribed telbivudine (Tyzeka). The nurse would consult the prescriber if what is noted?
    a. ALT increased from 287 to 350 IU/L in the past year
    b. Evidence of active HBV replication
    c. HBV, acute episode, recently diagnosed
    d. Patient is 17 years old

▶ 27. The nurse would be concerned about administering live flu vaccine to which patient?
    a. 7-year-old boy with a seizure disorder
    b. 12-year-old girl receiving aspirin for its cardioprotective effects
    c. 28-year-old man with type 1 diabetes
    d. 38-year-old woman with multiple sclerosis

28. It would be logical that which population(s) should not receive the LAIV (FluMist) because it is a live attenuated virus and is administered by spraying into the respiratory tract? (Select all that apply.)
    a. Children or adolescents receiving aspirin therapy
    b. Children younger than 5 years of age who have had recurrent episodes of wheezing with respiratory infections
    c. People who are HIV-positive
    d. People prescribed disease-modifying antirheumatic drugs for rheumatoid arthritis
    e. People with asthma

29. The nurse is aware that the most significant factor in determining the effectiveness of oseltamivir (Tamiflu) in treating influenza is
    a. administration with food.
    b. influenza A is the causative organism.
    c. starting therapy as soon as symptoms occur.
    d. vaccination for influenza has already been administered.

30. Which new assessment finding would be most significant if noted in an infant who is receiving inhaled ribavirin for RSV?
    a. Coarse rhonchi (gurgles) in upper airways
    b. Pulse 120 beats/min
    c. Respirations 30 breaths per minute
    d. Wheezing throughout lung fields

DOSE CALCULATION QUESTIONS

31. The recommended dose of acyclovir for immunocompetent children under 12 years is 15-20 mg/kg/day divided in three doses. What is the safe dose range for a child who weighs 44 pounds?

32. Foscarnet 7.2 grams is prescribed. The drug must be diluted in how much fluid if it is to be infused via a peripheral IV line?

CASE STUDIES

Case Study 1

A 32-year-old female patient with chronic HCV has just had boceprevir added to therapy with interferon alfa and ribavirin.

1. What instructions should the nurse provide regarding administration of this drug?

2. Why is it important to discuss sexual activity with this patient?

3. How should the nurse respond?

4. What intervention would be most important for the school nurse to emphasize when discussing with the teacher prevention of becoming infected with influenza from active cases or live vaccine?

Case Study 2

The public health nurse receives a call from a school nurse questioning whether a child who received intranasal LAIV (FluMist) should be in school. The nurse is concerned because the child's teacher is pregnant.

94

Antiviral Agents II: Drugs for HIV Infection and Related Opportunistic Infections

STUDY QUESTIONS

Matching

Match the drug to its mechanism of action.

1. ___ Efavirenz
2. ___ Enfuvirtide
3. ___ Maraviroc
4. ___ Raltegravir
5. ___ Ritonavir
6. ___ Zidovudine

a. Binds with CCR5, thereby blocking viral entry into CD4 cells.
b. Prevents the HIV envelope from fusing with the cell membrane of CD4 cells, thereby blocking viral entry and replication.
c. Suppresses synthesis of viral DNA, thereby blocking growth of the viral DNA strand.
d. Binds directly to HIV reverse transcriptase disrupting the active center of the enzyme, thereby suppressing enzyme activity.
e. Prevents insertion of HIV DNA genetic material into the DNA of CD4 cells, thereby stopping HIV replication.
f. Inhibits CYP3A4 metabolism, thereby raising lopinavir levels and enhancing antiviral actions.

CRITICAL THINKING, PRIORITIZATION, AND DELEGATION QUESTIONS

7. The nurse is teaching a patient about the need for multiple-drug therapy for HIV. Which statement, if made by the patient, would indicate a need for further teaching?
   a. "If I don't take all of the drugs as prescribed, the virus is more likely to become resistant to drugs."
   b. "The higher the number of viruses in my body, the greater the chance one will become resistant."
   c. "The virus recognizes the antibiotic and is able to change to prevent being destroyed."
   d. "When the HIV is changing RNA into DNA within the host cell, genetic changes can occur spontaneously."

8. The prescriber has informed a patient who has been prescribed a nucleoside/nucleotide reverse transcriptase inhibitor (NRTI) of the risk of hepatic steatosis. The patient asks the nurse "What is hepatic steatosis?" The nurse should explain that this is a possible severe adverse effect involving
   a. fatty degeneration of the liver.
   b. increased secretions of glands.
   c. infection of the liver.
   d. stools that are foamy and float.

✴ 9. An HIV-positive patient is prescribed trimethoprim-sulfamethoxazole for a urinary tract infection (UTI). A priority nursing action is to monitor which laboratory test(s)? (Select all that apply.)
a. AST and ALT
b. BUN and creatinine
c. CBC and differential
d. Electrolytes
e. Lipids
f. PT and INR

10. A patient has received instructions regarding administration of didanosine (Videx EC). Which statement made by the patient would indicate the patient understood the directions?
a. "I can sprinkle the powder on applesauce."
b. "I need to notify the prescriber if I cannot swallow this capsule whole."
c. "I should keep the medicine in my bathroom medicine cabinet so I remember to take it every morning."
d. "I should take this drug with meals."

11. Which nursing assessment finding would be most significant if a patient was receiving didanosine?
a. Flatulence
b. Headache
c. Itching
d. Vomiting

✴12. A patient who is prescribed highly active antiretroviral therapy (HAART) including rilpivirine reports loss of interest in usual activities. Which nursing action is of greatest priority?
a. Asking about difficulties complying with therapy.
b. Assessing for thoughts of harming self.
c. Identifying reasons for loss of interest.
d. Providing a safe environment.

13. A patient receiving HAART develops a sore throat and cough. The nurse should consult the prescriber immediately if the therapy includes which drug?
a. Abacavir (Ziagen)
b. Didanosine (Videx)
c. Stavudine (Zerit)
d. Zidovudine (Retrovir)

14. When planning nursing interventions and teaching for the most common adverse effects of efavirenz (Sustiva), which nursing problem should be the focus for the nurse?
a. Circulation
b. Nutrition
c. Safety
d. Skin integrity

15. When a patient who is receiving nevirapine (Viramune) or delavirdine (Rescriptor) complains of conjunctivitis or muscle and joint pain, it would be a priority to assess for
a. dizziness.
b. nausea.
c. paresthesias.
d. rash.

16. An HIV-positive patient who has recently been prescribed HAART, including the NNRTI efavirenz, calls the prescriber's office and reports experiencing drowsiness and dizziness. An appropriate recommendation by the telephone triage nurse is for the patient to do what?
a. Discontinue all drugs and make an appointment to be seen as soon as possible.
b. Discontinue taking efavirenz, but continue the other drugs in the regimen.
c. Use safety precautions and take efavirenz at bedtime.
d. Use safety precautions and take efavirenz with food.

17. Weight-bearing exercise and adequate calcium intake are most important if HAART includes a
a. fusion inhibitor.
b. nucleoside/nucleotide reverse transcriptase inhibitor (NRTI).
c. nonnucleoside reverse transcriptase inhibitor (NNRTI).
d. protease inhibitor (PI).

18. The nurse would be most concerned that a patient may not adhere to HAART therapy with which class of antiviral drugs if the patient verbalized that body image is an important priority?
a. Fusion inhibitor
b. Nucleoside/nucleotide reverse transcriptase inhibitor (NRTI)
c. Nonnucleoside reverse transcriptase inhibitor (NNRTI)
d. Protease inhibitor (PI)

19. The nurse is aware that the HIV-seropositive community often shares the belief that garlic supplementation decreases HIV reproduction and boosts the immune system. This belief can be particularly dangerous if the patient is prescribed which drug?
a. Indinavir
b. Lopinavir
c. Nelfinavir
d. Saquinavir

20. Patients who are prescribed protease inhibitors (PI) should be instructed to not self-prescribe the herbal product St. John's wort. What is the possible effect of this combination?
    a. Increase in metabolism and excretion of the PI
    b. Increase in likelihood of suicidal ideation
    c. Increase in likelihood of toxicity from the PI
    d. MAO inhibitor effects of the St. John's wort

21. What is not a known reaction if a patient who is taking the oral solution of lopinavir/ritonavir is also prescribed metronidazole (Flagyl)?
    a. Difficulty breathing
    b. Headache
    c. Hypertension
    d. Nausea and vomiting

22. A hospitalized HIV-positive patient who is prescribed indinavir (Crixivan) complains of sharp, colicky flank pain. In addition to notifying the prescriber, which nursing intervention would be most appropriate?
    a. Assess bowel sounds.
    b. Elevate the head of the bed.
    c. Increase VS to every 4 hours.
    d. Strain urine.

23. Which drug must be taken 12 hours apart from rilpivirine?
    a. Buffered aspirin (Bufferin)
    b. Calcium carbonate (TUMS)
    c. Omeprazole (Prilosec)
    d. Ranitidine (Zantac)

24. What are known adverse effects of raltegravir (Isentress)? (Select all that apply.)
    a. Facial edema and angioedema
    b. Flulike symptoms
    c. Loss of bone density
    d. Painful rash that blisters followed by shedding of the epidermis
    e. Teratogenesis

*25. It would be of greatest priority to consult the prescriber of enfuvirtide (Fuzeon) if the patient experienced
    a. headache.
    b. pain and tenderness at injection site.
    c. positive pregnancy test.
    d. muscle weakness in legs and arms.

26. Which action, when administering enfuvirtide (Fuzeon), would increase the risk of a severe injection-site reaction?
    a. Injecting the drug deep into a muscle.
    b. Not adequately cleaning the injection site.
    c. Reconstituting the drug in sterile water.
    d. Refrigerating the solution for 2 hours after reconstituting.

27. An HIV-positive patient who is receiving HAART, including maraviroc (Selzentry), reports to the nurse that he has vomited and is experiencing severe abdominal pain. Assessment reveals a generalized pruritic rash. Which action is appropriate?
    a. Obtain an order for diphenhydramine (Benadryl) for the itching.
    b. Withhold all prescribed drugs and contact the prescriber.
    c. Withhold all food and fluids until the source of the abdominal pain is identified.
    d. Withhold the maraviroc (Selzentry) and contact the prescriber.

28. What is the most important role of the nurse when treatment failure occurs?
    a. Identifying factors that may have contributed to treatment failure
    b. Identifying the patient's immune status
    c. Supporting the patient emotionally
    d. Teaching the new drug regimen

29. Principles of treating HIV-seropositive pregnant women include (Select all that apply.)
    a. prophylaxis is recommended for the infant/neonate.
    b. benefits of treatment normally outweigh risks.
    c. HAART should not be used during pregnancy.
    d. the drugs are not teratogenic.
    e the drug regimen should only include one drug at a time.

30. When emptying a urinal from an HIV-seropositive patient, the nurse splashes urine on intact skin. What should the nurse do?
    a. Go to the emergency department (ED) at the end of the shift for bloodwork.
    b. Immediately go to the ED for initiation of postexposure prophylaxis (PEP).
    c. Make an appointment with a primary care provider to discuss if postexposure prophylaxis (PEP) is appropriate.
    d. Report the incident immediately to a supervisor.

31. Which assessment finding would best indicate that HAART is currently effective?
    a. CD4 T count 400 cells/mm³
    b. Neutrophils 2750/mm³
    c. Plasma HIV RNA below 20-75 copies/mL
    d. WBC 5000/mm³

32. Current recommendations state that antiretroviral therapy for patients with chronic asymptomatic HIV disease should start when the CD4 count drops below what level?
    a. 200 cells/mm³
    b. 350 cells/mm³
    c. 500 cells/mm³
    d. 850 cells/mm³

DOSE CALCULATION QUESTIONS

33. IV zidovudine 120 mg is to be diluted to 4 mg/mL. How much 5% dextrose for injection should be added to the drug?

34. What is the recommended dose of enfuvirtide (Fuzeon) for an 8-year-old child who weighs 44 lb?

CASE STUDY

A 35-year-old male patient has been HIV-seropositive for 12 years. His HAART includes zidovudine. When being interviewed by the nurse during a routine clinic appointment, he complains of declining vision, headaches, and daily temperature elevations. Physical examination findings include multiple enlarged lymph nodes and several white retinal patches.

1. What complications of HIV are likely to be occurring?

2. The patient is diagnosed with CMV retinitis. The treatment of choice for CMV retinitis caused by cytomegalovirus (CMV) is ganciclovir. What concern does the nurse have about the addition of ganciclovir to a drug regimen including zidovudine?

3. The prescriber wants to begin with intravenous therapy. What strategies can the nurse employ when administering intravenous ganciclovir to reduce the risk of and identify possible damage to the patient's renal system?

4. The patient tells the nurse that he has no job or insurance at present. What would the nurse be concerned about?

95

Drug Therapy of Sexually Transmitted Diseases

STUDY QUESTIONS

True or False

For each of the following statements, enter T for true or F for false.

1. ___ More than 1 million cases of *Chlamydia trachomatis* in the U.S. each year are not reported/treated.

2. ___ Annual screening for *Chlamydia trachomatis* is recommended for all sexually active women younger than 25 years.

CRITICAL THINKING, PRIORITIZATION, AND DELEGATION QUESTIONS

3. Where does the nurse obtain the most accurate information about nursing care of sexually transmitted diseases/infections (STDs/STIs)?
   a. The Centers for Disease Control and Prevention
   b. Drug manufacturers
   c. The U.S. Food and Drug Administration
   d. Textbooks

✳ 4. A neonate was delivered vaginally to a mother with an active *Chlamydia trachomatis* infection. Relating to this exposure, what is the priority system when caring for the neonate?
   a. Gastrointestinal
   b. Ophthalmic
   c. Renal
   d. Respiratory

5. Why would doxycycline not be prescribed for a female patient for whom pregnancy status is unknown?
   a. It can damage fetal bones.
   b. It causes nausea.
   c. It is hepatotoxic.
   d. It is not effective 25% of the time.

6. A friend tells the nurse that a sexual partner has informed her that he has gonorrhea. She has a refillable prescription of ciprofloxacin (Cipro) for recurrent cystitis. She tells the nurse she knows that she has used this drug in the past for gonorrhea. What is the most important reason why the nurse should discourage using this ciprofloxacin?
   a. The nurse's friend is likely to develop an allergic reaction to ciprofloxacin (Cipro).
   b. The law requires reporting of gonorrhea infections.
   c. This drug is no longer effective against *Neisseria gonorrhoeae*.
   d. The dose is too low to treat gonorrhea.

7. A patient who is receiving intramuscular (IM) ceftriaxone 1 g once a day for disseminated gonococcal infection complains of a stiff neck. Which of these nursing actions should be performed first?
   a. Assess for history of arthritis.
   b. Complete the nursing assessment.
   c. Consult the prescriber.
   d. Document the finding.

✳ 8. The throat culture of a 6-year-old boy is positive for *Neisseria gonorrhoeae*. What is the nursing priority in this situation?
   a. Assessing for eye exudate.
   b. Calculating the dose of ceftriaxone to be administered.
   c. Ensuring the safety of the child.
   d. Removing the child from his home.

9. A patient is admitted to the hospital with a diagnosis of pelvic inflammatory disease (PID). She asks the nurse why her prescriber has recommended hospitalization and intravenous (IV) antibiotics instead of oral antibiotic therapy at home. What is the basis of the nurse's response?
   a. Inadequately treated PID is more likely to cause scarring of the uterine (fallopian) tubes.
   b. PID is very contagious, and the patient needs to be in isolation.
   c. The recommended antibiotic for PID is available only by IV route.
   d. Women who have PID have a higher incidence of cervical cancer.

10. A 32-year-old woman develops septic arthritis. When obtaining a history, it is important to evaluate for which previous infection?
   a. *Chlamydia trachomatis*
   b. *Neisseria gonorrhoeae*
   c. *Treponema pallidum*
   d. *Trichomonas vaginalis*

✳11. The nurse is caring for a neonate whose mother has an active infection with *Neisseria gonorrhoeae*. A priority nursing outcome for the neonate relating to possible infection during vaginal delivery is that the neonate will
   a. blink in response to direct light shone in the eyes.
   b. breast-feed for 10-15 minutes at least every 3 hours without becoming dyspneic.
   c. have clear breath sounds.
   d. not experience conjunctival discharge.

12. The recommended treatment for acute epididymitis is different depending on the age of the patient because usually
   a. older men have developed a resistance to the antibiotic used for younger men.
   b. the method and organism of infection is different.
   c. younger men have better kidney functioning.
   d. younger men are less likely to adhere to multi-dose therapy.

13. The nurse teaches that the primary cause of recurrent STIs caused by the same organism is failure to
   a. prescribe the correct antibiotic.
   b. seek treatment early in the disease.
   c. take the medication as prescribed.
   d. treat the sexual partner.

14. A 35-year-old woman reports a yellow-green vaginal discharge. She is diagnosed with trichomoniasis and prescribed metronidazole (Flagyl). It is important for the nurse to teach the patient the importance of not consuming
   a. alcohol.
   b. antacids.
   c. grapefruit juice.
   d. milk.

15. Why does clindamycin cream (Clindesse) require only one dose vaginally to treat bacterial vaginosis?
   a. Bacterial vaginosis is not a serious infection.
   b. Clindamycin has a half-life of several days.
   c. The cream adheres to the vaginal mucosa for several days.
   d. The medication immediately kills the infecting microbes.

16. What is a major goal of therapy with famciclovir (Famvir) for genital herpes?
   a. Analgesia
   b. Decreasing length of active episodes
   c. Eradication of the virus
   d. Prevention of superinfections during outbreaks

DOSE CALCULATION QUESTIONS

17. A 7-lb neonate develops *Chlamydia trachomatis* pneumonia following intrapartal exposure. The recommended safe dose of erythromycin succinate for neonates is 50 mg/kg/day divided into 4 doses. What is the safe dose of this drug?

18. Ceftriaxone, 1 g every 12 hours, is prescribed IV for a patient with disseminated gonococcal infection (DGI). It is available to be mixed with 50 mL of D$_5$½ NSS to be administered over 30 minutes. What is the rate of infusion in mL/hr?

CASE STUDY

A sexually active 19-year-old woman presents to the emergency department with a 2-week history of dull bilateral abdominal pain, low back pain, and mucopurulent vaginal discharge with increased pain today. She denies fever, nausea, vomiting, diarrhea, and urinary symptoms. She reports irregular periods since age 13 years. Her last menstrual period was 2 months ago. She does not use any measure of birth control. She was treated at the health department 3 months ago for an "infection" and states that she took the medication when she remembered and did not return for a follow-up examination. She has had two sexual partners in the past 6 months, one of whom was also treated for an infection 3 months ago at the health department. She is unsure whether he was adherent to his treatment plan or whether he is symptomatic at this time. She has no known medication allergies and takes no medication on a regular basis.

Her vital signs are: BP 110/72 mm Hg, pulse 88 beats/min, respirations 20 /min, and temperature 99.4° F. The physician orders a CBC, sedimentation rate, rapid plasma reagin, serum pregnancy, and a catheterized urinalysis. The physician performs abdominal and pelvic examinations and obtains cervical cultures for gonorrhea and chlamydia and specimens for saline and KOH wet preps. The physical examination reveals a soft abdomen, right and left lower quadrant tenderness without rebound, and normal bowel sounds. The pelvic exam reveals mucopurulent vaginal discharge and mild right and left adnexal tenderness with bimanual exam. The laboratory results reveal Hgb 11.1, WBC 7.0, and negative results for urinalysis and pregnancy tests.

After review of the medical history, physical exam, and laboratory results (excluding the cultures), the physician makes a diagnosis of PID. Orders include administering ceftriaxone 250 mg IM now and prescriptions for doxycycline 100 mg twice a day for 14 days, metronidazole 500 mg twice a day for 14 days, and Tylenol #3 1 tablet every 3-4 hours as needed for pain. The patient is told that she will be notified regarding the results of the cultures.

1. Why is it important to determine whether the patient is pregnant before administering doxycycline or tetracycline?

2. The patient is to be observed for 30 minutes after administration of the cephalosporin injection and then discharged home. She is given instructions for bedrest for 2 days with a reexamination in 24-48 hours if the signs and/or symptoms increase or persist. What teaching regarding the prescribed medication and follow-up care should the nurse provide to this patient?

3. Why is it important for the patient to avoid all forms of alcohol?

4. The patient is instructed to inform her sexual partners of the need for examination. The patient's phone number and address are verified for notification purposes. She is also advised that the culture results will be reported to the health department if they are positive, and the health department will then follow up with her. The patient states that she does not understand why she has to inform her sexual partners of her infection and why she has to take all of the medication if she is feeling better in a couple of days. What information and instructions can the nurse provide to the patient to help her understand the importance of adherence to her treatment plan?

5. After completing the teaching, the patient's verbalizations reflect that she still does not recognize the significance of her infection or importance of adhering to therapy. How might this alter the plan of care for this patient?

96

Antiseptics and Disinfectants

STUDY QUESTIONS

Matching

Match the term with its description.

1. ___ Anything used to prevent an infection or disease
2. ___ Harsh chemical used to decontaminate objects
3. ___ Kills germs
4. ___ Prevents germs from reproducing
5. ___ Reduction of contamination to a level compatible with public health standards
6. ___ Anti-infective cleanser that can be applied to living tissue
7. ___ Complete destruction of all microorganisms

a. Antiseptic
b. Disinfectant
c. Germicidal
d. Germistatic
e. Prophylactic
f. Sanitization
g. Sterilization

True or False

It is acceptable to use an alcohol-based handrub to cleanse the hands instead of soap and water in which of the following situations?

8. ___ After contact with an unknown powder present on a patient
9. ___ After eating
10. ___ After removing gloves

11. ___ After setting up a patient for lunch who is in isolation for VRE
12. ___ After setting up a patient for lunch who is in isolation for TB
13. ___ After taking linens into a patient's room
14. ___ After using the restroom
15. ___ Before taking a pulse
16. ___ When the hands have been exposed to wound drainage

CRITICAL THINKING, PRIORITIZATION, AND DELEGATION QUESTIONS

17. Which is an example of sterilization?
    a. Autoclaving surgical instruments
    b. Gowning before entering a room where a patient is in protective isolation
    c. Personal respiratory equipment for tuberculosis (TB)
    d. Standard precautions

18. Which is least significant in preventing a surgical incision-site infection?
    a. Preoperative scrubbing of surgical site with an antiseptic
    b. Preoperative scrubbing of scrub nurses' hands
    c. Rigorous disinfection of operating room and fixtures before surgery
    d. Sterilization of surgical instruments

19. To ensure effectiveness of ethyl alcohol (ethanol) as an antiseptic, the nurse should do what?
    a. Apply the alcohol directly to open wounds after medicating the patient for pain.
    b. Use alcohol in combination with other antimicrobial agents (chlorhexidine).
    c. Use an alcohol with a concentration greater than 75%.
    d. Use a gel that prolongs evaporation of the alcohol.

*20. The priority reason for not wiping a subcutaneous heparin injection site with an isopropyl alcohol pad immediately after injecting the medication is to avoid what?
    a. Bruising
    b. Neutralizing the heparin
    c. Poor absorption of the heparin
    d. Significant pain

21. Alcohol hand sanitizers are not effective against which organisms because they produce spores? (Select all that apply.)
    a. *Bacillus anthracis*
    b. *Clostridium difficile*
    c. Methicillin-resistant *Staphylococcus aureus* (MRSA)
    d. *Mycobacterium tuberculosis*
    e. Vancomycin-resistant enterococci (VRE)

22. When the nurse is preparing to cleanse a wound, which preparation would be most appropriate and effective?
    a. Glutaraldehyde (Cidex)
    b. Iodine solution
    c. Iodine tincture
    d. Povidone-iodine (Betadine)

23. Why is hexachlorophene no longer recommended as a preoperative scrub? (Select all that apply.)
    a. It can be absorbed through intact skin.
    b. It can depress the central nervous system (CNS) causing stupor and death.
    c. It can encourage the growth of gram-negative bacteria.
    d. It does not stop bacteria from replicating.
    e. It frequently damages the liver.

24. What is the surgical scrub that is fast-acting and antibacterial and remains active on the skin after rinsing?
    a. Benzalkonium chloride (BAC)
    b. Chlorhexidine (Hibiclens)
    c. Hexachlorophene (PHisoHex)
    d. Povidone-iodine (Betadine)

*25. The operating room nurse is preparing to apply BAC as a surgical scrub. Before applying the solution, it is a priority for the nurse to do what?
    a. Rinse the skin with water and alcohol.
    b. Shave the area.
    c. Wash the skin with soap.
    d. Warm the solution.

26. The nurse should scrub the hands and forearms with an antimicrobial soap for surgical scrub asepsis for how long?
    a. 1-2 minutes
    b. 2-6 minutes
    c. 6-8 minutes
    d. 8-10 minutes

27. The nursing professor is orienting student nurses to the intensive care unit. Hygiene instructions should include which directive?
    a. Alcohol handrub should be used when the hands are visibly dirty.
    b. All forms of jewelry are not allowed.
    c. Do not wear artificial nails.
    d. Trim natural nails to no more than one-half inch beyond the fingertip.

CASE STUDY

The delivery room nurse needs to prepare used instruments for disinfection with glutaraldehyde (Cidex) before being sent for sterilization.

1. What steps should the nurse take before soaking the instruments?

2. How long do the instruments need to soak?

3. What precautions does the nurse need to take when disinfecting with glutaraldehyde (Cidex)?

4. Describe the handwashing technique the nurse would use after completing this disinfection process.

97
Anthelmintics

STUDY QUESTIONS

True or False

For each of the following statements, enter T *for true or* F *for false.*

1. ___ Helminthiasis is the most common affliction of humans.
2. ___ Anthelmintics treat parasitic worm infestations.
3. ___ Parasitic worm infestation always causes symptoms.
4. ___ When individual treatment is impractical, improved hygiene may be the most valuable intervention.
5. ___ The sooner drug treatment is started after infestation, the less reproduction of the worm occurs in the body.
6. ___ Helminthiasis can involve the liver, lymphatic system, and blood vessels.
7. ___ Treatment may be deemed not needed if there is a high probability of reinfestation or the patient cannot afford the drug.
8. ___ Roundworms can cause pancreatitis by blocking the pancreatic duct.
9. ___ Pinworms live in the human body for 7-10 days.

CRITICAL THINKING, PRIORITIZATION, AND DELEGATION QUESTIONS

10. A patient has just started treatment with mebendazole (Vermox) for hookworm infestation. The nurse assesses for the most common complication of hookworm infestation, which may be what?
    a. Feculent vomiting
    b. Pale conjunctiva
    c. Perianal itching
    d. Rectal prolapse

11. A patient who has been treated with mebendazole (Vermox) for trichinosis is now prescribed prednisone. What is the purpose of this medication?
    a. Kill larvae that have migrated.
    b. Prevent calcification of dead larvae in skeletal muscle.
    c. Prevent migration of larvae.
    d. Reduce inflammation during larval migration.

12. Nursing examination of a missionary who was admitted after becoming ill in Haiti reveals severe scrotal and peripheral edema. What other assessment finding, if present, suggests possible nematode infestation?
    a. Limited range of motion of joints
    b. Multiple bruises
    c. Swollen lymph nodes
    d. Weak hand grasps

13. A patient who works for the World Health Organization (WHO) and whose job duties include worldwide travel, complains of recent noticeable decreased visual acuity. Because of the possibility of contracting onchocerciasis from fly bites, the nurse should assess for recent travel to which area(s) in the patient's history? (Select all that apply.)
    a. Argentina
    b. Guatemala
    c. Kenya
    d. Mexico
    e. Peru
    f. Rwanda
    g. Venezuela

14. It would be a priority to report which diagnostic test result to the prescriber treating a patient for intestinal roundworms?
    a. AST 5 IU/L
    b. BUN 15 mg/dL
    c. hCG 3400 IU/L
    d. INR 1

15. To prevent complications from therapy with praziquantel (Biltricide) prescribed for tapeworms, the nurse teaches the patient to
    a. avoid hazardous activity.
    b. chew the tablet completely before swallowing.
    c. monitor daily urine output.
    d. take the medication on an empty stomach.

16. The nurse is administering albendazole (Albenza) to an older adult patient who has been diagnosed with the larval form of the pork tapeworm. Which laboratory result would warrant consultation with the prescriber regarding administration of the medication?
    a. ALT 175 international units/L
    b. BUN 25 mg/dL
    c. Creatinine 1.4 mg/dL
    d. Potassium 3.8 mg/dL

∗17. A resident has just prescribed diethylcarbamazine (Hetrazan) for an infection with *Wuchereria bancrofti*. Which symptom, occurring after the start of administration of the drug, would be the priority concern for the nurse?
    a. Dizziness
    b. Headache
    c. Nausea
    d. Confusion

DOSE CALCULATION QUESTIONS

18. Mebendazole (Vermox) 500 mg once a day is prescribed. How many 100-mg tablets should be administered at each dose?

19. What is the safe dose of albendazole (Albenza) for a 27-kg child if the recommended dose is 7.5 mg/kg?

CASE STUDIES

Case Study 1

The father of a 2½-year-old child who attends day care notices that his son has been restless, is not sleeping well, has been scratching the perineal area, and has been wetting the bed. The father calls the pediatric office and is told by the nurse to put a loop of transparent tape in the child's anal area in the early morning before the child awakens. The nurse further instructs the father to remove the tape later in the morning, put it in a plastic bag, and bring it to the office. On examination of the tape sample, the pediatric nurse practitioner (PNP) diagnoses enterobiasis pinworms.

1. What is the probable mode of transmission of the parasite in this case?

2. The PNP prescribes mebendazole (Vermox) for the entire family. What did the prescriber need to determine before prescribing the drug for the entire family?

3. How could the pinworm infestation have been transmitted from the child to other family members?

4. What teaching can the nurse provide these family members to prevent future infestation and spread of pinworms?

5. The entire family is adherent to the prescribed therapy. Why is there little problem with adherence with this therapy?

6. The parents are embarrassed and do not want to notify the day care of the child's infection. How should the nurse respond?

Case Study 2

A nurse is caring for victims exposed to contaminated floodwaters who have been brought into a makeshift clinic in a temporary shelter.

7. The nurse knows that which segments of the population would be more at risk for helminthiasis?

8. Several children are experiencing vomiting and massive diarrhea. The nurse should be assessing for what symptoms of these possible fluid and electrolyte imbalances?
   a. Dehydration

   b. Potassium

   c. Magnesium

   d. Sodium

9. Some patients are diagnosed with threadworm infestation and treated with ivermectin (Stromectol). What follow up care should the patients expect to determine if the infestation has been adequately treated?

10. What can the nurse do in this situation to prevent spread of these infections?

98

Antiprotozoal Drugs I: Antimalarial Agents

STUDY QUESTIONS

Completion

1. Malaria deaths are most likely in _____ children.

2. Malaria eradication has not been successful because the transmitting insect and the parasite have become _____ to the drugs.

3. Malaria is transmitted by the _____ _____.

4. Malaria kills more people than any other infection except _____.

5. Infection in the human begins with sporozoites invading the _____.

6. The liver releases merozoites that infect _____.

7. _____ malaria is the most common form.

8. Falciparum malaria does not _____ because it does not form hypnozoites that remain in the liver.

9. _____ _____ _____ is the term for fever and dark urine associated with falciparum malaria.

Matching

Match the type of treatment with its definition.

10. ___ Prophylaxis
11. ___ Prevention of relapse
12. ___ Treatment of an acute attack

    a. Clinical cure
    b. Radical cure
    c. Suppressive therapy

CRITICAL THINKING, PRIORITIZATION, AND DELEGATION QUESTIONS

✳13. What is the most important action by the nurse to prevent transmission of malaria?
    a. Administer drugs at the correct time.
    b. Place the patient in strict isolation.
    c. Practice universal precautions.
    d. Use a mask during all patient contact.

14. The repeating episodes of fever, chills, and profuse sweating that are characteristic of malaria are due to what?
    a. Infection at the site of the mosquito bite
    b. Ingestion of blood by the mosquito
    c. Red blood cell (RBC) rupture
    d. Toxicity of the suppressant drugs

✳15. Prompt treatment of suspected cases of falciparum malaria is most urgent if the patient experiences what symptom?
    a. Chills
    b. Dark urine
    c. High fever
    d. Sweating

✳16. To prevent a serious complication, what is the most significant priority in the nursing care of a patient who has malaria caused by *Plasmodium falciparum*?
    a. Assessing for crackles and respiratory distress
    b. Assessing vital signs every 4 hours
    c. Performing glucometer checks every 2 hours
    d. Monitoring for elevations in liver function studies

✳17. A patient with falciparum malaria is at risk for hypoglycemia. It is a priority to assess the patient for what?
    a. Cold, clammy skin
    b. Hot, dry skin
    c. Hunger and thirst
    d. Nausea and vomiting

18. Primaquine is not used for relapse prevention of infection with malaria caused by *P. falciparum*. Why?
    a. It is a drug that is only used prophylactically to prevent infection of erythrocytes.
    b. *P. falciparum* is resistant to primaquine.
    c. The infection is mild, and relapses will decrease and disappear over time without treatment.
    d. There are no hypnozoites in the liver to be eradicated.

19. A patient asks why prophylactic chloroquine (Aralen) is taken only once a week. What is the basis of the nurse's response?
    a. Absorption is very slow after oral administration.
    b. Deposits in tissue are slowly released into the blood.
    c. It is administered IM as a depot preparation.
    d. It remains fat-soluble and cannot be excreted by the kidneys.

✳20. It is a priority to monitor urine color during treatment with primaquine if laboratory results for an adult female patient include what?
    a. Hemoglobin 8 g/dL
    b. Hematocrit 40%
    c. RBC 4.9×10^6/mcL
    d. Reticulocytes 2%

✳21. It is a priority to teach patients who are prescribed quinine for malaria to report which effect?
    a. Fatigue
    b. Headache
    c. Palpitations
    d. Pallor

22. Primaquine and quinine should not be administered to persons with G6PD deficiency because this deficiency
    a. causes cinchonism.
    b. increases hemolysis.
    c. increases the risk of hypotension.
    d. prevents the drugs from working.

23. Quinine is categorized as pregnancy category C. This means that the nurse should
    a. administer the drug to a pregnant woman if prescribed, because there are no known risks to the human fetus.
    b. administer the drug to a pregnant woman if the risk of not treating with the drug is greater than the risk of the drug itself.
    c. administer the drug to a pregnant woman and carefully assess for any adverse effects.
    d. not administer the drug until the pregnancy status of the woman has been determined.

24. The priority assessment when administering IV quinidine gluconate is monitoring what?
    a. ECG
    b. Electrolytes
    c. Respirations
    d. Urine output

25. Which change, if noted in a patient receiving mefloquine, is a reason for the nurse to withhold the drug and contact the prescriber?
    a. Headache
    b. Heartburn
    c. Lack of interest in things normally found to be pleasurable
    d. Nausea

26. Because of adverse effects, developmentally, which American patient would be least likely to adhere to atovaquone/proguanil (Malarone) therapy?
    a. 15-year-old girl
    b. 35-year-old man
    c. 55-year-old man
    d. 75-year-old woman

27. Tetracycline is prescribed for a female patient who has chloroquinolone-resistant malaria. Which laboratory test result would warrant withholding the drug and contacting the prescriber?
    a. ALT 60 international units/L
    b. Creatinine 1 mg/dL
    c. hCG 90 milli-international units/mL
    d. RBC 4.2×10^6/mcL

DOSE CALCULATION QUESTIONS

28. Quinidine gluconate 0.02 mg/kg/min continuous infusion is ordered for a patient who weighs 165 lb. The drug is supplied as 800-mg quinidine gluconate diluted in 50 mL of 5% dextrose in water. What rate/hr, rounded to tenths of mL, should be programmed into the IV pump?

29. Clindamycin 20 mg/kg/day in three divided doses is the recommended for a child with malaria. What is acceptable dosing for a child who weighs 55 lb?

CASE STUDY

A 45-year-old man has just returned from Africa after 4 years of service with the World Health Organization (WHO). During that time, he had been taking chloroquine (Aralen) prophylactically to prevent malaria in case he was bitten by an infected *Anopheles* mosquito.

1. What does this treatment actually accomplish?

2. What other measures should he have been taught to decrease the risk of malarial infection?

3. Before his service in Africa was completed, the patient quit taking the chloroquine because he was experiencing nausea and vomiting. Soon after, he started experiencing episodes of high fever followed by chills, and then diaphoresis occurring every 2 days. He was diagnosed with vivax malaria and was unable to perform his work due to

the frequency and intensity of the symptoms. The patient is prescribed a 3-day treatment of chloroquine for his acute attack of malaria. What teaching could the nurse provide to decrease adverse effects and to prevent serious effects?

4. The patient tells the nurse that he knows that missionaries took intravenous (IV) quinine in the past. He asks why he wasn't prescribed that drug. What information can the nurse share about the decrease in use of quinine?

5. The patient was advised that he should return home for treatment with primaquine to prevent relapse. Why was the patient not treated in Africa where he could continue his work?

6. When the patient completes his acute treatment, he asks why he cannot continue taking the chloroquine to prevent recurrence of the malaria symptoms. What is the basis of the nurse's response to this question?

99
Antiprotozoal Drugs II: Miscellaneous Agents

STUDY QUESTIONS

Matching

Match the term with its description.

1. ____ Amebiasis
2. ____ Cryptosporidiosis
3. ____ Giardiasis
4. ____ Leishmaniasis
5. ____ Toxoplasmosis
6. ____ Trichomoniasis

a. Infection is acquired most commonly by eating undercooked meat.
b. Transmission is fecal-oral, often by ingesting water contaminated with livestock feces.
c. Principal site of infestation is the intestine; may migrate to the liver, where abscesses may form.
d. Usual site of infestation is the genitourinary tract.
e. Disease is acquired through the bite of sand flies.
f. Infestation usually occurs by drinking contaminated water.

CRITICAL THINKING, PRIORITIZATION, AND DELEGATION QUESTIONS

✳ 7. A farmer is hospitalized after developing cryptosporidiosis during treatment with high-dose prednisone for exacerbated chronic obstructive pulmonary disease (COPD). What is the nursing priority for this patient?
   a. Activity intolerance
   b. Fatigue
   c. Fluid volume deficit
   d. Imbalanced nutrition

8. Which symptom, if present in a patient who is receiving iodoquinol (Yodoxin) for amebiasis, would be of most concern to the nurse?
   a. Anal itching
   b. Blurred vision
   c. Facial pustules
   d. Palpable thyroid

9. The nurse teaches a patient who is prescribed metronidazole (Flagyl) that it is very important to report which possible adverse effect of the drug to the prescriber?
   a. Darkening of the urine
   b. Metallic taste
   c. Mouth ulcers
   d. Paresthesias

10. An emergency department (ED) nurse is providing discharge teaching to a patient who is breastfeeding her infant who is prescribed metronidazole (Flagyl) for giardiasis. It is important for the nurse to teach this patient to feed her baby formula and discard her pumped breast milk throughout the time the medication is being taken and for how long afterward?
   a. 1 day
   b. 3 days
   c. 1 week
   d. 2 weeks

11. A patient who has been prescribed metronidazole (Flagyl) asks why he should not drink alcohol. The nurse's response is based on the fact that alcohol combined with metronidazole can cause what?
   a. Bradycardia
   b. Dangerous CNS depression
   c. Dysrhythmias
   d. Psychotic reaction

12. The nurse notes yellowish discoloration of the sclera of an immunocompetent 7-year-old girl who is receiving nitazoxanide (Alinia) for giardiasis. What should the nurse do?
   a. Administer the medication and continue nursing care.
   b. Review the most recent BUN and creatinine.
   c. Withhold the medication and review laboratory tests.
   d. Withhold the medication and contact the prescriber.

✳13. Which result, if noted in the urine of a patient who is receiving suramin sodium (Germanin) for early East African sleeping sickness, would be a priority to report to the prescriber?
   a. Multiple casts
   b. pH 5.7
   c. Protein 2 mg/dL
   d. Specific gravity 1.015

14. The drug handbook states that melarsoprol (Arsobal) has Herxheimer-type reactions as a frequent adverse effect. The nurse observes for this immune reaction, which presents as
   a. a maculopapular rash.
   b. flulike symptoms.
   c. lesions on the oral and conjunctival mucosa.
   d. tingling around the mouth and throat.

▶15. Which laboratory test result would warrant withholding eflornithine (Uridyl) prescribed for late-stage African sleeping sickness and consulting the prescriber?
   a. ALT 338 international units/L
   b. BNP 260 picograms/mL
   c. BUN 32 mg/dL
   d. CPK 80 ng/mL

✳16. A patient is admitted with American trypanosomiasis (Chagas' disease). If nifurtimox (Lampit) is prescribed, it would be of greatest priority to inform the prescriber of the patient's history of
   a. asthma.
   b. bowel obstruction.
   c. type 2 diabetes mellitus.
   d. G6PD deficiency.

DOSE CALCULATION QUESTIONS

17. Drug orders for a 140-lb patient include IM pentamidine isethionate (Pentam 300) 220 mg once a day for 7 days. The recommended dose is 4 mg/kg/day. Is the prescribed dose safe and therapeutic?

18. A 65-lb child with amebiasis is prescribed iodoquinol 375 mg every 8 hours for 20 days. Is this
dose safe?

CASE STUDIES

Case Study 1

The nurse works in a busy family practice. A 17-year-
old female patient presents to the office with complaints
of stabbing right upper quadrant (RUQ) pain, anorexia,
chills, and diarrhea for 10 days.

1. What subjective information would be helpful to
collect before the primary care practitioner (PCP)
sees the patient?

The patient was on a camping trip in the White Mountains
of New Hampshire a few weeks ago. She experienced
nausea and fatigue toward the end of trip, and the symptoms have gotten worse since coming home. She denies
alcohol and tobacco use and sexual activity and is currently experiencing a menstrual period. She has lost 4 lb
in the last 2 weeks. Assessment findings include T 102.7°
F, pulse 98 beats/min; BP 100/64 mm Hg; dry mucous
membranes, abdominal guarding, and weakness. The PCP
orders a CBC and differential, electrolytes, and a CT scan
of the abdomen. The PCP diagnoses amebiasis. Because
the patient states that she will have difficulty being com-
pliant with three times a day dosing with metronidazole,
the PCP prescribes tinidazole (Tindamax) 2 g once a day
for 3 days.

2. During teaching regarding the adverse effects of
this drug, the nurse should explain the importance
of contacting the prescriber if what symptoms occur?

3. Based on the patient's exposure to the organism,
symptoms, and developmental considerations,
what other teaching should the nurse provide?

4. One duty is to review laboratory tests and notify
the PCP of results. The nurse is reviewing laboratory results for the patient with amebiasis. Abnormal results include WBC 12,800/mm³, sodium
137 mEq/L, potassium 3.6 mEq/L, and multiple
small abscesses in the liver on CT scan. Which test
result is most important to promptly review with
the PCP and why?

5. The PCP asks the nurse to have the patient come
in immediately. After explaining the laboratory
test results, the patient agrees to be faithful for a
course of metronidazole followed by iodoquinol.
What teaching should the nurse provide?

Case Study 2

A patient who has a history of diabetes, seizure disorder, atrial fibrillation, and bipolar disorder is prescribed
metronidazole (Flagyl) for amebiasis. The patient's home
medication regimen lists metformin (Glucophage) 500 mg
twice a day, phenytoin (Dilantin) 100 mg three times a
day, warfarin (Coumadin) 2.5 mg once a day on Monday
and Thursday and 2 mg once a day on the rest of the days,
and lithium carbonate (Eskalith) 300 mg three times a day.

6. What are the possible effects on drug levels of the
interaction of each of these drugs with metronidazole (Flagyl)?

7. The nurse should assess for which symptoms of
these drug reactions?

8. What are interventions the nurse should employ if
symptoms occur?

100
Ectoparasiticides

STUDY QUESTIONS

Matching

Indicate if the statement applies to pediculosis (P), scabies (S), or both (B).

1. ____ Do not live on pets
2. ____ Burrows visible as dotted lines on skin
3. ____ Common site of adult infestation is in webs between fingers
4. ____ Intense itching
5. ____ Lice infestation
6. ____ Mite infestation
7. ____ Scratching may result in secondary infection
8. ____ Transmission possible via contact with inanimate objects
9. ____ Treatment differs by site of infestation
10. ____ Usually treated with topical drugs

CRITICAL THINKING, PRIORITIZATION, AND DELEGATION QUESTIONS

11. If retreatment with permethrin (Nix) is needed for head lice, the experts recommend that it should be done in how many days after the last treatment?
    a. 1 day
    b. 7 days
    c. 9 days
    d. 14 days

12. What could be associated with a severe reaction when malathion (Ovide) has been prescribed for head lice?
    a. Absorption of the lotion through scratches on the scalp
    b. Administration concurrently with drugs that inhibit the P-450 hepatic cytochrome system
    c. Failure to use the fine-toothed comb to remove nits after application
    d. Smoking while applying the lotion

13. Which treatment for head lice must be applied at least twice to be effective?
    a. Benzyl alcohol (Ulesfia)
    b. Ivermectin (Stromectol)
    c. Lindane (Kwell)
    d. Permethrin (Nix)

14. Lindane is no longer recommended except in cases resistant to safer drugs. Why is this true? (Select all that apply.)
    a. It causes neonatal gasping syndrome.
    b. It is the most expensive product.
    c. Rinsing off the drug can contaminate ground water.
    d. Systemic absorption can cause seizures.
    e. Treatment usually involves reapplication once a week for 3 weeks.

DOSE CALCULATION QUESTIONS

15. The recommended dose range of ivermectin (Stromectol) is 20-40 mcg/kg. What is the recommended dose range in mg for a 30-lb child? A 44-lb child?

16. Ivermectin (Stromectol) 9000 micrograms is prescribed. How many 3-mg tablets should be administered?

CASE STUDY

A second-grade teacher consults the school nurse about a girl in her class. The child is one of three siblings attending the elementary school. The child has very long hair, and over the past week, the child has been constantly scratching her head. She has scratched her head so much that her hair is tangled and almost impossible to brush, and her scalp is bleeding. The school nurse notes small white spots on her hair shaft close to the scalp. Examination under the microscope reveals nits. The nurse contacts the girl's parents to report these nits (eggs), telling them that it is probably *Pediculus humanus capitis* (head lice).

1. How should the school nurse handle the possibility that other children in the school may be infested?

2. The girl's parents are quite upset about the lice. They want to know how their child could have gotten "these bugs" and how to tell whether others in the family have them. How should the nurse respond?

3. The parents were told by a friend to cut all of their daughter's hair off to get rid of the lice. What are the reasons why the nurse would not want the parents to do this?

4. The parents contact the pediatrician, who orders permethrin (Nix) shampoo. What should the office nurse include in the explanation for using this product?

5. What is the purpose of the fine-toothed comb in head lice treatment?

6. The child's father tells the nurse that when he had head lice as a child, his prescriber had his parents apply lindane (Kwell) shampoo. He wants to know why that is not used anymore. What would the nurse tell him?

101

Basic Principles of Cancer Chemotherapy

STUDY QUESTIONS

Completion

1. In America, only_____ _____ causes more death than cancer.

2. Cancer is the leading cause of death in women age _____ to _____ years.

3. _____ cancer is one of the most common locations of cancer in men.

4. The most common treatment for solid tumors is _____.

5. _____ drugs are the class of anticancer drugs used most often.

6. The enzyme telomerase, which is active in most cancer, allows cancer cells to _____ _____.

CRITICAL THINKING, PRIORITIZATION, AND DELEGATION

7. Which characteristic best describes cancer cell reproduction?
   a. Abnormal
   b. Rapid
   c. Slow
   d. Unregulated

8. A patient is admitted for surgical removal of a cancerous tumor of the colon. He is concerned about the prospect of living with a colostomy and asks the nurse why the prescriber cannot just give him some drugs to kill the cancer. What is the basis of the nurse's response? (Select all that apply.)
   a. Solid tumors are disseminated.
   b. Solid tumors have fewer cells that are actively dividing.
   c. Solid tumors have fewer cells in the G_0 phase.
   d. Solid tumors have poor blood supply at the core.
   e. Solid tumors have normal DNA.

9. The spouse of a cancer patient asks why some tumors become resistant to chemotherapy. Which statement would not be included in the explanation?
   a. A transport molecule may be produced to transport drugs out of the cancer cell.
   b. Cancer cells in the G_0 phase have time to repair drug-induced damage before it does serious harm.
   c. Chemotherapy drugs alter the cancer cell's DNA, making the cell resistant.
   d. Drug-resistant mutant cells have a competition-free environment because of the death of drug-sensitive cells.

10. The father of a child with leukemia is concerned about his son's fear and discomfort during chemotherapy. He asks the nurse why the child cannot receive one large dose of a single powerful drug instead of multiple doses of different drugs. After teaching, which statement, if made by the father, suggests that that this parent needs further explanation?
    a. "Different drugs kill cancer cells in different ways."
    b. "It is especially important for my son to receive multiple doses because one of the drugs that my son is getting only kills cancer cells at a particular point of cell reproduction."
    c. "If multiple drugs are used, the cancer is less likely to develop resistance to all of them."
    d. "My son will not experience adverse effects if he receives multiple drugs administered at different times."

11. The nurse would expect what when two or more anticancer chemotherapeutic agents are used together?
    a. The drugs' adverse effects primarily affect different organs.
    b. The drugs are less effective than if used alone.
    c. The drugs can be mixed in the same intravenous solution.
    d. The drugs have the same mechanism of action.

12. A patient with brain cancer asks the nurse why they are putting the drug into her back instead of into a vein. The basis of the nurse's response should be that this route
    a. allows higher doses of chemotherapy to be used.
    b. allows the drug to get to the tumor cells.
    c. prevents many adverse effects.
    d. prevents drug-resistant mutation of the cancer cells.

▶13. The nurse is caring for a 62-year-old patient who developed pancreatitis during chemotherapy after mastectomy. Most recent laboratory results include RBC 2.8 10^6/mL, WBC 4100/mm³, neutrophils 18,000/mm³, and platelets 147,000/mm³. What is an expected nursing diagnosis, based on these laboratory results?
    a. Activity intolerance
    b. Decreased cardiac output
    c. Impaired gas exchange
    d. Ineffective cerebral tissue perfusion

▶14. The nurse is caring for a chemotherapy patient who has neutropenic precautions. The nurse washes her hands and dons a gown, mask, and gloves before entering the patient's room. The patient refuses care by the nurse until the nurse washes her hands at the sink in the room and puts on new gloves. What should the nurse do?
    a. Explain that she is more likely to transmit an infection if she takes off her current gloves while in the room.
    b. Explain that she washed her hands just outside the door before entering the room.
    c. Rewash her hands in the room and put on new gloves.
    d. Rewash her hands, put on new gown, gloves, and mask inside the room.

15. For a cancer patient who is receiving chemotherapy, which food would be least likely to cause an infection if the patient develops neutropenia?
    a. Commercially canned fruit
    b. Vegetables from the patient's garden
    c. Rare meat
    d. Yogurt

16. The nurse is administering subcutaneous insulin to a chemotherapy patient who is experiencing bone marrow suppression. Which technique would be best for the nurse to use to prevent an adverse effect from the bone marrow suppression?
    a. Administer the insulin via an existing IV port.
    b. Apply pressure to the site following injection.
    c. Delay the administration of insulin until after the patient has eaten his meal.
    d. Wipe the injection site with Betadine after injection.

17. A patient receiving chemotherapy develops hyperuricemia. A nursing priority addresses the effect of the urate crystals on which body part?
    a. Blood
    b. Joints
    c. Kidneys
    d. Liver

▶18. When administering a known vesicant chemotherapeutic agent, which information is most important for the nurse to know?
   a. If the patient has been premedicated with an antiemetic
   b. Stop infusion immediately if extravasation occurs
   c. The mechanism of action of the drug
   d. Whether gloves are needed during administration

CASE STUDIES

Case Study 1

A 28-year-old female patient is admitted to the oncology unit with a diagnosis of suspected Hodgkin's disease. The diagnosis is confirmed after a biopsy. The patient is started on treatment, which consists of external radiation treatments and chemotherapy. The patient asks the nurse, "How does cancer spread?"

1. What information can the nurse provide about the characteristics of cancer cells that promote growth and metastasis?

2. The patient asks why people are more likely to get cancer if they have a family history of cancer. How are genetics linked to cancer?

3. The nurse is discussing strategies to minimize the adverse effects of chemotherapy, including mouth ulcer (stomatitis). The patient asks why these drugs cause mouth ulcers if they are given intravenously. How should the nurse respond?

4. What interventions can the nurse suggest to minimize the effects of chemotherapy on the patient's GI tract?

Case Study 2

A nurse has just lost his sister to breast cancer. Before she died, his sister challenged him to use his nursing knowledge and energy to prevent cancer suffering and death. The nurse networks with fellow nurses to identify what they can do to work toward fulfilling his sister's wishes.

5. What actions could the nurse take?

102

Anticancer Drugs I: Cytotoxic Agents

STUDY QUESTIONS

True or False

For each of the following statements, enter T for true or F for false.

1. ____ Cytotoxic cancer drugs kill cancer cells and healthy cells.
2. ____ Cells in the G_0 are phase are most likely to be killed by cytotoxic drugs.
3. ____ It is critical that phase-specific cytotoxic drugs be administered on a specific timetable as prescribed.
4. ____ Cell-cycle phase–nonspecific drugs are equally effective during any phase of the cell cycle.
5. ____ Bifunctional alkylating agents are more effective than monofunctional agents.
6. ____ Alkylating agents are considered cell-cycle phase–nonspecific.

7. ___ Most antimetabolites are M-phase–specific.

8. ___ Folic acid analogs are effective because folic acid is toxic to cancer cells.

9. ___ Failure to give sufficient leucovorin at the right time when administering high doses of methotrexate coupled with leucovorin rescue can kill the patient.

10. ___ Antitumor antibiotics are used to treat infections associated with neutropenia caused by cancer drugs.

CRITICAL THINKING, PRIORITIZATION, AND DELEGATION QUESTIONS

▶ 11. Which teaching would be appropriate relating to a common, serious adverse effect of every category of cytotoxic drugs?
a. "Change positions slowly to prevent dizziness or fainting."
b. "Night driving may not be safe."
c. "It's important to perform weight-bearing exercise."
d. "Use an electric razor to avoid cutting yourself."

✳ 12. Which diagnostic test result would be of greatest priority when a patient is receiving cytotoxic drugs for cancer?
a. Absolute neutrophil count 476/mm^3
b. Platelets 130,000/mm^3
c. Reticulocytes 3.2%
d. WBC 11,000/mm^3

13. Which administration strategy would be most likely to ensure that phase-specific anticancer drugs are present when cancer cells will be harmed by the drug?
a. Combined with other drugs
b. Frequent intervals with prolonged infusion
c. Rapid infusion of large doses
d. Small doses spaced at least 4 weeks apart

14. Cell-cycle phase–nonspecific drugs may not kill cells in G_0 phase because the
a. cell has time to repair damage.
b. cell is not cancerous if it is in G_0 phase.
c. cell is reproducing.
d. cell's DNA is not harmed.

15. The nurse is teaching a patient who has been prescribed oral cyclophosphamide. Which statement, if made by the patient, suggests a need for further teaching?
a. "I need to notify my doctor if I develop a fever higher than 100.4° F."
b. "I need to take the drug 1 hour before or 2 hours after meals."
c. "I should drink at least 65 ounces of fluids every day, especially water."
d. "I should notify my doctor if my skin color changes."

16. Why is mesna (Mesnex) prescribed with nitrogen mustard alkylating agents?
a. It decreases nausea and vomiting.
b. It inhibits production of enzymes that repair DNA.
c. It potentiates drug action.
d. It prevents damage to the urinary tract.

✳ 17. It is of greatest priority for the nurse to consult with the oncologist before administering cisplatin if the patient reports which symptom since the last infusion?
a. Headache
b. Nausea
c. Ringing in his ears
d. Urinary frequency

18. What is most likely to worsen symptoms of peripheral sensory neuropathy associated with oxaliplatin (Eloxatin)?
a. Dehydration
b. Exposure to cold
c. Fatigue
d. Sweating

▶ 19. How long should a female patient of childbearing age be instructed to use two reliable forms of birth control when prescribed methotrexate?
a. During therapy
b. During therapy and through at least 1 month after therapy
c. During therapy and through at least 6 weeks after therapy
d. During therapy and through at least 6 months after therapy

✳ 20. Which diagnostic test result, if it is a change from a previous result, would be of greatest priority to report to the prescriber of methotrexate?
a. ALT 55 international units/L
b. BUN 22 mg/dL
c. Creatinine clearance 45 mL/min
d. Hemoglobin 10.8 g/dL

✳21. A patient with laryngeal cancer is receiving massive doses of methotrexate and leucovorin (folinic acid, citrovorum factor). Which action is of greatest priority?
   a. Administering the prescribed ondansetron (Zofran) 30 minutes before the start of the methotrexate infusion
   b. Administering the leucovorin exactly as prescribed
   c. Infusing the methotrexate over exactly the prescribed time interval
   d. Monitoring for electrolyte imbalances because of the high risk of diarrhea or vomiting

22. Which statement by a patient who has been taught about prevention of adverse effects of methotrexate therapy suggests understanding of the teaching?
   a. "A new cough should be reported to the doctor."
   b. "Drinking cranberry juice will help protect my kidneys from damage by methotrexate."
   c. "Drinking grapefruit juice can prevent my liver from breaking down this drug."
   d. "I should increase my fluid intake to 4 glasses each day."

23. The nurse teaches a patient that dexamethasone is prescribed for patients who are being treated with pemetrexed (Alimta) to prevent which condition?
   a. Anemia
   b. Nausea
   c. Rash
   d. Stomatitis

▶24. Which symptoms of adverse effects of the liposomal formulation of cytarabine (ara-C) would be of most concern to the nurse?
   a. Anorexia, nausea, and bruising
   b. Headache, fever, and vomiting
   c. Mouth ulcers, inflamed conjunctiva, and nausea
   d. Nausea, vomiting, and fever

25. Which adverse effects of fluorouracil (Adrucil) are reasons to reevaluate use of the drug? (Select all that apply.)
   a. Blistering of the palms and soles
   b. Dark spots on the skin
   c. Diarrhea
   d. Loss of hair
   e. Mouth ulcers

✳26. Which symptom, if occurring in a patient receiving mercaptopurine (Purinethol), would be of greatest priority to the nurse?
   a. Constipation
   b. Diarrhea
   c. Hair loss
   d. Petechiae

27. A patient who is receiving an infusion of liposomal doxorubicin (Doxil) reports back pain and chest tightness within minutes of the start of the infusion. The nurse stops the infusion. The symptoms abate, and the patient's vital signs are within normal limits. What is the appropriate nursing action in this situation?
   a. Administer an antidote.
   b. Consult with the prescriber STAT.
   c. Hold the drug until the next scheduled dose.
   d. Restart the infusion at a slower rate and monitor for return of symptoms.

28. The nurse should warn patients that they may experience a blue-green discoloration of their urine and the whites of their eyes if they receive which antitumor antibiotic?
   a. Epirubicin (Ellence)
   b. Idarubicin (Idamycin)
   c. Liposomal daunorubicin (DaunoXome)
   d. Mitoxantrone (Novantrone)

✳29. The nurse is preparing to administer bleomycin to a patient with testicular cancer. It would be of greatest priority to report which diagnostic test result to the prescriber?
   a. Erythrocyte sedimentation rate (ESR) 10 mm/hr
   b. Hematocrit (Hct) 38%
   c. Peak expiratory flow (PEF) 54% of best
   d. Platelets 180,000/mm³

✳30. An adolescent patient is scheduled to receive vincristine (Oncovin) for Hodgkin's lymphoma. Developmentally, which adverse effect is most likely to be a priority concern for this patient?
   a. Alopecia
   b. Constipation
   c. Nausea
   d. Paresthesias

✳31. Which nursing action would be of greatest priority when administering an infusion of paclitaxel (Taxol)?
   a. Monitor urine output.
   b. Monitor vital signs.
   c. Prepare for possible vomiting.
   d. Reposition patient every 2 hours.

▶32. Which assessment finding is most significant if a patient is receiving docetaxel (Taxotere)?
   a. Blood pressure 147/90 mm Hg
   b. Eight-hour output of 850 mL of very dark amber urine
   c. Expiratory wheezing
   d. Two-plus pitting edema of the ankles

▶33. The spouse of a patient who received cabazitaxel (Jevtana) reports that the patient has been up all night with diarrhea. The patient is currently in bed and is too weak to stand up. The spouse asks the nurse what to do. What is the most appropriate response?
   a. Administer 1 tsp of bismuth salicylate (Pepto-Bismol) after each unformed stool.
   b. Allow the patient to rest.
   c. Have the patient take frequent sips of a sports drink with sugar and electrolytes.
   d. Seek medical care now for the patient.

DOSE CALCULATION QUESTIONS

34. Filgrastim (Neupogen) is prescribed 5 mcg/kg/day. The patient weighs 132 lb. What dose should be administered?

35. What is the maximum recommended lifetime dose of doxorubicin (Adriamycin) for a patient who is 72 inches tall and weighs 220 lb, when the cumulative lifetime dose should be kept below 550 mg/m^2?

CASE STUDIES

Case Study 1

A 41-year-old patient is admitted to the outpatient area for her first course of intravenous fluorouracil (Adrucil) chemotherapy for metastatic breast cancer.

1. What techniques should the nurse use when administering this drug to prevent personal harm?

2. What administrative techniques should the nurse use to prevent patient injury from this drug?

Case Study 2

The nurse is preparing to administer doxorubicin (Adriamycin) to a 38-year-old patient with ovarian cancer.

3. Developmentally, what effect of this drug would be a priority for the nurse to prepare this patient to experience?

4. What things should the nurse assess and teach the patient to report relating to the risk of cardiotoxicity?

5. Ramipril (Altace) 2.5 mg daily is prescribed. What should the nurse include in teaching about this drug?

103

Anticancer Drugs II: Hormonal Agents, Targeted Drugs, and Other Noncytotoxic Anticancer Drugs

STUDY QUESTIONS

True or False

For each of the following statements, enter T *for true or* F *for false.*

1. ____ Hormonal agents lack serious adverse effects.
2. ____ Chemotherapy and hormonal therapy are drugs added to cancer treatment to improve the response to other therapy.
3. ____ For hormonal agents to be effective, the tumor must have receptors for the hormone being blocked.
4. ____ Tamoxifen is not recommended for breast cancer prevention for women older than 60 years because they have a lower incidence of breast cancer than women ages 40-59 years.
5. ____ Antidepressant drugs Prozac, Paxil, and Zoloft slow metabolism of tamoxifen by the liver causing tamoxifen toxicity.
6. ____ The likelihood of infusion reactions to trastuzumab (Herceptin) increases with each subsequent dose of the drug.

CRITICAL THINKING, PRIORITIZATION, AND DELEGATION QUESTIONS

7. Which nursing action would be most likely to support patient adherence to taking antiestrogen drug therapy for breast cancer?
   a. Demonstrating administration techniques
   b. Emphasizing benefits of therapy
   c. Identifying patient concerns
   d. Teaching mechanism of action of the drugs

✳ 8. A 58-year-old patient has been taking tamoxifen to prevent breast cancer. Which question would be of greatest priority for the nurse to ask?
   a. "Has anyone in your family ever had breast cancer?"
   b. "Have you ever been told that your cholesterol is high?"
   c. "Have you experienced a broken wrist, hip, or backbone?"
   d. "Have you had any vaginal bleeding after the drug was started?"

9. Which teaching would be appropriate for the most common adverse effect of tamoxifen?
   a. Adequate hydration
   b. Dress in layers
   c. Safe use of OTC analgesics
   d. Small, frequent meals

✳ 10. Which possible adverse effect would be of greatest priority to report to the prescriber of a selective estrogen receptor modulator (SERM)?
   a. Calf pain and swelling
   b. Hot flushes and night sweats
   c. Longer menstrual cycles
   d. Nausea without vomiting

11. What is the expected effect on tamoxifen levels of also taking a CYP2D6 inhibitor such as fluoxetine (Prozac)?
   a. Decreased fluoxetine levels
   b. Decreased tamoxifen levels
   c. Increased fluoxetine levels
   d. Increased tamoxifen levels

✳ 12. Which laboratory test result would be of greatest priority to report to the prescriber if a patient is prescribed toremifene (Fareston)?
   a. Calcium 8.8 mg/dL
   b. Magnesium 2.2 mEq/L
   c. Potassium 2.7 mEq/L
   d. Sodium 147 mEq/L

13. A 38-year-old patient with breast cancer asks why she has been prescribed tamoxifen instead of anastrozole (Arimidex). Which statements could be included in the explanation by the nurse?
    a. Anastrozole blocks production of estrogen by the ovaries, causing severe menopausal symptoms.
    b. Anastrozole can cause endometrial cancer.
    c. Tamoxifen is more effective and has fewer adverse effects.
    d. Tamoxifen activates receptors increasing bone density and healthy lipid levels.

14. The nurse would consult the prescriber of trastuzumab (Herceptin) immediately if the patient suddenly developed which symptom?
    a. Crackles throughout the lung fields
    b. Generalized weakness
    c. Headache with sensitivity to light
    d. Temperature greater than 100.4° F (38° C)

15. Which action should the nurse perform first if a patient who is receiving the first dose of trastuzumab (Herceptin) complains of shortness of breath?
    a. Assess lung sounds.
    b. Elevate the head of the bed.
    c. Notify the prescriber.
    d. Stop the drug infusion.

16. What would suggest possible cardiotoxicity from trastuzumab (Herceptin)? (Select all that apply.)
    a. BNP 850 picograms/mL
    b. Echocardiogram showing ejection fraction of 60%
    c. Pulse 58 beats/min
    d. Shift of point of maximal impulse (PMI) to the left
    e. Slight increase in pulse with deep inspiration

17. The prescriber of a potentially cardiotoxic drug asks the nurse, "What is the patient's weight?" What information is the prescriber seeking?
    a. Actual weight in kilograms
    b. Body mass index (BMI)
    c. Change in weight in the past 24 hours
    d. How weight relates to ideal body weight

18. Which herb has been known to increase metabolism of lapatinib (Tykerb) and possibly decrease effectiveness?
    a. Echinacea
    b. Feverfew
    c. Garlic
    d. St. John's wort

▶ 19. Which symptom suggests hypercalcemia from metastasis of breast cancer to bone?
    a. 4+ deep tendon reflexes (DTR)
    b. Bilateral weak hand grasps
    c. Negative Babinski's reflex
    d. Positive Homans' sign

20. A patient who is receiving leuprolide for advanced prostate cancer is at risk for new-onset diabetes. Which symptom suggests that the patient is experiencing hyperglycemia?
    a. Anorexia
    b. Diaphoresis
    c. Frequent urination
    d. Xeroderma

21. Which injection interval should the nurse question if a patient is prescribed Leuprolide depot injection?
    a. Once a month
    b. Once every 4 months
    c. Once every 6 months
    d. Once every 12 months

22. Which instruction should be included in teaching for a patient who has been prescribed nilutamide (Nilandron)?
    a. Change positions slowly to prevent dizziness or fainting.
    b. Limit your fluid intake in the evening so you do not need to get up to go to the bathroom.
    c. Night driving may not be safe.
    d. Use an electric razor to prevent cutting yourself.

23. Which new symptom since starting nilutamide (Nilandron) is most likely a reason to withhold the drug and consult the prescriber?
    a. Dyspnea
    b. Gynecomastia
    c. Insomnia
    d. Nausea

24. A patient who is prescribed high-dose ketoconazole (Nizoral) for prostate cancer has experienced prolonged vomiting. It would be of highest priority to monitor which laboratory tests?
    a. Complete blood count and differential
    b. Electrolytes
    c. Lipids
    d. Urinalysis

25. Which drugs are commonly used for premedication before infusing sipuleucel-T (Provenge)? (Select all that apply.)
    a. Acetaminophen
    b. Aspirin
    c. Diphenhydramine
    d. Epinephrine
    e. Ibuprofen

26. Which value should be reported to the prescriber immediately when a patient is prescribed docetaxel (Taxotere) or cabazitaxel (Jevtana)?
    a. ANC 875/mm^3
    b. Hb/Hct 13.2/37%
    c. Platelets 400,000/mm^3
    d. WBC 11,000/mm^3

27. The teaching plan for patients receiving cetuximab should include the importance of reporting sudden onset of which symptom to the oncologist?
    a. Fever
    b. Irritability
    c. Nausea
    d. Difficulty breathing

28. Which assessment finding suggests that a patient who is receiving panitumumab (Vectibix) is experiencing hypomagnesemia?
    a. Constipation
    b. Tremors
    c. Fever
    d. Hypotension

29. Which OTC drug can decrease absorption of gefitinib? (Select all that apply.)
    a. Acetaminophen (Tylenol)
    b. Calcium carbonate (TUMS)
    c. Diphenhydramine (Benadryl)
    d. Omeprazole and sodium bicarbonate (Zegerid OTC)
    e. Ranitidine (Zantac)

30. The nurse notes a 2-lb weight gain in 24 hours when assessing a hospitalized patient who has been receiving imatinib (Gleevec) for chronic myeloid leukemia (CML). It is of greatest priority for the nurse to assess which body system at this time?
    a. Cardiopulmonary status
    b. Gastrointestinal status
    c. Musculoskeletal status
    d. Neurologic status

31. What is the most common symptom of long QT syndrome and should be reported to the prescriber of nilotinib (Tasigna)?
    a. Dizziness with position changes
    b. Palpitations with significant exertion
    c. Shortness of breath with significant exertion
    d. Unexplained fainting

32. Which assessment finding would be of greatest concern to the nurse caring for a male patient who is prescribed sunitinib (Sutent) for advanced renal cell carcinoma?
    a. 10 mm Hg increase in BP over baseline
    b. Large bruises at venipuncture sites
    c. Dizziness with position changes
    d. Hemoglobin 13.2 g/dL

33. Which symptom, if occurring 12-24 hours after the first infusion of rituximab (Rituxan), suggests possible drug-induced tumor lysis syndrome (TLS)?
    a. Constipation, epigastric pain, and cool, clammy skin
    b. Muscle spasms and tingling around the mouth
    c. Anorexia, vomiting, altered mental status, and muscle cramps
    d. Weakness and thirst

34. A patient is receiving rituximab (Rituxan). The nurse should teach the patient to report which symptom that suggests a critical adverse effect warranting immediate medical attention?
    a. Dizziness and throat tightness
    b. Muscle aches and pains
    c. Stomatitis and widespread rash
    d. Vomiting and diarrhea

35. The nurse teaches a patient who is receiving ibritumomab tiuxetan (IT) linked with yttrium-90 that the most severe neutropenia and thrombocytopenia will occur at what point in therapy?
    a. After the first treatment
    b. At the time of the last dose
    c. 7-9 weeks after treatment
    d. 10-15 weeks after treatment

36. Teaching should include prompt reporting of abdominal pain, chest pain, shortness of breath, change in mental status, and blood in sputum when a patient is receiving treatment with which drug?
    a. Bevacizumab (Avastin)
    b. Bortezomib (Velcade)
    c. Gemtuzumab ozogamicin (Mylotarg)
    d. Rituximab (Rituxan)

37. What is a symptom of the most common serious adverse effect of vorinostat (Zolinza)?
    a. Anorexia
    b. Fatigue
    c. Frequent watery stool
    d. Dyspnea

38. If a patient experiences hypothyroidism from ipilimumab (Yervoy) therapy, what symptoms would the nurse expect to find?
    a. Weight gain, fatigue, and cold intolerance
    b. Weight loss, fatigue, and cold intolerance
    c. Weight gain, fatigue, and heat intolerance
    b. Weight loss, fatigue, and heat intolerance

39. To prevent some of the most common adverse effects of interferon alfa-2a (Intron-A), the nurse teaches the patient about administering which drugs?
    a. Acetaminophen (Tylenol)
    b. Dexamethasone (Decadron)
    c. Diphenhydramine (Benadryl)
    d. Ondansetron (Zofran)

40. The oncology nurse has just completed infusing aldesleukin (Proleukin) when the patient suddenly becomes very short of breath. Which action should the nurse perform first?
    a. Assess the patient's vital signs.
    b. Flush the IV.
    c. Elevate the head of the bed.
    d. Notify the oncologist.

41. Nursing preparation for administration of bacille Calmette-Guerin (BCG) vaccine includes
    a. accessing a central venous line.
    b. assessing the intravenous site for patency.
    c. inserting a urethral catheter.
    d. identifying the appropriate landmarks for IM infusion.

42. The nurse teaches a patient who is receiving BCG vaccine to use precautions to protect from contamination with excreted urine for 6 hours after the end of therapy, including cleaning the toilet with what?
    a. Alcohol
    b. Ammonia
    c. Bleach
    d. Peroxide

43. What is the greatest nursing priority when a patient is experiencing neuropsychiatric effects from interferon alfa-2b?
    a. Completing drug therapy with interferon alfa-2b
    b. Compliance with antipsychotic drugs
    c. Establishing reality
    d. Preventing injury

DOSE CALCULATION QUESTIONS

44. Fulvestrant 500 mg is to be administered as two 5-mL injections, one into each buttock, each over 1-2 minutes. The 5-mL syringe is marked in 2/10 increments. How long would it take to administer each injection if the nurse administers 2/10 mL (1 line) every 5 seconds? Is this acceptable?

45. A loading dose of cetuximab (Erbitux) 800 mg via IV infusion is prescribed for a patient who is 5'10" and 180 pounds. The recommended dose is 400 mg/m^2. Is the prescribed dose safe and therapeutic?

CASE STUDY

Abiraterone (Zytiga) and prednisone are prescribed for a patient with metastatic castration-resistant prostate cancer.

1. The nurse should teach the patient to report what symptoms of possible electrolyte imbalances?

2. What foods should the patient consume and avoid to decrease the risk of these imbalances?

3. What are possible effects of a decrease in glucocorticoid production?

4. What symptoms should the nurse teach the patient to report because they suggest possible liver damage from the abiraterone?

5. What over-the-counter drug can rise to toxic levels if taken when prescribed this therapy? What are the possible effects?

104
Drugs for the Eye

STUDY QUESTIONS

Matching

Match the term or drug with its description.

1. ____ Block muscarinic receptors preventing pupil constriction
2. ____ Progressive optic nerve damage with eventual impairment of vision
3. ____ Contracts the ciliary muscle facilitating outflow of aqueous humor
4. ____ Decrease production of aqueous humor
5. ____ Dilate pupil by activating alpha$_1$-adrenergic receptors
6. ____ Facilitates outflow of aqueous humor in part by relaxing the ciliary muscle; may increase pigmentation of eyelid
7. ____ Maximally effective doses reduce aqueous flow by 50%; should be reserved for patients who have been refractory to preferred medications
8. ____ Inhibit the breakdown of acetylcholine, causing miosis, focusing of the lens for near vision, and reduction of IOP
9. ____ Paralysis of ciliary muscle
10. ____ Constriction of the pupil
11. ____ Widening of the pupil
12. ____ Cause fluid to move from the eye into the plasma, thereby causing a rapid and marked reduction of IOP
13. ____ May delay optic nerve degeneration and may protect retinal neurons from death
14. ____ IOP increases rapidly and to dangerous levels

a. Phenylephrine
b. Brimonidine
c. Anticholinergic drugs
d. Beta-adrenergic blocker
e. Carbonic anhydrase inhibitor
f. Cholinergic (muscarinic) agonist
g. Cholinesterase inhibitor
h. Acute angle-closure glaucoma
i. Cycloplegia
j. Miosis
k. Mydriasis
l. Osmotic agents
m. Primary open-angle glaucoma (POAG)
n. Prostaglandin analog

Completion

15. Age-related macular degeneration (ARMD) causes loss of _____ vision.

16. _____ are yellow deposits under the retina that occur with ARMD.

17. Vision loss occurs in advanced _____ and _____ ARMD.

18. Patients who take vitamins to prevent ARMD should also ensure adequate intake of copper to prevent copper deficiency _____.

CRITICAL THINKING, PRIORITIZATION, AND DELEGATION QUESTIONS

*19. What is the priority action for prevention of blindness from POAG?
a. Administer eye medications as ordered.
b. Explain the importance of following recommendations for eye screening.
c. Identify individuals at high risk for glaucoma.
d. Teach the common symptoms of glaucoma.

*20. The nurse works in emergency department triage. Which patient would be of greatest priority for receiving immediate care?
a. Patient who sees halos around lights.
b. Patient who experiences itching and watering of eyes.
c. Patient who has sensitivity to light.
d. Patient who has severe eye pain that started 10 minutes ago.

21. Even though systemic effects of topical timolol (Timoptic), echothiophate (Phospholine Iodide), and pilocarpine eye drops are uncommon, which finding would be a reason for the nurse to contact the prescriber before administering the drops? (Select all that apply.)
a. Audible wheezing
b. Blood pressure 170/100 mm Hg
c. Clouding of lens of eye
d. Keyhole appearance to pupil
e. Pulse 50 beats/min

22. What should the nurse do if a brown discoloration of the iris is noted on a patient who has hazel eyes and is receiving latanoprost (Xalatan)?
a. Administer the medication and note the finding.
b. Assess for symptoms of a migraine headache.
c. Teach the patient proper eye cleansing hygiene.
d. Withhold the medication and contact the prescriber.

23. It is important for the nurse to teach orthostatic blood pressure precautions when a patient is prescribed which drug for POAG?
a. Apraclonidine (Iopidine)
b. Bimatoprost (Lumigan)
c. Brimonidine (Alphagan)
d. Latanoprost (Xalatan)

24. The drug handbook lists retinal detachment as an uncommon but serious adverse effect of pilocarpine eye drops. The nurse determines that the patient needs more teaching if the patient includes which issue in the list of things to be reported immediately to the ophthalmologist?
a. Floaters in the field of vision
b. Halos around lights
c. Light flashes
d. Painless loss of part of his vision

25. Which symptom(s), if reported by a patient who is prescribed echothiophate (Phospholine Iodide), would suggest possible development of cataracts? (Select all that apply.)
a. Difficulty reading small print
b. Eye pain
c. Floaters in the field of vision
d. Halos around lights
e. Itching and discharge from eyes

▶26. A patient who has been prescribed oral acetazolamide (Diamox Sequels) for refractory POAG and experiences the adverse effects of severe vomiting and diarrhea should be monitored by the nurse for what?
a. Calcium greater than 11 mg/dL
b. Capillary blood glucose greater than 100 mg/dL
c. Potassium less than 3.5 mEq/L
d. Sodium greater than 145 mEq/L

27. It is of greatest priority to monitor for what finding when a patient is administered an IV osmotic agent for acute angle-closure glaucoma?
a. Bowel sounds
b. Urine output
c. Pain in eyes
d. Vision changes

28. Which adverse effects of mydriatic drugs are serious and warrant withholding the drug and consulting the prescriber? (Select all that apply.)
a. Blurred vision
b. Headache
c. Palpitations
d. Sensitivity to light
e. Sudden eye pain

29. The nurse can help decrease the progression of ARMD by teaching patients at risk to
a. have preventive laser surgery.
b. use adequate light when reading.
c. take supplements of vitamins C and E, beta carotene, zinc, and copper.
d. wear sunscreen and UV-protective sunglasses in bright light.

✱30. It is of greatest priority for the nurse to teach a patient who had vitreous humor injection of pegaptanib (Macugen) to immediately seek medical care if what occurs?
   a. Blurred vision
   b. Conjunctival redness
   c. Halos around lights
   d. Light sensitivity

31. Because of effects of the drug, patients who are prescribed verteporfin should be taught to
   a. protect skin from sunlight.
   b. assess for fever.
   c. report eye discharge.
   d. expect some ocular pain.

32. A patient asks the nurse why the prescriber does not advise using the ocular decongestant tetrahydrozoline (Visine) for allergic conjunctivitis. What would be included in the nurse's explanation?
   a. Benefits take several days to develop.
   b. Rebound congestion is likely.
   c. The drug can cause cataracts.
   d. The drug can elevate IOP.

DOSE CALCULATION QUESTIONS

33. Acetazolamide is available in 250-mg immediate-release tablets. How many tablets should the nurse administer if the dose is 0.5 g?

34. Mannitol is prescribed preoperatively for a 165-lb patient with acute closed-angle glaucoma. The drug is prescribed 0.25g/kg as a 20% solution. The drug is to be infused over 30 minutes one hour prior to surgery. How many grams of mannitol will the patient receive?

CASE STUDY

A 62-year-old patient is seen by her ophthalmologist at the direction of her primary care physician (PCP). She has a history of chronic obstructive pulmonary disease (COPD), psoriasis, and breast cancer. She is accompanied by her adult son and is reluctant to seek care because she says her eyes are "fine." A topical anesthetic is placed in the eye, and the ophthalmologist measures her IOP to be 23 mm Hg. Tropicamide (Tropicacyl) drops are applied, and the patient is sent to wait until mydriatic and cycloplegic effects occur.

1. What are mydriatic and cycloplegic effects, and what are their purposes in this situation?

2. After further examination, the patient is diagnosed with POAG. Her son asks how she could have this disease, glaucoma, and not be aware of it? How should the nurse respond?

3. The patient is prescribed latanoprost (Xalatan) 1 drop to each eye at bedtime. The prescription is denied by the patient's insurer. The prescriber changes the order to betaxolol 1 drop in each eye twice a day. Why had the prescriber originally chosen latanoprost instead of betaxolol for this patient?

4. What teaching should the nurse provide the patient regarding the betaxolol prescription and her glaucoma?

5. The patient returns to the ophthalmologist to have her IOP checked. Her IOP measures at 25 mm Hg. The prescriber adds brimonidine (Alphagan) 1 drop instilled in each eye 3 times a day and dorzolamide (Trusopt) 1 drop 3 times a day. The patient asks why the prescriber did not just order the additional drops of latanoprost (Xalatan). How should the nurse respond?

6. What teaching should the nurse provide about therapy with brimonidine and dorzolamide?

105

Drugs for the Skin

STUDY QUESTIONS

Completion

1. The _____ is the outermost layer of the skin.

2. All cells of the epidermis arise from the _____ _____.

3. The cytoplasm of dead epidermal cells is converted to _____.

4. The outer layer of the epidermis is called the stratum _____.

5. _____ determines skin color and protects the skin from damage from UV rays.

6. Skin collagen, blood vessels, and nerves are found in the _____.

7. Sebaceous glands secrete an oily composite known as _____.

8. Subcutaneous tissue is primarily composed of _____.

9. _____ _____ are lesions of acne commonly called *blackheads*.

10. _____ _____ develop when pores become blocked with sebum and scales below the skin surface.

11. Under the influence of _____, sebum production and turnover of follicular epithelial cells are increased, leading to the development of acne.

12. Common misconceptions regarding nondrug treatment of acne include that vigorous _____ and avoiding certain _____ can cure or prevent acne.

CRITICAL THINKING, PRIORITIZATION, AND DELEGATION QUESTIONS

13. The nurse is teaching the parents of a 2½-year-old child about administration of topical glucocorticoid therapy prescribed for their son's eczema. Which statement, if made by a parent, would suggest the need for further teaching?
    a. "I should apply a thick film when using the cream on his chin."
    b. "I should not cover the area of the skin where the cream was applied unless the doctor tells me to."
    c. "It is important that I only apply the cream to areas with the rash."
    d. "The cream can help stop itching so my child won't scratch it and get infected."

14. A patient who was admitted for a knee replacement asks the nurse to get an order for "cortisone cream" because she has an irritated area of skin under her breast. It is most important for the nurse to do what?
    a. Explain that cortisone cream should not be used in moist areas.
    b. Insist that the nurse apply the cream.
    c. Keep the area covered with a dressing.
    d. Assess the area and communicate findings to the prescriber.

✳15. The nurse is teaching an adolescent about expected and adverse effects of applying prescribed salicylic acid. The priority teaching would be instructing the patient to report which symptom?
    a. Ringing in the ears
    b. Flaking skin
    c. Headache
    d. Itching in the area where the drug was applied

16. A patient who has recently been prescribed benzoyl peroxide calls the telephone triage nurse in a dermatology office because she has been experiencing scaling and swelling at the site of application. What would an expected protocol for the nurse's response normally include?
    a. Continue to use the benzoyl peroxide and try an oil-based moisturizer to relieve the severe dryness.
    b. Continue to use the benzoyl peroxide as prescribed because this is an expected therapeutic effect.
    c. Continue to use the benzoyl peroxide, but use it less often.
    d. Stop using the benzoyl peroxide.

17. When taking a history from a new patient being seen for acne, it is a priority to alert the prescriber that the adolescent has a history of
    a. asthma.
    b. ear infections.
    c. Hashimoto's thyroiditis.
    d. tendonitis.

18. A 56-year-old patient asks what the nurse can tell her about using tretinoin (Retin-A) to prevent wrinkles. The nurse could share the research that suggests that tretinoin
    a. causes the skin to feel softer.
    b. eliminates deep wrinkles.
    c. prevents sunburn.
    d. repairs sun-damaged skin.

19. A patient has been prescribed adapalene (Differin) for acne. Which statement(s) would the nurse include in teaching? (Select all that apply.)
    a. An increase in acne lesions is common early in therapy.
    b. Apply a sunscreen, such as zinc oxide, before applying the cream.
    c. Expect a decrease in blackheads, whiteheads, and inflamed lesions.
    d. Stop the drug if a burning sensation or peeling of the skin occurs.
    e. Use a sunscreen and wear protective clothing.

20. It is important to teach patients who have been prescribed azelaic acid (Azelex) to apply the cream (Select all that apply.)
    a. after washing.
    b. evenly but avoiding the eyes, nose, and mouth.
    c. only to active lesions.
    d. to every area that is red.

＊21. Which effects should the nurse teach the patient to report to the prescriber when prescribed isotretinoin for severe acne? (Select all that apply.)
    a. Back pain and muscle stiffness
    b. Burns easily when out in sun
    c. Frequent nosebleeds
    d. Missed menstrual period
    e. No longer interested in normally pleasurable activities
    f. Peeling of skin from palms and soles
    g. Severe headache followed by transient blurred vision

▶22. The oral contraceptive Estrostep is prescribed for acne treatment for a 17-year-old female patient who also desires contraception. Developmentally, which effect of the estrogen component of this drug is most likely to be a concern to this patient?
    a. Anorexia
    b. Nausea
    c. Swollen breasts
    d. Weight gain

23. A patient has been prescribed Ortho Tri-Cyclen and spironolactone (Aldactone) for contraception and treatment of acne that has been resistant to topical treatments. It is important to instruct the patient to report which symptom that suggests hyperkalemia related to this therapy?
    a. Weakness and nausea
    b. Bone pain and constipation
    c. Cool, clammy skin
    d. Thirst and flushed skin

24. Why does the nurse teach patients to use sunscreens that contain avobenzone?
    a. It is effective on prominent body parts such as the nose.
    b. It is the only ingredient that absorbs UVA1 rays.
    c. It is currently available in a clear formula.
    d. It is most efficient in reflecting the sun's rays.

25. Recent research suggests that psoriasis is caused by what?
    a. An inflammatory disorder
    b. Excessive production of sebum
    c. Excessive reproduction of keratinocytes
    d. Poor hygiene

26. A patient asks the nurse why he should not use a high-potency glucocorticoid on his face. The basis of the nurse's response is that the face is especially prone to what effect of topical glucocorticoids?
    a. Acne-like eruptions
    b. Changes in pigmentation
    c. Sensitivity to sunlight
    d. Thinning of the skin

27. A patient is admitted with fatigue, nausea, vomiting, and constipation. Lab test results include Na$^+$ 136 mEq/L, K$^+$ 3.5 mEq/L, and Ca^{++} 12 mg/dL. The nurse notes red patches with silvery, flaking scales on a patient's knees, elbows, and scalp. It is important for the nurse to determine the dose and frequency of medication if this patient is being treated for psoriasis with which drug?
    a. Anthralin
    b. Calcipotriene (Dovonex)
    c. Tars
    d. Tazarotene (Tazorac)

28. A 28-year-old patient is prescribed anthralin. Which statement, if made by the patient, suggests a need for additional teaching?
    a. "I need to be especially careful to wash my hands after applying the cream."
    b. "It is best if I put the cream on at bedtime."
    c. "I need to cover the cream so that it does not stain my clothing."
    d. "I need to contact my prescriber if the area around my psoriasis becomes red."

29. Which laboratory result for a 57-year-old female patient who is receiving methotrexate for psoriasis would be of most concern to the nurse?
    a. Alanine aminotransferase 35 international units/L
    b. Hemoglobin 12 g/dL
    c. Platelet count 2000/mm^3
    d. White blood cell (WBC) count 9000/mm^3

30. The nurse would be especially vigilant about monitoring the cardiovascular system of a patient who has severe psoriasis being treated with acitretin (Soriatane) and who has a history of what condition?
    a. Chronic obstructive pulmonary disease (COPD)
    b. Diabetes mellitus (DM)
    c. Gastroesophageal reflux disease (GERD)
    d. Osteoarthritis (OA)
    e. Degenerative joint disease (DJD)

31. A history of which condition would be a contraindication for treatment of psoriasis with adalimumab (Humira), etanercept (Enbrel), infliximab (Remicade), and ustekinumab (Stelara)?
    a. Bipolar disorder
    b. Gastroesophageal reflux disease (GERD)
    c. Hypothyroidism
    d. Active tuberculosis (TB)

∗32. The priority nursing intervention to prevent squamous cell carcinoma is teaching patients to
    a. avoid chronic exposure of the skin to sunlight.
    b. examine moles for irregular borders.
    c. report rough, scaly, red-brown papules to the primary care provider.
    d. use sunscreen.

33. The nurse in a long-term care facility is administering topical fluorouracil (Carac) to an actinic keratosis lesion. Which assessment suggests that therapy has achieved the desired effect and treatment can be stopped?
    a. Burning and vesicle formation
    b. Complete healing of lesion
    c. Erosion, ulceration, and necrosis
    d. Severe inflammation and stinging

34. What is an important nursing teaching for patients using diclofenac gel (Solaraze) or imiquimod cream (Aldara)?
    a. Minimize exposure to sunlight.
    b. Cover the treated area with an occlusive dressing.
    c. Discontinue treatment if redness or itching occurs.
    d. Be aware that the medications may stain clothing.

∗35. Which laboratory result for a 27-year-old patient, who has an appointment to receive podophyllum (Podocon-25) for genital warts, would be most important for the nurse to report to the gynecologist administering the treatment?
    a. Alanine aminotransferase 35 international units/L
    b. hCG positive
    c. Hemoglobin 14 g/dL
    d. White blood cell (WBC) count 5000/mm^3

36. What is the primary action of deodorant?
    a. Cover odor with a pleasant fragrance
    b. Decrease flow of apocrine but not eccrine sweat glands
    c. Inhibit release of acetylcholine
    d. Inhibit the growth of surface bacteria

37. The principle of treatment for seborrheic dermatitis is suppression of
    a. cellular reproduction.
    b. growth of yeasts.
    c. histamine release.
    d. scalp oil production.

DOSE CALCULATION QUESTIONS

38. Infliximab (Remicade) 150 mg is prescribed. The drug is diluted in 250 mL of 0.9% NaCl to be infused over 3 hours. What is the rate of infusion in mL/hr?

39. Ustekinumab (Stelara) is supplied in solution of 45 mg/0.5 mL. Prescribed is 90 mg. What is the correct dosage?

CASE STUDIES

Case Study 1

The nurse identifies that body image is a priority concern when collecting data from a 46-year-old female patient who is being seen in the dermatology practice. The patient has heard of using tretinoin (Renova) to prevent aging of the skin. She asks if this drug really works.

1. What information can the nurse provide?

2. The patient is concerned about cost and asks if tretinoin is better than face creams that you can buy in the drugstore. What does research suggest on this topic?

3. The patient and prescriber agree that tretinoin (Renova) is appropriate for this patient. What information can the nurse provide when the patient asks how this differs from the tretinoin (Retin-A Micro) prescribed for her son's acne?

4. What teaching should the nurse provide about use of tretinoin products?

5. The patient reports that she has always used a sunscreen of at least SPF 30 and reapplies it regularly because she enjoys activities out in the sun. What teaching about skin protection should the nurse provide to this patient?

Case Study 2

An 18-year-old female high school senior is being seen at the dermatology office after treatment with antibiotics, benzoyl peroxide, tretinoin (Retin-A Micro), and adapalene (Differin) over the past 2 years have failed to provide acceptable results.

6. What data needs to be collected when the prescriber is considering treatment with isotretinoin?

7. The dermatologist has decided to prescribe isotretinoin and has asked the office nurse to reinforce teaching regarding this drug. What are some nursing diagnoses that should be included when planning teaching relating to this patient, diagnosis, and treatment?

8. How should the nurse respond to the patient's question of how isotretinoin therapy differs from tretinoin?

9. Because patients do not always remember what is explained to them, what teaching methods besides oral explanation should the nurse provide to this patient?

10. What teaching must the nurse provide this patient regarding the iPLEDGE program?

106

Drugs for the Ear

STUDY QUESTIONS

Completion

1. The visible outside part of the ear is called the _____ or _____.

2. The auditory canal and auricle make up the _____ _____.

3. The malleus, incus, and stapes transmit sound vibrations from the _____ to the _____ ear.

4. The _____ _____ allows air pressure within the middle ear to equalize with air pressure in the environment.

5. The _____ _____ provide our sense of balance.

True or False

For each of the following statements, enter T *for true or* F *for false.*

6. ____ Ear wax (cerumen) should be removed from the auditory canal every time we bathe.

7. ____ Acute otitis media (AOM) can be caused by blockage of the eustachian tube.

8. ____ Presence of ear pain (otalgia) suggests serious complications have occurred.

9. ____ In an otherwise healthy child with AOM, it is more important to treat the pain than the infecting microbe.

10. ____ AOM primarily occurs in children ages 5-12 years.

CRITICAL THINKING, PRIORITIZATION, AND DELEGATION QUESTIONS

11. The nurse is caring for a 2-year-old child. When bathing the child, the nurse notes sticky, crusting exudate filling the right external ear canal. The nurse would use which term when documenting this finding?
    a. Otalgia
    b. Otitis media
    c. Otorrhea
    d. Otosclerosis

12. Which assessment finding in a child receiving amoxicillin would be a reason for the parent to contact the prescriber?
    a. Allergy to clarithromycin
    b. Diarrhea
    c. Facial rash that is maculopapular and does not itch
    d. Multiple intensely itchy vesicles on the chest and back

13. What is the most significant reason why prophylactic antibiotic therapy for recurrent otitis media is not currently recommended?
    a. It increases the development of antibiotic resistance.
    b. It involves the use of drugs that stain the teeth.
    c. It frequently causes diarrhea.
    d. It is too expensive.

14. Recommendations for acute otitis externa include instilling into the ear canal a 2% solution of the acid found in
    a. alcohol.
    b. oranges.
    c. peroxide.
    d. vinegar.

15. The nurse is doing telephone triage in a primary care office. A patient calls complaining of ear pain. Which information would warrant the patient being seen immediately? (Select all that apply.)
    a. Elderly diabetic patient
    b. Immunocompromised patient
    c. Pain when the outer ear is touched
    d. Purulent otic discharge
    e. Uses cotton swabs regularly to clean ear canal

16. Which vaccination has been shown to decrease the risk of AOM?
    a. DTaP
    b. MMR
    c. OPV
    d. PVC

17. Amoxicillin-clavulanate is used for antibiotic-resistant AOM because the clavulanate
    a. allows for a lower dose of amoxicillin.
    b. decreases incidence of adverse effects.
    c. increases antibacterial action against *Streptococcus pneumoniae.*
    d. prevents destruction of the antibiotic by bacterial enzymes.

DOSE CALCULATION QUESTIONS

18. A child who was born prematurely and weighs 10 lb at 3 months is prescribed amoxicillin 200 mg to be administered twice a day for AOM. The pharmacy supplies an oral suspension of 250 mg/mL. Is the dose safe for a 3-month-old child? How much amoxicillin should be administered?

19. Amoxicillin 750 mg is prescribed for a 38-kg child. Is the dose appropriate? How many mL should be administered if the drug is available as 500 mg/10 mL ?

CASE STUDIES

Case Study 1

A pregnant woman has brought her 2½-year-old son to the pediatrician because he was fussy all last night. The pediatric nurse practitioner (PNP) diagnoses AOM, but does not prescribe an antibiotic.

1. What factors did the PNP consider when deciding whether to treat with an antibiotic?

2. The patient's mother is upset and complains to the office nurse that she always received a prescription in the past when her older child had an ear infection. What should the nurse include in the explanation of why antibiotics are not being prescribed?

3. What drug treatment should be provided for this child?

4. What symptoms should the nurse teach the patient's mother to report regarding the need for the child to be brought back for reevaluation?

5. The nurse notes that this child has had multiple episodes of otitis media. What teaching can the nurse provide that may decrease the incidence of otitis media for this child and the new sibling when born?

Case Study 2

A female pediatric patient has been prescribed Cipro HC drops for otitis externa.

6. What information should the nurse include when teaching about administration of these drops?

7. What technique should the nurse use to evaluate the learning if the child's parents do not appear to understand oral instruction?

8. The patient's parents ask if they can use old drops from a previous infection. What should the nurse include in the response?

9. The nurse notes that the patient has had repeated episodes of otitis externa. What teaching can the nurse provide that might decrease the number of episodes?

107

Miscellaneous Noteworthy Drugs

STUDY QUESTIONS

Matching

Match the class of the drug used to treat pulmonary artery hypertension (PAH) with the drug(s).

1. ___ Derivative of prostacyclin that promotes vascular relaxation, suppresses growth of vascular smooth muscle cells, and inhibits platelet aggregation
2. ___ Reduces pulmonary arterial pressure by causing dilation of pulmonary blood vessels
3. ___ Inhibits calcium ion influx into vascular smooth muscle
4. ___ Reduce pulmonary vascular resistance and may have a favorable impact on vascular remodeling
5. ___ Prevents thrombosis
6. ___ Reduce fluid retention, and thereby reduce cardiac preload

    a. Ambrisentan and bosentan
    b. Amlodipine, felodipine, and nifedipine
    c. Epoprostenol, iloprost, and treprostinil
    d. Furosemide and hydrochlorothiazide
    e. Sildenafil and tadalafil
    f. Warfarin

CRITICAL THINKING, PRIORITIZATION, AND DELEGATION QUESTIONS

▶ 7. What is the priority nursing instruction to a patient
✳ with PAH who is receiving iloprost (Ventavis)?
    a. Change positions slowly.
    b. Cough and deep-breathe.
    c. Do not cross your legs.
    d. Use pursed-lip breathing.

8. Which of these laboratory test results, if identified for a female patient who is receiving bosentan (Tracleer), should the nurse report to the prescriber immediately?
    a. ALT 60 IU/mL
    b. Creatinine 1.4 mg/dL
    c. Hbg 12.8/ Hct 37
    d. hCG positive

9. Which drug for type 2 diabetes mellitus is contraindicated when a patient is prescribed bosentan (Tracleer)?
    a. Glimepiride
    b. Glipizide
    c. Glyburide
    d. Metformin

10. The most recent ALT result for a patient receiving bosentan (Tracleer) is 95 international units/L. What should the nurse do if it is time to administer the drug?
    a. Administer the drug as prescribed.
    b. Assess for nausea, vomiting, fever, jaundice, and fatigue.
    c. Withhold the drug and consult with the prescriber regarding a dose decrease or interruption.
    d. Withhold the drug and consult with the prescriber regarding discontinuing the drug.

11. Which statement, if made by a patient who has just been prescribed sildenafil (Revatio) for PAH, would warrant teaching to prevent a possible fatal reaction?
    a. "I know I should exercise more but I often do not have enough energy."
    b. "I use aspirin when I get a headache because I also heard that it is good for my heart."
    c. "I use the little tablets that dissolve under the tongue that the doctor prescribed for my wife when I get chest pain."
    d. "My hearing is not as good as it used to be."

▶12. The nurse is administering intramuscular (IM)
  * dexamethasone to a pregnant patient who is at risk
    for premature delivery of the fetus. The patient's
    skin is hot and dry, and the patient is voiding 200
    to 300 mL every hour. Which diagnostic test result
    is of greatest priority for the nurse to monitor in
    this situation?
    a. BUN
    b. Creatinine
    c. Glucose
    d. Urine specific gravity

▶13. The risk of what is of greatest priority if a
  * premature neonate needed beractant (Survanta)?
    a. Ineffective airway clearance
    b. Deficient fluid volume
    c. Hypothermia
    d. Ineffective breast-feeding

14. For maximal therapeutic results, dornase alfa (Pul-
    mozyme) should be administered to patients with
    cystic fibrosis at which time?
    a. After chest physiotherapy
    b. After meals
    c. Before chest physiotherapy
    d. Before meals

15. The nurse is caring for a 15-year-old female pa-
    tient who has been admitted in a sickle cell crisis.
    The patient complains of severe joint pain (10 of
    10). The nurse notes that the patient is sitting qui-
    etly in bed conversing with her parents. Intrave-
    nous morphine 0.5 mg and oral ibuprofen 200 mg
    are ordered every 3 hours as needed. The patient
    has not had any analgesic medication in the past 3
    hours. What should the nurse do?
    a. Administer the ibuprofen.
    b. Administer the morphine.
    c. Assess for other physiologic indicators of pain.
    d. Provide nonpharmacologic pain relief mea-
       sures.

16. A 16-year-old patient with sickle cell anemia has
    been prescribed hydroxyurea (Droxia). Which
    nursing problem would be of most concern relat-
    ing to this drug therapy?
    a. Adherence to prescribed regimen
    b. Body image
    c. Infection
    d. Tissue perfusion

17. A patient has come to the outpatient oncology
    clinic for an infusion of rasburicase (Elitek).
    Which symptom suggests that the patient may be
    experiencing methemoglobinemia?
    a. Cyanosis
    b. Fever
    c. Nausea and vomiting
    d. Rash

18. A patient with chronic kidney disease (CKD)
    who receives hemodialysis is prescribed calcium
    carbonate (PhosLo) to lower blood phosphate. To
    achieve maximum binding of phosphate and mini-
    mal absorption of the calcium, the drug should be
    administered in which way?
    a. First thing in the morning
    b. At least 1 hour before meals
    c. At least 2 hours after meals
    d. With meals

19. The nurse is caring for a patient who is prescribed
    sevelamer HCl (Renagel) to prevent hyperphos-
    phatemia of CKD. Which respiratory change
    suggests that the patient may be experiencing
    metabolic acidosis?
    a. Hyperventilation
    b. Diminished lung sounds
    c. Lower lobe crackles (rales)
    d. Sonorous gurgles (rhonchi)

20. Which laboratory test result would be of most
    concern to the nurse when a patient is prescribed
    gamma-hydroxybutyrate (GHB) (Xyrem) for cata-
    plexy associated with narcolepsy?
    a. BNP 1750 picograms/mL
    b. hCG 12 mIU/mL
    c. HDL 85 mg/dL
    d. INR 1.1

21. When a patient is receiving riluzole (Rilutek) for
    amyotrophic lateral sclerosis (ALS), it is most im-
    portant for the nurse to assess for which symptom
    of the underlying condition?
    a. Dizziness
    b. Nausea and vomiting
    c. Respiratory distress
    d. Weakness

22. Which question is of greatest priority when a patient is prescribed tetrabenazine (Xenazine) for treatment of chorea associated with HD?
    a. "Are you concerned about weight gain when you take medications?"
    b. "Are you having any thoughts about doing anything to harm yourself?"
    c. "Do you experience dizziness when you stand up?"
    d. "Have you had any difficulty voiding?"

23. Which data would warrant consulting the prescriber before administering milnacipran (Savella)?
    a. BP 100/64 mm Hg
    b. eGFR 42 mL/min
    c. INR 0.9
    d. Pulse 62 beats/min

24. Which drugs for hereditary angioedema (HAE) have a possible adverse effect of anaphylaxis? (Select all that apply.)
    a. Berinert
    b. Cinryze
    c. Firazyr
    d. Kalbitor
    e. Winstrol

DOSE CALCULATION QUESTIONS

25. The recommended dose of belimumab is 10 mg/kg. What is the dose for a patient with systemic lupus erythematosus (SLE) who weighs 137.5 lb?

26. A patient is prescribed 0.2 mg/kg of rasburicase. What is the dose for a patient weighing 165 lb? The reconstituted drug is further diluted in 50 mL 0.9% normal saline to infuse over 1 hour. The infusion pump is calibrated in mL/hr. What rate of infusion should be programmed into the pump?

CASE STUDY

A 22-month-old African-American pediatric patient is admitted to a pediatric hospital because of fever, irritability, jaundice, and unremitting malaise. Laboratory test results reveal anemia and presence of hemoglobin S, confirming the diagnosis of sickle cell disease. The patient's parent asks the nurse why the patient's eyes are so yellow.

1. What would be the logical explanation for jaundice in sickle cell disease?

2. The parent has heard of a new drug, hydroxyurea, and asks why it has not been prescribed for the child. What is the best explanation?
    a. The drug has adverse effects.
    b. The drug has only been approved for patients who are age 18 and older.
    c. The drug is an orphan drug.
    d. The drug is only used as a last resort.

3. The parent asks the nurse if anything can be done to keep the child from experiencing sickle cell crises. How should the nurse respond?

108
Dietary Supplements

STUDY QUESTIONS

Matching

Match the dietary product to its primary use.

1. ___ Benign prostatic hyperplasia
2. ___ Reduce triglycerides
3. ___ Depression
4. ___ Increase pain-free walking distance
5. ___ Prophylaxis of migraine
6. ___ Treat vertigo
7. ___ Treat symptoms of menopause
8. ___ Stimulate immune function
9. ___ Promote sleep
10. ___ Treat constipation

a. Black cohosh
b. Echinacea
c. Feverfew
d. Garlic
e. Ginger root
f. Ginkgo biloba
g. Flaxseed
h. St. John's wort
i. Saw palmetto
j. Valerian

True or False

For each of the following statements, enter T for true or F for false.

11. ___ Natural products are always better and safer than synthetic products.
12. ___ Products marketed as dietary supplements do not require rigorous evaluation before marketing.
13. ___ The FDA cannot remove a dietary supplement from the market even if there is evidence that it causes harm.
14. ___ Dietary supplement labels can insinuate that they provide health benefits.
15. ___ Dietary supplements have been found to contain harmful ingredients such as arsenic, mercury, and lead.

16. ___ Dietary supplements have been found to not contain the stated ingredients in the amount listed on the label.
17. ___ Dietary supplement labels may claim to treat a specific disease without adequate research supporting the claim.
18. ___ There is conflicting evidence that dietary supplements are effective or safe.

CRITICAL THINKING, PRIORITIZATION, AND DELEGATION QUESTIONS

19. Current Good Manufacturing Practices (CGMPs) are designed to ensure that dietary supplements
    a. list their active and inert ingredients.
    b. meet the needs of all socioeconomic groups.
    c. are generic formulations, not brand name.
    d. are used to promote health.

✳20. The priority teaching when a patient chooses to use a dietary supplement is that it is best to
    a. always buy the more expensive brand.
    b. take the herb with at least 8 ounces of water.
    c. use products that have the seal of approval from the USP.
    d. use the lowest dose possible.

✳21. What is a priority nursing action when a nurse discovers that a patient self-prescribes herbal products?
    a. Assess for drug interactions and adverse effects of the product.
    b. Be an advocate for the patient's right to make choices.
    c. Convince the patient to stop taking the products.
    d. Teach the patient the importance of informing all health care providers of all products being used.

22. A patient who is taking metronidazole is at risk for a disulfiram-like (Antabuse) reaction if also taking an herbal product in which form?
    a. Decoctions
    b. Extracts or tinctures containing alcohol
    c. Solid extracts
    d. Teas and infusions

＊23. Which laboratory test would be a priority for the nurse to monitor if a patient with heart failure was prescribed warfarin and self-prescribes coenzyme Q-10, saw palmetto, resveratrol, ginger, garlic, and/or ginkgo biloba?
    a. ALT
    b. CBC
    c. INR
    d. Sodium

24. Research suggests which possible effect of cranberry juice?
    a. Increasing excretion of bacteria
    b. Making urine acidic, which kills bacteria
    c. Preventing bacteria from adhering to the bladder wall
    d. Preventing kidney stones

▶25. Based on German studies, it is important for the nurse to teach women prescribed antihypertensives and taking black cohosh for hot flashes and insomnia to
    a. avoid prolonged exposure to the sun.
    b. change positions slowly.
    c. drink adequate amounts of fluids.
    d. stop taking the herb if headache occurs.

26. Pregnant nurses should wear gloves if they are administering which herbal supplement?
    a. Aloe
    b. Feverfew
    c. Ginger
    d. Saw palmetto

27. What is true about echinacea? (Select all that apply.)
    a. It can aggravate autoimmune disorders.
    b. It can produce an allergic reaction in patients allergic to ragweed the first time it is taken.
    c. It can suppress the immune system with long-term use.
    d. It decreases the severity of the common cold.
    e. It prevents symptoms of the common cold.

28. The nurse is assessing a new admission. The patient lists echinacea, garlic, and kava among the products that she uses regularly. On first observation, the nurse notes that the patient's skin has a yellowish color. What is the most appropriate action for the nurse to take next?
    a. Continue to assess the patient.
    b. Document jaundice in the nurses' notes.
    c. Notify the health care provider of the findings STAT.
    d. Tell the patient to stop taking the herbal products.

29. A patient who regularly takes feverfew to prevent migraine headaches stopped taking the herb before elective surgery. The nurse should assess the patient for what?
    a. Bleeding
    b. Flatulence
    c. Insomnia
    d. Nausea

30. A patient who is prescribed glipizide (Glucotrol) for type 2 diabetes mellitus and celecoxib (Celebrex) for inflamed joints informs the nurse that she has started taking ginger because she read in a magazine that it helps arthritis. It is a priority to teach the patient to be alert for possible hypoglycemia symptoms, including
    a. dry, itchy skin.
    b. headache.
    c. loss of appetite.
    d. palpitations and sweating.

＊31. It is a priority to inform patients with which disorder that ginkgo biloba can aggravate their condition?
    a. Diabetes mellitus
    b. Hay fever
    c. Hypertension
    d. Seizures

32. What is an appropriate outcome for a 12-year-old child relating to probiotics prescribed during a rotavirus infection?
    a. Soft, formed stool
    b. No bacterial growth in urine
    c. Temperature 98° F to 99° F
    d. No adventitious lung sounds

＊33. What is a priority concern for the nurse when a patient with multiple medical disorders self-prescribes St. John's wort?
    a. Effect on other prescribed drugs
    b. Constipation
    c. Photosensitivity
    d. Potency of the preparation

34. The nurse is aware that which herbal supplement has been associated with liver failure?
    a. Black cohosh
    b. Ginger
    c. Kava
    d. Valerian

✳35. The nurse is caring for a patient who admits to using mail order ma huang (ephedra) for weight loss. It is a priority for the nurse to do what?
    a. Assess mental status.
    b. Monitor vital signs.
    c. Not administer any other sedatives.
    d. Weigh the patient daily.

CASE STUDIES

Case Study 1

A 52-year-old man is admitted with chest pain. Assessment findings include height 5' 8", weight 220 lb, waist circumference 42", BP 145/86 mm Hg, and pulse 78 beats/min. Lab results include triglycerides 380 mg/dL, LDL 240 mg/dL, and HDL 34 mg/dL. He is diagnosed with gastroesophageal reflux disease (GERD) and metabolic syndrome. He informs his health care provider that he wants to try natural therapy and has heard that garlic can help many things. The health care provider asks the nurse to discuss garlic therapy with this patient.

1. What are possible positive effects of garlic supplementation for this patient?

2. The health care provider recommends enteric-coated garlic supplements. What can the nurse teach the patient to ensure that the product that he purchases contains effective amounts of allicin?

3. The patient insists on using raw garlic. What information should the nurse provide about raw garlic therapy?

4. Why is it important for the patient to inform all health care providers and his pharmacist that he is using garlic therapy?

Case Study 2

An 85-year-old woman with atrial fibrillation is being treated with digoxin (Lanoxin) and warfarin (Coumadin). At times, she is fatigued and forgetful. Her friend suggests that she take ginkgo biloba to give her more energy.

5. What possible complications can occur with this combination of drugs and herbs?

6. What teaching should the nurse provide this patient regarding the use of herbal products?

7. The patient informs the nurse that she is not going to get her annual flu shot because she has purchased a bottle of echinacea. How should the nurse respond?

109

Management of Poisoning

STUDY QUESTIONS

Matching

Match the chelating agent and the metal(s) it binds with. (Select all that apply.)

1. ___ Arsenic
2. ___ Copper
3. ___ Ethylene glycol (antifreeze)
4. ___ Gold
5. ___ Iron
6. ___ Lead
7. ___ Mercury

   a. Deferoxamine (Desferal)
   b. Dimercaprol (BAL in oil)
   c. Edetate calcium disodium (Calcium EDTA)
   d. Fomepizole (Antizole)
   e. Penicillamine (Depen)
   f. Succimer (Chemet)

CRITICAL THINKING, PRIORITIZATION, AND DELEGATION QUESTIONS

✳ 8. What is the initial priority of nursing care of a patient with a suspected ingestion of a poison?
   a. Administering an antidote
   b. Assessing airway, breathing, and circulation
   c. Identifying the poison
   d. Preventing absorption of poison that has not been absorbed

9. A person with an unknown medical history arrives at the emergency department (ED) after ingesting an unidentified poison. The patient is comatose when arriving at the ED. An intravenous (IV) line of normal saline is infusing, respirations are unlabored at 17 breaths per minute, and BP is 118/72 mm Hg. Which assessment findings suggest hypoglycemia? (Select all that apply.)
   a. Capillary refill 2-3 seconds
   b. Diaphoresis
   c. DTR 2+
   d. Dry mucous membranes
   e. Pulse 108 beats/min

10. The nurse knows that the most accurate and efficient method of identifying the poison and the dose is what?
   a. Analysis of urine, blood, and gastric contents
   b. Evaluation of patient symptoms
   c. Examining the container
   d. Interviewing the caregiver

11. What is the purpose of an antidote to a poison?
   a. Increase renal excretion of the poison.
   b. Prevent absorption of the poison.
   c. Remove residual poison from the gastrointestinal (GI) tract.
   d. Counteract the effects of a poison.

12. Charcoal is most effective in binding with poisons in the GI tract and preventing absorption if administered
   a. after the patient has vomited.
   b. for fat-soluble poisons.
   c. within 30 minutes of poison ingestion.
   d. with milk.

13. The nurse is assessing a 3-year-old patient who is receiving 0.5 L/hr of polyethylene glycol (GoLYTELY) via nasogastric (NG) tube after having ingested 60 tablets of adult iron supplement. Which assessment finding would be of most concern to the nurse?
   a. BP 80/52 mm Hg
   b. Dark brown emesis
   c. Pulse 120 beats/min
   d. 475 mL of yellow-tinged liquid stool in past hour

▶ 14. A child has ingested several bottles of children's chewable aspirin (acetylsalicylic acid). The ED resident informs the nurse that treatment will include enhancing renal excretion of the drug. The nurse would question orders for all substances except
   a. acetic acid.
   b. ammonium chloride.
   c. citric acid.
   d. sodium bicarbonate.

►15. A patient has been treated for poisoning by hemo-perfusion, which passes blood over an absorbent resin. The nurse should monitor the patient for
a. bleeding.
b. dehydration.
c. hyperglycemia.
d. seizures.

16. A patient is being treated for acute ferric iron poisoning with deferoxamine (Desferal). The nurse knows that this drug works by
a. binding with iron in the blood, causing excretion in the urine.
b. binding with iron in the GI tract, preventing absorption.
c. flushing the GI tract.
d. inducing vomiting.

►17. A nurse assesses the vital signs of a patient who is being treated for ferric iron poisoning with IV deferoxamine (Desferal). Which finding suggests that the administration rate of the drug might be too rapid?
a. Blood pressure 150/85 mm Hg
b. Pulse 112 beats/min
c. Respirations 15/min
d. Temperature 100.4° F (38° C)

18. The nurse is teaching a patient who has been prescribed deferasirox (Exjade) for iron overload associated with beta-thalassemia. Which statement, if made by the patient, suggests a need for additional instruction?
a. "I need to have bloodwork done as directed to make sure that the drug dose and my kidneys are okay."
b. "I need to crush the tablet and mix it with a full glass of juice."
c. "I should stop taking this drug if I have a fever higher than 99° F."
d. "If I take this with a drug for heartburn, it won't be absorbed."

19. Which would be an appropriate technique when the nurse is administering dimercaprol (BAL in oil)?
a. Deep injection into the dorsogluteal muscle
b. Subcutaneous injection into abdominal fat
c. Subcutaneous injection above the vastus lateralis
d. Z-track injection into the ventrogluteal muscle

20. The nurse is caring for a 3-year-old child who weighs 15 kg and is scheduled to receive an intramuscular dose of edetate calcium EDTA for lead poisoning. The child's urinary output has averaged 15 mL/hr for the last 4 hours. What should the nurse do?
a. Administer the drug and continue nursing care.
b. Consult the prescriber regarding the need for additional fluids.
c. Withhold the medication and consult the prescriber.
d. Withhold the medication and assess for renal failure.

21. The nurse would withhold calcium EDTA and contact the prescriber if which laboratory test result occurs?
a. Albumin 5 g/dL
b. Amylase 190 international units/L
c. Protein total 8.3 g/dL
d. Protein in urine 287 mg/dL

22. To detect serious adverse effects, it is most important for the nurse to monitor the results of which laboratory test when caring for a patient with Wilson's disease who is receiving penicillamine (Depen)?
a. Alanine aminotransferase
b. Blood urea nitrogen
c. Complete blood count and differential
d. Creatinine

23. A child who was admitted after ingesting antifreeze is treated with fomepizole (Antizol). Which symptom suggests that the child's body is attempting to compensate for metabolic acidosis?
a. Decreased urine output
b. Increased urine output
c. Rapid, deep respirations
d. Shallow breathing

24. The nurse teaches parents that dialing 1-800-222-1222 will connect them with what?
a. A local poison center
b. The national poison center
c. A pharmacist
d. A specially trained nurse

DOSE CALCULATION QUESTIONS

25. Naloxone 1 mg is prescribed IV as an antidote to heroin overdose. Available is naloxone 0.4 mg/mL. What is the amount of naloxone to be administered?

26. Calcium EDTA 1 ampule is diluted in 500 mL of normal saline solution. It is to be infused in 90 minutes. What rate in mL/hr should be programmed into the IV pump?

CASE STUDY

A 4-year-old girl, who has been playing outside in her yard, comes in the house and says she doesn't feel well. Her parents notice a purple stain on their daughter's face. Knowing that they do not have any grape juice in the house, the parents ask their daughter what she has eaten. The child tells them about some berries she found in the yard. The parents call the poison control center, and the child is rushed to the ED of the hospital.

1. When the nurse questions the parents, they describe "weeds" growing at the back of the yard with blueberry-size purple berries that their daughter may have ingested. What should be done to identify the ingested substance?

2. The stomach contents contain a noncaustic neurotoxin. What data can the nurse collect to assist the emergency physician with deciding if charcoal, gastric lavage, or whole bowel irrigation is the best approach for this poisoning?

3. The parents are sure that the ingestion of the poison occurred less than 30 minutes ago. Gastric lavage and aspiration is ordered. What is the nurse's role?

4. Why is the child positioned on the left side with her head down?

5. The child is stabilized and observed overnight. What instruction should the nurse provide this family before discharge?

110

Potential Weapons of Biologic, Radiologic, and Chemical Terrorism

STUDY QUESTIONS

True or False

For each of the following statements, enter T *for true or* F *for false.*

1. ___ Anthrax spores can live outside of a host for many years.

2. ___ Respiratory anthrax can cause hemorrhage and inflammation of the meninges of the brain.

3. ___ Approximately 20% of patients who contract cutaneous anthrax die despite antibiotic therapy.

4. ___ Intravenous antibiotics kill anthrax bacteria and spores.

5. ___ Research has proven that raxibacumab neutralizes deadly anthrax toxins in humans.

6. ___ Antibiotic treatment of cutaneous anthrax is not likely to prevent skin lesions and necrosis.

7. ___ Inactivated vaccine for anthrax cannot be administered to immunocompromised patients.

8. ___ Anthrax vaccination can be administered before and immediately after exposure.

9. ___ Bubonic plague is not transmitted person to person.

10. ___ Smallpox vaccine involves pricking the skin with the live virus.

11. ___ Early treatment with antibiotics is often effective when treating smallpox.

CRITICAL THINKING, PRIORITIZATION, AND DELEGATION QUESTIONS

12. Which symptom would be a priority to report to the prescriber if a patient is suspected of being exposed to *Bacillus anthracis?*
    a. Blurred vision
    b. Diarrhea
    c. Hemoptysis
    d. Malaise

13. Which statement, if made by a patient receiving ciprofloxacin for cutaneous anthrax, would indicate understanding of drug therapy teaching?
    a. "I must take all of the prescription as directed because if I do not, serious illness and death could occur."
    b. "I should take the antibiotic until the scabs fall off."
    c. "If I start the antibiotic immediately, there is a chance that I will not experience itchy vesicles."
    d. "My prescription needs to be changed if I get pregnant."

14. The community health nurse, who works in areas known to have the presence of *B. anthracis*, promotes routine vaccination with anthrax vaccine (BioThrax) for people with which occupation?
    a. Police officer
    b. Postal worker
    c. Receptionist
    d. Sheep farmer

▶ 15. Intramuscular streptomycin 0.5 g twice a day is prescribed for a 150-lb man who has been diagnosed with tularemia. Nursing assessments before administration of the drug include BP 140/72 mm Hg, pulse 88 beats/min, respirations 24/min, moist cough, and end inspiratory crackles in upper lobes. What should the nurse do?
    a. Administer the drug and consult the prescriber regarding the low dose.
    b. Administer the drug as one injection in the dorsogluteal site.
    c. Wear a high-efficiency particulate mask when administering the drug.
    d. Withhold the drug and consult the prescriber.

16. A patient is admitted with a diagnosis of pneumonic plague. Which precaution would be best to prevent spread of this infection?
    a. Contact precautions
    b. Droplet precautions
    c. Immediate vaccination of the patient
    d. Prophylactic vaccination of staff

17. Which symptoms most specifically suggest a smallpox infection?
    a. Headache, high fever, chills, and rigors
    b. Multiple red spots on the tongue and buccal mucosa
    c. Painless ulcers with a necrotic core that develop black eschar
    d. Tender, enlarged, inflamed lymph nodes

18. The public health nurse is administering smallpox vaccine to police officers. Which statement, if made by a vaccination recipient, would indicate a need for further teaching?
    a. "I should keep the site covered to avoid spreading the live vaccine."
    b. "I should seek medical care if any drainage occurs from the vaccination site."
    c. "It is important that I not get pregnant for at least 4 weeks after receiving this vaccination."
    d. "This vaccination should be effective even if I was exposed to smallpox yesterday."

19. The Department of Health and Human Services has contracted to buy the modified vaccinia virus Ankara (MVA) instead of ACAM2000 in case of a terrorist attack with smallpox. Why has MVA been chosen?
    a. It is safe for immunocompromised people.
    b. It does not have a risk of postvaccine encephalitis or cardiac problems.
    c. It is the only drug approved by the FDA.
    d. It is less expensive and more effective than Dryvax.

20. The nurse is preparing to vaccinate a patient who has been exposed to the smallpox virus. The patient states that she is pregnant. What should the nurse do?
    a. Administer the vaccine.
    b. Administer cidofovir before administering the smallpox vaccine.
    c. Assess if the patient has been informed of benefits and risks of vaccination.
    d. Withhold the vaccine.

✳21. What is the highest nursing priority when caring for a patient with botulism poisoning?
    a. Effective breathing
    b. Impaired mobility
    c. Swallowing ability
    d. Visual acuity

22. The nurse is providing emergency care after a disaster at a nuclear power plant that caused the release of radioactive material. Which dose of potassium iodide should be administered to a patient who breast-feeds her infant?
    a. None
    b. 65 mg daily
    c. 130 mg daily
    d. 195 mg daily

▶23. To prevent magnesium deficiency when receiving zinc trisodium (Zn-DTPA), the nurse teaches a patient to include adequate amounts of which food?
    a. Eggs
    b. Liver
    c. Red meat
    d. Whole grains

24. Which statement, if made by a patient who has been prescribed Ca-DPTA therapy for americium poisoning, would suggest understanding of teaching?
    a. "I cannot receive these drugs if my kidneys are not functioning properly."
    b. "I need to take a pill every day for at least 2 months."
    c. "I should drink 100 ounces of fluid, especially water, each day."
    d. "I should try to empty my bladder at least once every 8 hours."

25. The nurse knows that adverse effects of ferric hexacyanoferrate (Prussian blue) used to increase excretion of nonradioactive thallium can cause hypokalemia, increasing the risk of toxicity of which medication?
    a. Acetaminophen
    b. Atenolol
    c. Digoxin
    d. Furosemide

DOSE CALCULATION QUESTIONS

26. A woman has potassium iodide 65-mg tablets. Her 2½-year-old daughter is exposed to radiation. How many tablets should she administer if the recommended dose is 32 mg?

27. Calcium trisodium Ca-DPTA solution 1 g in 5 mL 5% dextrose in water is to be administered over 3-4 minutes. How many mL should be administered every 10 seconds if the drug is administered over 3 minutes and 20 seconds?

CASE STUDIES

Case Study 1

People in the United States died from inhalation of anthrax spores in October 2001. The nation was on alert for terrorist attacks.

1. What are possible reasons for the infections not being promptly diagnosed and treated in time to prevent all deaths?

2. How can the nurse contribute to early recognition of infections caused by biologic agents?

3. People who were possibly exposed to *B. anthracis* were offered prophylactic drug therapy. What teaching should be provided by the community health nurses assisting with this mass prophylaxis?

Case Study 2

A patient has come to the ED because of exposure to an unknown powder.

4. If this person were exposed to anthrax bacilli, how can the infection spread to other people?

5. What precautions should the nurse take to prevent the spread of anthrax infection?

Case Study 3

The military nurse is participating in a drill imitating exposure of soldiers to mustard gas.

6. What would be the first action that the nurse should take?

7. How can the nurse prevent additional exposure to the agent for the soldiers and health care providers?

8. What questions about the episode would the nurse ask to determine which persons probably received the most exposure to the gas?

9. What symptoms would the nurse expect to occur first?

10. What should the nurse assess to determine if the most serious consequences could be occurring?

Case Study 4

Reports of ricin being used by terrorists cause a great deal of fear.

11. Why is ricin a logical weapon of bioterrorism?

12. What treatment would the nurse anticipate if a patient is admitted with inhalation of ricin?

13. What test would detect the early effects of ricin on the gastrointestinal tract?

Answer Key

Answers to the Case Studies can be reviewed online at http://evolve.elsevier.com/Lehne/.

CHAPTER 1

1. b
2. d
3. c
4. a
5. Selectivity
6. Low cost
7. Reversible action
8. Freedom from interactions
9. Possession of a simple generic name
10. Effectiveness
11. Ease of administration
12. Safety
13. Chemical stability
14. Predictability
15. c
16. a (The others are not within the scope of nursing practice.)

CHAPTER 2

1. d
2. b
3. f
4. g
5. a
6. e
7. c
8. b
9. d (Suggests possible anaphylactic reaction.)
10. c
11. d
12. b (These assessments are a priority, as well as being needed to determine if prescribed pain medication can safely be administered.)
13. d

CHAPTER 3

1. b
2. a
3. c
4. generic
5. chemical
6. generic
7. brand
8. Generic
9. generic
10. generic
11. d
12. b, c
13. a
14. b, d

CHAPTER 4

1. e
2. c
3. b
4. f
5. a
6. d
7. c
8. a
9. b
10. T
11. F
12. T
13. T
14. F
15. T
16. F
17. F
18. T
19. F
20. T
21. F
22. T
23. T
24. T
25. F
26. T
27. d (Continued administration of morphine would lead to respiratory arrest.)
28. b (The nurse must find out how much additional heparin is to be administered in order to prevent DVT; since the nurse has realized the error just after administration, assessment for DVT is not a priority; the incident report would be completed after provider notification.)
29. a

30. c
31. a (Most general anesthetics are excreted by exhalation.)
32. b, c, d
33. b
34. d

CHAPTER 5

1. T
2. F
3. T
4. T
5. T
6. T
7. F
8. F
9. T
10. T
11. F
12. T
13. T
14. T
15. a
16. a, d
17. b, d, e
18. b
19. b (Patients must be closely monitored for recurrence of opioid toxicity when the antagonist effects of naloxone fade; the half-life of naloxone is 2 hours and effects persist for about an hour.)
20. a

CHAPTER 6

1. T
2. F
3. T
4. F
5. F
6. T
7. a (Combining metronidazole and alcohol leads to acetaldehyde syndrome manifested by nausea, copious vomiting, flushing, palpitations, headache, sweating, thirst, chest pain, weakness, blurred vision, and hypotension; blood pressure

may ultimately decline to shock levels.)
8. d
9. c
10. d (By inhibiting the effects of clopidogrel, the use of omeprazole can lead to reduced antiplatelet effects and increase the risk of recurrent MI.)
11. b
12. c
13. c
14. a

CHAPTER 7
1. c
2. f
3. b
4. g
5. a
6. e
7. physically dependent
8. allergic
9. Carcinogenic
10. teratogenic
11. side effects
12. idiosyncratic
13. Iatrogenic
14. Toxicity
15. d
16. a, d, e
17. c (Suggests possible anaphylactic reaction.)
18. d
19. c (Statins can cause hepatotoxicity; liver injury is evidenced by elevations in serum transaminase levels.)
20. a
21. d
22. b
23. c
24. c
25. a
26. d

CHAPTER 8
1. body surface area
2. increase
3. Bioavailability
4. Tachyphylaxis
5. bleeding
6. intense; longer
7. c
8. d (Tolerance to nitroglycerin-induced vasodilation can develop over the course of a single day; the prescriber must be contacted to determine when the patch should be reapplied,

once the previous patch has been removed.)
9. c (G6PD deficiency affects the oxygen-carrying red blood cells; when persons with this deficiency take certain drugs, they develop hemolytic anemia [red blood cells are destroyed faster than the body can replace them].)
10. a
11. c (These are signs of hypokalemia.)

CHAPTER 9
1. T
2. F
3. T
4. F
5. T
6. F
7. T
8. T
9. F
10. T
11. d
12. f
13. a
14. g
15. b
16. c
17. h
18. e
19. d
20. a
21. b
22. c
23. c

CHAPTER 10
1. F
2. T
3. T
4. F
5. T
6. F
7. b
8. a
9. c (Normal respiratory rate for a newborn is 30-60 respirations per minute; a respiratory rate of 22/min is depressed.)
10. a
11. a, c
12. b
13. a
14. 227 mg is calculated safe dose. Yes, 225 mg is safe.
15. 4.5 mL

CHAPTER 11
1. F
2. T
3. F
4. F
5. T
6. T
7. F
8. T
9. T
10. c (Creatinine clearance is a more precise test used to help detect and diagnose kidney dysfunction.)
11. a
12. d
13. b (Methyldopa can cause orthostatic hypotension and bradycardia in older adults.)
14. c (Is an indicator of severe urinary retention requiring catheterization.)
15. b

CHAPTER 12
1. i
2. f
3. b
4. c
5. d
6. a
7. e
8. h
9. g
10. T
11. F
12. T
13. F
14. F
15. T
16. a, b, c
17. b
18. d
19. a, c, d
20. b

CHAPTER 13
1. e
2. b
3. d
4. c
5. a
6. skeletal muscle
7. pupillary constriction; focuses eye
8. bronchodilation; respiratory rate
9. slowing
10. motility (peristalsis); digestion
11. emptying (voiding)
12. skeletal muscle

13. c
14. b
15. a (Cholinesterase inhibitors can cause bradycardia.)
16. d
17. b (Principal adverse effects of doxazosin are hypotension, fainting, dizziness, somnolence, and nasal congestion.)
18. c
19. a (Flomax may increase the risk of cataract surgery-related complications due to relaxation of the smooth muscles of the iris.)
20. b (Inhibiting MAO increases the risk of triggering a hypertensive crisis.)

CHAPTER 14

1. a. administer
    b. consult
    c. consult
    d. consult
    e. administer
    f. consult
    g. administer
    h. administer
    i. consult
    j. consult
2. c, e
3. b (Prominent symptoms of muscarinic poisoning are profuse salivation, lacrimation [tearing], visual disturbances, bronchospasm, diarrhea, bradycardia, and hypotension. Severe poisoning can produce cardiovascular collapse.)
4. d
5. d
6. a
7. d (Compared with other drugs for OAB, trospium is notable for its low bioavailability, lack of CNS effects, and lack of metabolism-related interactions with other drugs.)
8. c
9. c, d
10. a, c
11. a
12. a, e
13. c
14. b (Patients should wash their hands immediately after application of GELNIQUE.)
15. 5-mL dose
16 a. 0.1 mg is safe dose
    b. 0.2 mL dose

CHAPTER 15

1. c
2. g
3. f
4. b
5. h
6. a
7. e
8. d
9. b
10. a, e
11. a, b
12. a (Neuromuscular blockade decreases protective reflexes [coughing, gagging]; in the period after surgery, the loss of muscle strength resulting from blockade can lead to aspiration.)
13. c
14. d
15. 2.5 tablets per dose
16. 2.8 mL of neostigmine

CHAPTER 16

1. c
2. b
3. e
4. d
5. a
6. a
7. d
8. c, d
9. c
10. c
11. a, d
12. d (Succinylcholine produces a state of flaccid paralysis; respiratory depression secondary to neuromuscular blockade is the major concern.)
13. 250 mg

CHAPTER 17

1. a
2. c
3. b
4. d
5. T
6. F
7. T
8. F
9. T
10. T
11. b, c, d
12. b
13. c, d
14. c, d
15. a
16. b, d
17. d, e

18. b
19. 45 mL/hr
20. Dilute the vial in at least 50 mL of diluent and infuse at a rate of 3 mL/hr.

CHAPTER 18

1. b
2. c
3. a
4. T
5. T
6. F
7. F
8. F
9. T
10. T
11. T
12. c
13. a
14. b
15. c (Terazosin can cause orthostatic hypotension [a drop in SBP of > 20 mm Hg] and reflex tachycardia [increased heart rate in response to stimulus conveyed through the cardiac nerves].)
16. d (Sildenafil, when used in combination with alpha blockers, may cause a severe drop in blood pressure, lightheadedness, dizziness, or fainting.)
17. a
18. b
19. c
20. b
21. a
22. a (Betaxolol, although pregnancy category C, crosses the placenta and may lead to bradycardia in the neonate; the normal pulse for a newborn is 100-160 bpm.)
23. c (While metoprolol is approved for treating heart failure, it can also cause heart failure if used incautiously.)
24. a, b, c, d, e
25. b
26. d (Blockade of beta$_2$ receptors in the lung can cause bronchoconstriction.)
27. c
28. d (Combining a beta blocker with a calcium channel blocker can produce excessive cardiosuppression.)
29. 6 seconds/push
30. 180 mL/hr

CHAPTER 19

1. peripheral adrenergic
2. Hypertension
3. direct-acting adrenergic receptor blockers
4. drowsiness; xerostomia
5. vasodilation
6. b
7. c (Clonidine is embryotoxic in animals. Because of the possibility of fetal harm, clonidine is not recommended for pregnant women. Pregnancy should be ruled out before clonidine is given.)
8. b
9. c (Reserpine produces sedation and a state of indifference to the environment. In addition, the drug can cause severe depression. These effects are thought to result from depletion of certain neurotransmitters [catecholamines, serotonin] from neurons in the brain.)
10. d
11. a, b
12. a
13. c
14. 2 tablets
15. 200 mL/hr

CHAPTER 20

1. a, d
2. b, c
3. a, c
4. c

CHAPTER 21

1. Dopamine agonists
2. Catechol-O-methyltransferase (COMT inhibitor)
3. Anticholinergic agents
4. Inhibitors of monoamine oxidase-B (MAOB inhibitor)
5. Levodopa
6. Amantadine
7. c
8. b
9. b
10. c
11. c
12. b
13. a
14. c, e
15. c
16. a (Ropinirole may cause increased hepatic enzymes.)
17. b

18. d (Ergot derivatives have been associated with valvular heart injury.)
19. a
20. c
21. b, d, e
22. 6 tablets
23. 2 orally disintegrating tablets

CHAPTER 22

1. F
2. F
3. T
4. F
5. F
6. T
7. T
8. F
9. F
10. T
11. F
12. T
13. T
14. d
15. a (With oral dosing, the most common cholinergic effects are nausea [47%], vomiting [31%], diarrhea [19%], abdominal pain [13%], and anorexia [17%].)
16. c
17. a, b, c
18. d
19. c
20. b
21. e (Estrogen/progesterone therapy may actually increase risk.)
22. None. The nurse needs to consult the prescriber and the pharmacist because IR and ER formulas are not interchangeable.
23. 2.5 mL—use 3-mL syringe without needle

CHAPTER 23

1. T
2. F
3. F
4. T
5. T
6. T
7. F
8. T
9. T
10. F
11. F
12. c, e
13. c
14. b

15. d (Interferon beta can suppress bone marrow function, thereby decreasing production of all blood cell types.)
16. d
17. d, e
18. c, e
19. a, c
20. b
21. d
22. c
23. 0.2 mL/dose
24. 115 mL/6 = 19 mL

CHAPTER 24

1. e
2. m
3. a
4. k
5. g
6. n
7. j
8. c
9. f
10. h
11. i
12. b
13. l
14. d
15. a, b, c
16. a
17. b
18. c, e
19. d
20. a
21. b
22. a (Between 2% and 5% of patients develop a morbilliform [measles-like] rash. Rarely, morbilliform rash progresses to toxic epidermal necrolysis or Stevens-Johnson syndrome, an inflammatory skin disease characterized by red macules, papules, and tubercles. If a rash develops, phenytoin should be stopped.)
23. b
24. b
25. a (To avoid transmitting infections, wash hands frequently with soap and water.)
26. a (Carbamazepine can cause vertigo. These reactions are common during the first weeks of treatment. Fortunately, tolerance usually develops with continued use. These effects can be minimized by initiating therapy at low doses and giving the largest portion of the daily dose

at bedtime [safety measures to prevent falls].)
27. c
28. d (A major risk factor for severe skin reactions is a genetic variation known as human leukocyte antigen [HLA]-B*1502, which occurs primarily in people of Asian descent.)
29. c
30. a (Valproic acid has been associated with fatal liver failure; inform patients about signs and symptoms of liver injury [reduced appetite, malaise, nausea, abdominal pain, jaundice] and instruct them to notify the prescriber if these develop.)
31. b
32. a
33. a (Severe overdose produces generalized CNS depression; death results from depression of respiration. Assessing vital signs evaluates respiratory status.)
34. c, d
35. c
36. c
37. a
38. d
39. b
40. c
41. d
42. c
43. Yes. Calculated safe/effective dose is 19.88 mg
44. 0.16 mL

CHAPTER 25

1. T
2. F
3. T
4. F
5. T
6. F
7. F
8. F
9. F
10. T
11. d (Centrally acting muscle relaxants can produce generalized depression of the CNS. Drowsiness, dizziness, and lightheadedness are common. Patients should be warned not to participate in hazardous activities [e.g., driving] if CNS depression is significant. In addition, they should be advised to

avoid alcohol and all other CNS depressants.)
12. c
13. a
14. b
15. 0.4 mL
16. No. The safe dose is 168 mg.

CHAPTER 26

1. T
2. T
3. T
4. F
5. F
6. T
7. F
8. F
9. T
10. T
11. F
12. a
13. c
14. d (When spinal anesthesia is used, the prescriber should be notified if the patient fails to void within 8 hours of the end of surgery; spinal anesthesia frequently causes headache. These "spinal" headaches are posture-dependent and can be relieved by having the patient assume a supine position. Due to headaches, asking the patient to sit up to attempt to void or having him/her go to the bathroom to void may not be possible.)
15. b, e
16. a (Systemic absorption of epinephrine can result in systemic toxicity [e.g., palpitations, tachycardia, nervousness, hypertension].)
17. d
18. b
19. c (When the tourniquet is loosened at the end of surgery, about 15% to 30% of administered anesthetic is released into the systemic circulation; it is at this point systemic adverse events can occur.)

CHAPTER 27

1. f
2. d
3. b
4. e
5. g
6. c
7. a

8. d
9. c
10. b
11. a (Depression of respiratory and cardiac function is a concern with virtually all inhalation anesthetics.)
12. d
13. c
14. b
15. c
16. d (The risk of malignant hyperthermia is greatest when an inhalation anesthetic is combined with succinylcholine.)
17. a (Isoflurane causes hypotension; hypotension results from vasodilation. Amlodipine lowers blood pressure through peripheral arterial dilation.)
18. b
19. d
20. a, b, d
21. a
22. b (Propofol can cause profound respiratory depression [including apnea].)

CHAPTER 28

1. T
2. F
3. T
4. T
5. F
6. F
7. T
8. d
9. b (Safety issue—fall risk with opioid analgesics. Do not keep patients in position or leave patients unattended in position from which they could fall.)
10. c
11. c (Signs of withdrawal include excessive crying, sneezing, tremor, hyperreflexia, fever, and diarrhea; fever and diarrhea may result in hypovolemia.)
12. d
13. b (The half-life of naloxone is approximately 2 hours. Dosing is repeated at 2- to 3-minute intervals until a satisfactory response has been achieved.)
14. d
15. a
16. c
17. a
18. a (The dose of fentanyl in the lozenge on a stick is sufficient to kill nontolerant

individuals—especially children.)

19. d
20. d
21. b
22. a
23. b
24. a
25. c
26. d
27. a, c
28. d
29. 0.6 mL. Push one line (0.2 mL) every 10 seconds. Total liquid is 6 mL; 5 lines/mL = 30 lines ("pushes") over 5 minutes (300 seconds). Push one line (0.2 mL) every 10 seconds.
30. 0.08 mL

CHAPTER 29

1. c
2. a
3. d
4. b
5. d
6. c
7. b
8. c
9. c
10. a
11. d
12. c
13. b
14. c (NSAIDs inhibit platelet aggregation.)
15. d (Severe respiratory depression can be reversed with naloxone; however, caution is required. Excessive dosing will reverse analgesia, thereby putting the patient in great pain.)
16. a
17. d (Respiratory depression is increased by concurrent use of other drugs that have CNS-depressant actions (e.g., alcohol, barbiturates, benzodiazepines.)
18. Yes, the rate will be safe.

CHAPTER 30

1. c
2. e
3. f
4. d
5. a
6. b
7. g
8. b, d, e
9. d
10. b

11. b (While all of these are a concern with a patient receiving meperidine, breathing [safety] is the priority.)
12. c (Ergotamine can cause peripheral vasoconstriction.)
13. a
14. a, c
15. d
16. b (Coronary vasospasm is the biggest concern in patients taking sumatriptan; however, about 50% of patients experience unpleasant chest symptoms, usually described as "heavy arms" or "chest pressure" rather than pain. These symptoms are transient and not related to ischemic heart disease.)
17. a
18. c
19. b (Propranolol can exacerbate symptoms of asthma.)
20. d
21. d
22. 1 mL
23. 2 tablets

CHAPTER 31

1. F
2. T
3. F
4. T
5. F
6. T
7. F
8. F
9. c
10. a
11. a (Laryngeal dystonia can impair respiration.)
12. d (Acute dystonia can be both disturbing and dangerous. Typically, the patient develops severe spasm of the muscles of the tongue, face, neck, or back.)
13. b (Dantrolene can reduce rigidity and hyperthermia associated with neuroleptic malignant syndrome.)
14. c
15. d (First-generation agents produce varying degrees of muscarinic cholinergic blockade, thus eliciting the full spectrum of anticholinergic responses. Monitoring intake and output is one means of assessing for urinary retention.)
16. c
17. a, e

18. a
19. a
20. c
21. b
22. c (Haloperidol should be used with caution in patients with dysrhythmia risk factors, including long QT syndrome, hypokalemia or hyperkalemia, or a history of dysrhythmias, heart attack, or severe heart failure.)
23. b, d
24. c (Clozapine produces agranulocytosis in 1% to 2% of patients. The overall risk of death is about 1 in 5000. The usual cause is gram-negative septicemia; high fever would be an indicator of such infection.)
25. a, c, d
26. 2 mL in 2 sites (right and left ventrogluteal muscles) because should not exceed 2-3 mL in this site
27. 0.08 mL every 10 seconds

CHAPTER 32

1. little interest; pleasure
2. dosage change
3. 1; 3
4. 4; 9
5. more adverse effects
6. stimulating; insomnia
7. heart
8. MAOI
9. antihistamines; sleep aids
10. headache; jaw pain; dental problems
11. tyramine
12. b (Patients with depression often think about or attempt suicide. During treatment with antidepressants, especially early on, the risk of suicide may actually increase. If mood deteriorates, or if thoughts of suicide intensify, the patient should see his or her prescriber immediately.)
13. d
14. c (If mood deteriorates, or if thoughts of suicide intensify, the patient should see his or her prescriber immediately; the answer "provide a safe environment" assumes the patient is in the hospital, which may not be the case.)
15. c
16. c (Because fluoxetine is highly bound to plasma proteins, it

can displace other highly bound drugs. Displacement of warfarin [an anticoagulant] is of particular concern. Monitor responses to warfarin closely.)

17. a
18. c
19. d
20. b (SNRIs can result in neonatal withdrawal syndrome, characterized by irritability, abnormal crying, tremor, respiratory distress, and possibly seizures.)
21. b
22. a
23. b (The combination of a TCA with an MAOI can lead to severe hypertension, owing to excessive adrenergic stimulation of the heart and blood vessels.)
24. a, c, e
25. a
26. b
27. c (Tranylcypromine is an MAOI and symptoms of hypertensive crisis include headache, tachycardia, palpitations, nausea, and vomiting.)
28. c, e
29. b
30. d
31. c (Patients should not take Wellbutrin if they have seizures; the most serious adverse effect of Wellbutrin is seizures.)
32. a
33. d
34. a
35. 2 CR tablets of 25 mg each
36. 2 capsules

CHAPTER 33

1. F
2. T
3. T
4. F
5. F
6. T
7. F
8. F
9. c (In a mixed episode, patients experience symptoms of mania and depression simultaneously. Patients may be agitated and irritable (as in mania), but may also feel worthless and depressed. The combination of high energy and depression puts them at significant risk for suicide.)
10. a

11. b
12. a, d
13. c (Diuretics promote sodium loss, and can thereby increase the risk of lithium toxicity.)
14. a, b, d
15. a (Administer the drug; a serum level at 6 mcg/mL is within the target range of 4-12 mcg/mL.)
16. a
17. d (Lamotrigine can cause life-threatening rashes, including Stevens-Johnson syndrome and toxic epidermal necrolysis; typical presentation includes blistering of mucous membranes, typically in the mouth.)
18. 2 capsules
19. 7.5 mL

CHAPTER 34

1. a
2. c
3. d
4. b
5. T
6. T
7. F
8. F
9. T
10. T
11. T
12. F
13. T
14. F
15. d, e
16. b
17. b
18. b (Flumazenil can reverse the sedative effects of benzodiazepines, but may not reverse respiratory depression.)
19. d (Safety is paramount as patients taking benzodiazepines in sleep-inducing doses may carry out complex behaviors, and then have no memory of their actions. Reported behaviors include sleep driving, preparing and eating meals, making phone calls, and having sexual intercourse. Additionally, when employed to treat anxiety, benzodiazepines sometimes cause paradoxical responses, including insomnia, excitation, euphoria, heightened anxiety, and rage.)
20. a
21. b, c, d

22. d
23. a
24. b
25. d (Severe barbiturate overdose produces generalized CNS depression; death results from depression of respiration.)
26. b, e
27. c
28. a
29. a
30. b, e
31. 2 tablets
32. First dose 2 mL, second dose 3 mL

CHAPTER 35

1. T
2. F
3. T
4. T
5. F
6. F
7. F
8. T
9. F
10. T
11. agoraphobia
12. generalized anxiety disorder (GAD)
13. social anxiety disorder
14. obsessive compulsive disorder (OCD)
15. posttraumatic stress disorder (PTSD)
16. panic disorder
17. b (An intoxicated person is considered legally incapable of consent.)
18. c
19. c, e
20. a (Alprazolam should be used with caution in those with pulmonary impairment.)
21. c
22. d (Overdose with a TCA can be life-threatening; the lethal dose is only 8 times the average daily dose.)
23. b (To reduce the risk of tyramine-induced hypertensive crisis, the following precautions must be taken: avoid foods rich in tyramine—which include yeast extracts, most cheeses, fermented sausages [e.g., salami, pepperoni, bologna], and aged fish or meat.)
24. a
25. b
26. c

27. 1 1/2 (1.5) tablets
28. 1.1–3.3 mg

CHAPTER 36

1. c
2. f
3. b
4. e
5. g
6. a
7. d
8. T
9. F
10. T
11. T
12. F
13. F
14. T
15. a, d
16. a
17. c
18. a
19. c
20. b
21. d
22. a
23. b
24. d
25. d (Guanfacine activates brainstem alpha$_2$-adrenergic receptors, and thereby reduces sympathetic outflow to the heart and blood vessels.)
26. 60 mg is a safe dose.
27. 6 gtt/min

CHAPTER 37

1. Tolerance
2. physically dependent
3. Psychological dependence
4. withdrawal syndrome
5. cross-tolerance
6. Cross-dependence
7. Dopamine
8. Chronic; relapsing
9. a, b, d
10. a, b, d
11. d
12. b
13. c
14. a

CHAPTER 38

1. T
2. F
3. F
4. F
5. T
6. T
7. F

8. F
9. T
10. F
11. F
12. T
13. b
14. e
15. a
16. c
17. d
18. a, c, e
19. d
20. b
21. a (Approximately 35% of cases of acute pancreatitis can be attributed to alcohol, making alcohol the second most common cause of the disorder. Symptoms of pancreatitis include severe abdominal pain radiating to the back; amylase is used to diagnose pancreatitis. Normal amylase ranges from 25-85 units/L.)
22. a, c, d
23. d
24. a
25. a
26. c
27. d
28. c
29. d (Acamprosate is used along with counseling and social support to help people who have stopped drinking large amounts of alcohol to avoid drinking alcohol again.)
30. d
31. 1/2 tablet
32. 1 mL (2 mL of drug + 1 mL diluent = 3 mL)

CHAPTER 39

1. T
2. F
3. F
4. T
5. T
6. F (10 seconds)
7. T
8. F
9. F
10. T
11. T
12. T
13. T
14. F
15. T
16. F
17. T
18. c

19. c
20. c
21. a
22. a, b
23. a
24. d (Postmarketing reports indicate that varenicline can cause serious neuropsychiatric effects, including mood changes, erratic behavior, and suicidality.)
25. a, b, c, d
26. 3 SR tablets
27. 1 tablet

CHAPTER 40

1. F
2. T
3. T
4. T
5. F
6. T
7. F
8. T
9. F
10. T
11. F
12. F
13. F
14. T
15. F
16. T
17. F
18. T
19. F
20. T
21. F
22. T
23. F
24. T
25. c (The desire to avoid symptoms of withdrawal may be sufficient to promote continued drug use.)
26. d (Following IV injection, effects of naloxone begin almost immediately and persist about 1 hour; respiratory depression will return when the effects of naloxone have worn off.)
27. b
28. a
29. d
30. d
31. b (Barbiturates reduce ventilation; doses only 3 times greater than those needed to induce sleep can cause complete suppression of the neurogenic respiratory drive. With severe overdose, barbiturates can cause apnea and death.)

32. a
33. d
34. c
35. c
36. a, b, c, d
37. d
38. b
39. 2 sublingual tablets
40. 4 mL

CHAPTER 41

1. b
2. e
3. d
4. a
5. c
6. T
7. F
8. F
9. F
10. T
11. F
12. T
13. T
14. F
15. 180,000
16. 1800
17. sodium; chloride
18. thick segment of the ascending limb of the loop of Henle
19. acids; bases; calcium; chloride; glucose; lipids; magnesium; potassium; sodium; uric acid; water (fluid)
20. c
21. c
22. a
23. a, b, d, e
24. c
25. c
26. a (This selection has the 20 mm Hg drop in SBP associated with orthostatic hypotension.)
27. a, b, c, d
28. c (Muscle weakness and cramping are symptoms associated with hypokalemia.)
29. b
30. d
31. c
32. d
33. b
34. b
35. b
36. b (Adolescents and young adults are particularly concerned about body image, perceived flaws, and appearing different from their peers.)
37. d
38. c, d

39. c (Some water-softening systems replace calcium and magnesium ions with sodium ions. The higher the concentration of calcium and magnesium, the more sodium needed to soften the water. Patients on a very low-sodium diet who are concerned about the amount of sodium in softened water may want to consider a water-purification system that uses potassium chloride instead.)
40. 0.5 (1/2) tablet
41. 30 seconds/line

CHAPTER 42

1. volume expansion
2. volume contraction
3. hypertonic contraction
4. isotonic contraction
5. twice (two times) the osmolality of sodium
6. metabolic alkalosis
7. Respiratory alkalosis
8. metabolic acidosis
9. d
10. b
11. c
12. a
13. a (In isotonic contraction, volume should be replenished slowly to avoid pulmonary edema.)
14. d
15. b
16. c
17. a (With the exception of the sustained-release tablets, solid formulations of KCl can produce high local concentrations of potassium, resulting in severe intestinal injury [ulcerative lesions, bleeding, perforation]; death has occurred.)
18. b (Serum levels of potassium are regulated primarily by the kidneys.)
19. a
20. d, e
21. b (The most serious consequence of hyperkalemia is disruption of the electrical activity of the heart.)
22. d
23. b (In the heart, excessive magnesium can suppress impulse conduction through the atrio-ventricular (AV) node. Accordingly, magnesium sulfate is

contraindicated for patients with AV heart block.)
24. a
25. 10,800 mL/24 hr
26. 675 mL/hr

CHAPTER 43

1. F
2. T
3. T
4. T
5. T
6. F
7. F
8. T
9. T
10. F
11. F
12. f
13. b
14. g
15. l
16. a
17. h
18. e
19. k
20. i
21. j
22. d
23. c
24. b
25. a, b, c
26. d
27. a
28. a (A cough that produces frothy sputum that may be tinged with blood is an indication of pulmonary edema.)
29. a, b, c, f
30. a

CHAPTER 44

1. d
2. e
3. g
4. f
5. b
6. a
7. i
8. h
9. c
10. d
11. c
12. a
13. c
14. b
15. a, c, d, e
16. d (A precipitous drop in blood pressure may occur following the first dose of an ACE

inhibitor. This reaction is caused by widespread vasodilation secondary to abrupt lowering of angiotensin II levels. First-dose hypotension is most likely in patients with severe hypertension, in patients taking diuretics, and in patients who are sodium-depleted or volume-depleted.)

17. c
18. a (Angioedema is a potentially fatal reaction that develops in up to 1% of patients. Symptoms, which result from increased capillary permeability, include giant wheals and edema of the tongue, glottis, and pharynx. Severe reactions should be treated with subcutaneous epinephrine.)
19. d
20. a
21. d (Aspirin, ibuprofen, and other NSAIDs may reduce the antihypertensive effects of ACE inhibitors.)
22. b
23. d
24. a
25. b
26. d
27. c
28. 2 tablets
29. 30 seconds

CHAPTER 45

1. vasodilation
2. veins (venous system)
3. arterioles
4. vasodilation; reduced arterial pressure; increased coronary perfusion
5. -ine
6. b (In the SA node, calcium channel blockade can cause bradycardia; in the AV node, blockade can cause partial or complete AV block; and in the myocardium, blockade can decrease contractility.)
7. a
8. a, c, e
9. b
10. b
11. d (Blockade of cardiac calcium channels can cause bradycardia, AV block, and heart failure.)
12. b
13. a
14. b
15. a

16. c
17. d
18. c
19. b
20. d (Caution is advised when using nifedipine in persons with kidney disease.)
21. 11 mL/hr
22. 20 mg is the safe dose for this patient.

CHAPTER 46

1. T
2. F
3. F
4. T
5. F
6. T
7. F
8. T
9. T
10. c (Principal adverse effects of hydralazine are hypotension, tachycardia; the risk of orthostatic hypotension is low.)
11. b
12. d
13. a
14. c
15. d (If an SLE-like reaction occurs, hydralazine should be withdrawn. Approximately 50% of patients have constitutional symptoms of fever, weight loss, and fatigue. Reporting fever as a priority over fatigue is important, as those with an SLE-like reaction may also develop pericarditis, of which low-grade fever is a sign.)
16. a
17. c
18. d
19. a
20. 0.3 mL/10 sec
21. 72 mL/hr

CHAPTER 47

1. n
2. m
3. j
4. d
5. b
6. k
7. l
8. o
9. g
10. h
11. a
12. i
13. c

14. f
15. e
16. c
17. d
18. a
19. a, b, c
20. b
21. c
22. d
23. a
24. c (The most disturbing side effect of alpha blockers is orthostatic hypotension. Hypotension can be especially severe with the initial dose. Significant hypotension continues with subsequent doses, but is less profound. Hypotension puts the patient at risk for falls.)
25. c
26. a (The major cause of treatment failure in patients with chronic hypertension is lack of adherence to the prescribed regimen. In this section, we consider the causes of nonadherence and discuss some solutions.)
27. b
28. d
29. c
30. b
31. a
32. a
33. c
34. b (Beta blockers can suppress glycogenolysis and mask early signs of hypoglycemia, and therefore must be used with caution.)

CHAPTER 48

1. e
2. d
3. c
4. b
5. a
6. c
7. f
8. e
9. b
10. a
11. h
12. d
13. g
14. c
15. b
16. a, c, d
17. b
18. c (Weakness is a symptom of hyperkalemia.)

19. d (Dopamine is administered by continuous infusion. Constant monitoring of blood pressure, the electrocardiogram [ECG], and urine output is required.)
20. b
21. a
22. a, c, d (All of these are signs and symptoms of drug-induced lupus-like syndrome.)
23. a
24. b
25. a
26. b
27. c
28. d
29. c (Hypokalemia increases the risk of digoxin-induced dysrhythmias.)
30. 4 mL/hr (calculates to 4.125 mL/hr)
31. Calculates to recommended dose of 52.5 mg—yes, 50 mg is safe.

CHAPTER 49

1. absence
2. abnormal
3. slower
4. faster
5. ventricular
6. c
7. a
8. b
9. c
10. b
11. a
12. a (Cardiac output affects all of the other diagnoses; therefore, without adequate cardiac output, fluid balance, tissue perfusion, and breathing cannot be adequately maintained.)
13. a
14. b
15. b
16. a
17. d
18. b
19. b
20. a
21. b (Cinchonism [overdose/toxicity] is characterized by tinnitus [ringing in the ears], headache, nausea, vertigo, and disturbed vision. These symptoms can develop with just one dose.)
22. a
23. b
24. a, b, c, e
25. c

26. d (A postvoid residual > 100 mL may necessitate urinary catheterization.)
27. b
28. a
29. d
30. b
31. a
32. a
33. c
34. a
35. c (Verapamil may produce a decrease in blood pressure below normal levels, which may result in dizziness or symptomatic hypotension.)
36. b
37. c
38. 18.75 mg/dose
39. 30 mL/hr

CHAPTER 50

1. hormones
2. liver
3. saturated
4. Lipoproteins
5. water-loving; fear of water
6. 100
7. 40
8. 30; 60
9. c
10. b
11. a
12. d
13. d (Statins are classified in Food and Drug Administration Pregnancy Risk Category X: the risks to the fetus outweigh any potential benefits of treatment.)
14. c (Elevated CK level is an indication of muscle damage. Rhabdomyolysis is the breakdown of muscle tissue that leads to the release of muscle fiber contents into the blood. These substances are harmful to the kidney and often cause kidney damage)
15. d
16. b
17. c
18. a
19. d
20. c
21. b
22. b
23. c
24. 3 tablets
25. 2 capsules

CHAPTER 51

1. oxygen; heart
2. preload; afterload
3. diastolic
4. aspirin
5. c (Anginal pain is precipitated when the oxygen supply to the heart is insufficient to meet oxygen demand. Cardiac oxygen supply is determined by myocardial blood flow.)
6. b
7. d
8. a
9. c
10. b
11. a
12. d
13. a
14. a
15. c
16. b
17. c
18. d
19. a, d
20. d
21. 2 inches
22. 3 mL/hr

CHAPTER 52

1. T
2. F
3. T
4. T
5. F
6. T
7. d
8. c (In heparin-treated patients, platelet aggregation is the major remaining defense against hemorrhage. A depressed platelet count means this defense is weakened; hence, heparin must be employed with caution.)
9. a
10. b
11. a
12. c
13. c
14. d
15. b
16. b
17. a, b, c, d, e
18. d (Spinal hematomas may occur in patients anticoagulated with drugs such as enoxaparin and who receive spinal anesthesia; these hematomas may result in long-term or permanent paralysis.)
19. a, b, c, d, e

20. c, d
21. b
22. d
23. b (Dabigatran dosing has not been determined for patients with an eGRF/[CrCl] < 15.)
24. a (12% of patients receiving bivalirudin experience hypotension; patients are advised to change positions slowly to minimize orthostatic hypotension.)
25. a
26. d
27. d
28. b
29. c
30. a
31. d (Neutropenia develops in 2.4% of patients receiving ticlopidine, and is sometimes severe. This reduces the body's ability to fight off infections.)
32. b, c, d
33. c
34. c
35. c (If treatment begins soon after symptoms start, heart attack deaths and heart damage can often be avoided.)
36. 5 mL
37. 12 mL/hr

CHAPTER 53

1. myocardial infarction
2. STEMI
3. ST segment
4. ST-elevation
5. advanced age; family history of MI; obesity; high serum cholesterol; hypertension; smoking; diabetes
6. atherosclerotic plaque
7. angiotensin II
8. troponins; creatine kinase
9. 90%
10. d
11. a, b, d, e
12. a, b
13. b
14. d (Patient with asthma or other similar diseases should not receive beta blockers, including metoprolol. Because of its relative beta₁ selectivity, however, metoprolol may be used with caution in patients with asthma who cannot tolerate other treatments. Since beta₁ selectivity is not absolute, a beta₂-stimulating agent should be administered concomitantly, and the lowest

possible dose of metoprolol used. In this instance, the nurse should clarify the dose [which totals 200 mg/day] with the prescriber.)
15. a
16. d
17. d
18. a
19. c
20. 0.8 mL
21. Adding 4.2 mL of diluent for a total of 5 mL and pushing 0.1 mL every 5 seconds will result in completing the drug administration in 4 minutes and 10 seconds.

CHAPTER 54

1. F
2. T
3. F
4. F
5. T
6. F
7. T
8. T
9. b
10. c
11. a
12. d
13. c
14. d
15. b
16. c
17. d (Symptoms of anaphylaxis include wheezing, tightness in the throat, shortness of breath, and swelling of the face. The treatment of choice is epinephrine, injected subQ, *after* stopping administration of the factor concentrate!)
18. a
19. a, c
20. c
21. 1125 units of factor VIII for this child
22. 2.25 mL desmopressin will be injected into 50 mL 0.9% NS and infused at 100 mL/hr

CHAPTER 55

1. a
2. j
3. l
4. i
5. g
6. h
7. d
8. c

9. f
10. b
11. e
12. m
13. k
14. a
15. d
16. c
17. b
18. e
19. d
20. b (Anemia is common in patients with chronic kidney disease.)
21. a
22. c, d
23. c
24. d
25. c
26. b
27. a
28. c
29. a (To minimize anaphylactic reactions, intravenous iron dextran should be administered following a small test dose [25 mg over 5 minutes] and observe the patient for signs and symptoms of anaphylaxis for at least 15 minutes.)
30. d
31. c (Epoetin has been associated with an increase in cardiovascular events. Among these are cardiac arrest, hypertension, HF, and thrombotic events, including stroke and MI.)
32. b (Because of its unique composition [ferumoxytol is a superparamagnetic form of iron oxide], the drug can interfere with magnetic resonance imaging [MRI] studies.)
33. a
34. c (Early manifestations of pernicious anemia include paresthesias of the hands and feet; if deficiency is prolonged, neurologic damage can become permanent.)
35. b
36. a, c, d
37. a (Hematopoietic growth factors have been associated with an increase in cardiovascular events.)
38. Yes, dose is safe and effective (50 mg in divided doses).
39. 0.2 mL

CHAPTER 56

1. brain; bone marrow; liver; heart; uterus; testes; blood vessels
2. cancer
3. cardiovascular events; death
4. 1
5. two
6. yeast
7. increase
8. clots
9. a (Epoetin has been associated with an increase in cardiovascular events. Among these are cardiac arrest, hypertension, HF, and thrombotic events, including stroke and MI.)
10. b
11. d
12. a (Darbepoetin is generally well-tolerated; the most common problem is hypertension.)
13. b
14. c
15. c (High levels of uric acid in the blood can cause solid crystals to form within joints. This causes joint inflammation.)
16. c
17. b
18. b
19. c
20. c
21. b, c
22. a (Oprelvekin causes retention of sodium and water by the kidney. As a result, about 48% of patients experience dyspnea.)
23. d (Eltrombopag may cause bone marrow fibrosis, hematologic malignancy, and thrombotic/thromboembolic events, and may pose a risk of bleeding; in addition, the drug may cause liver injury. Accordingly, safety is a priority in patients receiving this drug.)
24. b, e
25. 375 mcg = 38 mL/dose
26. 10 mL/hr

CHAPTER 57

1. T
2. T
3. T
4. F
5. T
6. F
7. T
8. F
9. T

10. T
11. T
12. F
13. F
14. a
15. a
16. d
17. b
18. d
19. c (Persons receiving insulin are at risk for hypoglycemia; sweating and confusion/altered level of consciousness are signs of hypoglycemia.)
20. b
21. b
22. a
23. a
24. a
25. d
26. c
27. a
28. c
29. b
30. d
31. d
32. c (If the swallowing reflex or the gag reflex is suppressed, nothing should be administered by mouth.)
33. d
34. b
35. a
36. a
37. c
38. b
39. c
40. d
41. c
42. a
43. a
44. c, d
45. c (Glucagon promotes the breakdown of glycogen to glucose, reduces conversion of glucose to glycogen, and stimulates biosynthesis of glucose.)
46. d
47. 24 mL/hr

CHAPTER 58

1. T
2. F
3. T
4. F
5. F
6. T
7. F
8. F
9. T
10. c

11. a (By the second trimester, the fetal thyroid gland is fully functional; hence, the fetus can supply its own hormones from then on. Therefore, to help ensure healthy fetal development, maternal hypothyroidism must be diagnosed and treated very early.)
12. a (In thyrotoxicosis the heartbeat is rapid and strong, and dysrhythmias and angina may develop.)
13. c
14. d
15. a, b, c, d, e
16. a
17. b
18. b
19. c
20. d (Thionamides can cause neonatal hypothyroidism and goiter. Accordingly, these drugs must be used judiciously during pregnancy. To minimize effects on the fetus, dosage should be kept as low as possible.)
21. d
22. b
23. c
24. c
25. No. Safe range is 32.7-40 mcg per day.
26. 1/2 tablet

CHAPTER 59

1. h
2. a
3. e
4. c
5. g
6. d
7. i
8. f
9. b
10. d
11. b
12. a (Mecasermin can cause a variety of adverse effects. The most common is hypoglycemia, which develops in nearly 50% of patients, usually during the first weeks of treatment. Diaphoresis and tremor are signs of hypoglycemia.)
13. d
14. b, c , d
15. c
16. b
17. c

18. d (Tolvaptan blocks vasopressin V$_2$ receptors in renal collecting ducts, and thereby increases renal excretion of free water, causing the sodium concentration in blood to rise.)
19. b (In a few patients treated with pegvisomant, serum levels of hepatic transaminases rise, indicating liver injury. Monitoring of hepatic function is recommended.)
20. 2 mg/dose
21. 0.08 mL

CHAPTER 60

1. c
2. a
3. b
4. F
5. T
6. T
7. F
8. T
9. F
10. F
11. T
12. F
13. T
14. F
15. a
16. b
17. a (Cushing's syndrome is characterized by hyperglycemia and glycosuria, among other symptoms.)
18. d
19. c
20. b (At times of stress, patients must increase their glucocorticoid dosage. Failure to increase the dosage can be fatal.)
21. d (With fludrocortisone, salt and water may retained in excess, resulting in expansion of blood volume. Patients should be monitored for weight gain.)
22. a
23. a
24. 0.5 (1/2) tablet
25. Yes. The safe dose is 24-30 mg.

CHAPTER 61

1. d
2. b
3. a
4. e
5. c
6. a
7. c
8. c

9. b
10. a, d
11. b
12. d (SERMs can increase the risk of endometrial cancer and thromboembolism.)
13. a (High-dose therapy during the first 4 months of pregnancy has been associated with an increased incidence of birth defects.)
14. d
15. d

CHAPTER 62

1. T
2. F
3. T
4. F
5. F
6. F
7. T
8. F
9. T
10. T
11. T
12. T
13. F
14. T
15. T
16. T
17. F
18. T
19. F
20. T
21. b (The principal concern with drospirenone is venous thromboembolism, which occurs more often than with other progestins. The thromboembolism can break apart, causing pieces to travel through the bloodstream, resulting in pulmonary embolism.)
22. d
23. c (Drospirenone is a structural analog of spironolactone, a potassium-sparing diuretic that blocks receptors for aldosterone; taken with NSAIDs, there is an increased risk of hyperkalemia.)
24. d
25. b (By increasing levels of clotting factors, OCs can decrease the effectiveness of warfarin; therefore, it is important patients adhere to blood testing schedules.)
26. a
27. b

28. c (Combination OCs have been associated with an increased risk of venous thromboembolism [VTE], arterial thromboembolism, and pulmonary embolism.)
29. d (OCs may precipitate gallbladder disease in women who already have gallstones or a history of gallbladder disease; right upper quadrant pain is a symptom of gallbladder disease.)
30. a
31. d
32. c
33. b
34. c
35. d
36. b, c, d
37. c
38. c
39. c
40. a, b, e

CHAPTER 63

1. c
2. a
3. b
4. F
5. F
6. T
7. T
8. F
9. F
10. T
11. T
12. F
13. F
14. F
15. T
16. c (Very rarely, clomiphene can cause ovarian hyperstimulation. Symptoms include low abdominal pain, pressure, weight gain, and swelling.)
17. c
18. d
19. b
20. b (Hyperstimulation syndrome following hCG therapy may cause pleural effusion.)
21. a
22. b
23. 0.5 (1/2) tablet
24. 2 mL in 2 sites (total 4 mL)

CHAPTER 64

1. F
2. F
3. T
4. T

5. F
6. a, b, c, d
7. d (Adverse effects of greatest concern when administering terbutaline are pulmonary edema; shortness of breath and foamy sputum are signs and symptoms of pulmonary edema.)
8. c (There is some concern that nifedipine may compromise uteroplacental blood flow.)
9. a
10. c
11. c
12. a, c, e
13. a (Because it poses a risk of severe hypertension, methylergonovine is considered a second-line drug for controlling postpartum hemorrhage.)
14. a, d, f, g
15. d, e
16. d (The pouch is removed when active labor occurs.)

CHAPTER 65

1. follicle-stimulating hormone (FSH); luteinizing hormone (LH)
2. anemia
3. ALT; AST; bilirubin
4. water; sodium (or salt)
5. irreversible
6. a (Androgens can lower plasma levels of high-density lipoprotein [HDL] cholesterol ["good cholesterol"] and elevate plasma levels of low-density lipoprotein [LDL] cholesterol ["bad cholesterol"]. These actions may increase the risk of atherosclerosis and related cardiovascular events.)
7. c (Edema can result from androgen-induced retention of salt and water. This complication is a concern for patients with heart failure and for those with a predisposition to developing edema from other causes.)
8. d
9. d
10. b
11. d
12. d
13. b (The 17-alpha-alkylated androgens can cause cholestatic hepatitis, jaundice, and other liver disorders. Rarely, liver cancer develops. Obtain periodic tests of liver function. Inform patients about signs of liver dysfunction [jaundice, malaise, anorexia, fatigue, nausea], and instruct them to notify the prescriber if these occur.)
14. c (Androgens can cause cholestatic hepatitis and other disorders of the liver. Since this patient does not report symptoms that are emergent in nature, it is a priority to gather all assessment data [history and physical] plus laboratory data, prior to calling the provider.)
15. 0.25 mL
16. 4 pellets

CHAPTER 66

1. F
2. F
3. T
4. F
5. F
6. T
7. F
8. F
9. F
10. T
11. T
12. F
13. F
14. b, d
15. c
16. d (If sildenafil and isosorbide are combined, life-threatening hypotension could result. Therefore, sildenafil is absolutely contraindicated for men taking nitrates.)
17. a (Although sildenafil is generally well-tolerated, it can be dangerous for men taking certain vasodilators, specifically alpha-adrenergic blockers, nitroglycerin, and other nitrates used for angina pectoris.)
18. d
19. b (Vardenafil can prolong the cardiac QT interval, and might therefore pose a risk for serious dysrhythmias.)
20. a
21. a
22. a, b, c, e
23. c
24. d (Dutasteride is classified in FDA pregnancy risk category X. It can be absorbed through the skin, so pregnant women should not handle the drug.)
25. b (Terazosin may be dangerous for men with reduced blood pressure.)
26. b (Doxazosin's principal adverse effects are hypotension, fainting, and dizziness.)
27. c

CHAPTER 67

1. d
2. c
3. e
4. i
5. b
6. g
7. a
8. f
9. j
10. h
11. c
12. e
13. a
14. d
15. b
16. gamma globulins; immunoglobulins
17. B lymphocytes (cells); T lymphocytes (cells)
18. d
19. b
20. c
21. d
22. c
23. a
24. c
25. b
26. c

CHAPTER 68

1. f
2. g
3. c
4. d
5. l
6. h
7. e
8. j
9. k
10. b
11. a
12. i
13. a
14. d
15. b
16. c (Swelling of lips is symptomatic of anaphylactic reaction.)
17. b
18. d, e
19. a
20. b, d, e

21. c (Children with severe immunodeficiency should NOT be given MMR. Severe immunodeficiency may result from immunosuppressive drugs [e.g., glucocorticoids, cytotoxic anticancer drugs], certain cancers [e.g., leukemia, lymphoma, generalized malignancy], and advanced HIV infection.)
22. d
23. a, c, d
24. a
25. a
26. c
27. d
28. b
29. a, e
30. b, d
31. a
32. d (Rotarix may carry a small risk of intussusception, a rare, life-threatening form of bowel obstruction that occurs when the bowel folds in on itself, like a collapsing telescope. Bloody, mucus-like bowel movement, sometimes called a "currant jelly" stool, is a symptom.)
33. d

CHAPTER 69

1. hyperglycemia
2. azathioprine (Imuran)
3. 6:00 PM (1800)
4. 12 weeks
5. fat
6. antacids
7. c (Immunosuppressive drugs inhibit immune responses which poses increased risk of infection.)
8. d
9. d
10. b
11. a (Renal damage occurs in up to 75% of patients taking cyclosporine. Injury manifests as reduced renal blood flow and reduced glomerular filtration rate.)
12. d (Signs of anaphylaxis include flushing, respiratory distress, hypotension, and tachycardia. If anaphylaxis develops, discontinue the infusion and treat with epinephrine and oxygen.)
13. c, d, e
14. a, b, d
15. b

16. d (Like tacrolimus, NSAIDs can injure the kidneys. Accordingly, NSAIDs should be avoided.)
17. c
18. a (Owing to the risk of infection, patients taking sirolimus should avoid sources of contagion. In addition, for 12 months after transplant surgery, patients should take medicine to prevent *Pneumocystis* pneumonia.)
19. a
20. b (The full range of glucocorticoid adverse effects can be expected in persons taking prednisone, including osteoporosis with resultant fractures.)
21. b
22. a, b, d
23. 2.7 mL
24. 14 mL/hr

CHAPTER 70

1. T
2. T
3. T
4. F
5. T
6. T
7. F
8. T
9. T
10. F
11. b
12. d
13. d
14. a
15. c
16. c
17. d (Antihistamines should be avoided late in the third trimester, because newborns are particularly sensitive to the adverse actions of these drugs; in this case, the sedating effects. The normal respiratory rate for a newborn is 30-60 breaths per minute.)
18. c, d
19. d
20. 5 mL
21. No. 25 mg of the drug would be infused in 50 seconds.

CHAPTER 71

1. 8 days
2. 1 week
3. 2
4. Reye's syndrome
5. vinegar
6. acetaminophen

7. Acetylcysteine
8. 2000 mg
9. b (The most common side effects are gastric distress, heartburn, and nausea. Occult GI bleeding occurs often.)
10. d
11. a
12. b
13. d
14. c (Smoking increases platelet aggregation; caution should be exercised when treating patients who smoke cigarettes with aspirin alone—the preferred drug to decrease platelet aggregation in smokers is Plavix.)
15. a (The aspirin hypersensitivity reaction begins with profuse, watery rhinorrhea and may progress to generalized urticaria, bronchospasm, laryngeal edema, and shock. Maintaining a patient's airway is the highest priority.)
16. c
17. a
18. d
19. b
20. a (The principal risks to pregnant women are [1] anemia [from GI blood loss], and [2] postpartum hemorrhage. A uterus that has not contracted down well [boggy] is the main cause of postpartum hemorrhage.)
21. b
22. c
23. c
24. d
25. b
26. b (Celecoxib can impair renal function, thereby posing a risk to patients with hypertension, edema, heart failure, or kidney disease. A daily weight increase is a marker of fluid accumulation.)
27. c (There is strong evidence that coxibs increase the risk of MI, stroke, and other serious cardiovascular events.)
28. a
29. b
30. a (Acetylcysteine causes allergic reactions [rash, itching, angioedema, bronchospasm, hypotension], most often in response to the first dose.

Fortunately, these reactions tend to be mild and self-limiting.)
31. a (Use of aspirin in children under 18 is associated with Reye's syndrome; characteristic symptoms are encephalopathy and fatty liver degeneration.)
32. 400 mL/hr
33. 1.2 mL/dose

CHAPTER 72
1. b
2. c
3. e
4. d
5. a
6. c (Because of their mineralocorticoid activity, glucocorticoids can cause sodium and water retention and potassium loss.)
7. d (By suppressing host defenses [immune responses and phagocytic activity of neutrophils and macrophages], glucocorticoids can increase susceptibility to infection.)
8. b
9. a, b, c, d, e
10. a, c, e
11. b
12. c
13. a
14. a
15. a, d, e
16. 0.2 mL/15 sec
17. Yes. Safe dose is up to 11.25 mg per day or 5.625 mg per dose.

CHAPTER 73
1. b
2. c
3. a
4. c, e
5. b
6. c (When symptoms flare, patients may be given 10 to 20 mg/day until symptoms are controlled, followed by gradual drug withdrawal over 5 to 7 days.)
7. a
8. d
9. d
10. c
11. a
12. a
13. d (Retinal damage, which is rare, is the most serious toxicity. Retinopathy may be irreversible and can produce blindness.)
14. b

15. c
16. d
17. c (Infliximab may pose a risk of heart failure. Exercise caution in patients with existing heart failure, and monitor them closely for disease progression.)
18. b
19. d
20. a (Rituximab can cause severe infusion-related hypersensitivity reactions. The immediate reaction and its sequelae include hypotension, bronchospasm, angioedema, hypoxia, pulmonary infiltrates, myocardial infarction, and cardiogenic shock.)
21. b, d
22. No. The safe dose is 20 mg.
23. 0.6 mL

CHAPTER 74
1. F
2. T
3. T
4. F
5. T
6. T
7. a
8. a
9. b (The most serious toxicity is a rare but potentially fatal hypersensitivity syndrome, characterized by rash, fever, eosinophilia, and dysfunction of the liver and kidneys. To prevent renal injury, fluid intake should be sufficient to maintain a urine flow of at least 2 L/day.)
10. c
11. c (Allopurinol can inhibit hepatic drug-metabolizing enzymes, thereby delaying the inactivation of other drugs. This interaction is of particular concern for patients taking warfarin, whose dosage should be reduced.)
12. b
13. a (During premarketing trials, pegloticase triggered anaphylaxis in 6.5% of patients. Symptoms include wheezing, perioral or lingual edema, hemodynamic instability, and rash.)
14. 1 1/2 tablets per dose
15. 125 mL per hour

CHAPTER 75
1. parathyroid hormone; vitamin D; calcitonin

2. hypercalcemia
3. clot
4. lethargy; depression
5. tetany, convulsions, spasm of the pharynx, spasm of other muscles (or spasm of the pharynx and other muscles)
6. increases
7. whole grains (or bran); spinach (or rhubarb, Swiss chard, beets)
8. vitamin D
9. tetracycline; fluoroquinolones; thyroid hormone; phenytoin; bisphosphonates
10. a (Calcium is critical to function in skeletal, nervous, muscular, and cardiovascular systems. However, maintenance of normal levels is a priority in the cardiovascular system, as calcium plays a role in myocardial contraction, vascular contraction, and blood coagulation.)
11. a
12. c
13. h (For severe hypercalcemia, initial therapy consists of replacing lost fluid with IV saline.)
14. d (Hypocalcemia increases neuromuscular excitability. As a result, tetany, convulsions, and spasm of the pharynx and other muscles may occur.)
15. a
16. b
17. d
18. b, e
19. d
20. d (Parenteral calcium may cause severe bradycardia in patients taking digoxin.)
21. b, c, e
22. a, c
23. d
24. c, e
25. a (Esophagitis, sometimes resulting in ulceration, is the most serious adverse effect of alendronate. The cause of injury is prolonged contact with the esophageal mucosa, which can occur if alendronate fails to pass completely through the esophagus, as would be the case in dysphagia.)
26. d
27. b
28. b
29. c, d
30. a

31. c
32. b
33. d (Raloxifene increases the risk of thromboembolic events. Because inactivity promotes DVT, patients should discontinue raloxifene at least 72 hours before prolonged immobilization and should not resume the drug until full mobility has been restored.)
34. d (Raloxifene is classified in FDA pregnancy risk category X—the potential for fetal harm outweighs any possible benefits of use during pregnancy.)
35. b
36. c
37. b (Denosumab increases the risk of serious infections; patients who develop signs of severe infection should seek immediate medical attention. Flank pain and fever may indicate UTI or infection of the abdomen.)
38. b, c, d, e
39. d
40. b
41. 2 to 10 minutes
42. 1.7 mL

CHAPTER 76

1. l
2. f
3. k
4. e
5. j
6. a
7. c
8. i
9. d
10. h
11. b
12. g
13. c (Symptoms of asthma result from a combination of inflammation and bronchoconstriction. Accordingly, treatment must address both components.)
14. c
15. a
16. d
17. b, c, d
18. d (Like oral glucocorticoids, inhaled glucocorticoids can promote bone loss—at least in premenopausal women. Fortunately, the amount of loss is much lower than the amount caused by oral glucocorticoids.)
19. b

20. a (The selectivity of the beta$_2$-adrenergic agonists is only relative, not absolute. Accordingly, these drugs are likely to produce some activation of beta$_1$ receptors in the heart. If dosage is excessive, stimulation of cardiac beta$_1$ receptors can cause angina pectoris and tachydysrhythmias.)
21. d (Following withdrawal of oral glucocorticoids [or transfer to inhaled glucocorticoids], several months are required for recovery of adrenocortical function. Throughout this time, all patients—including those switched to inhaled glucocorticoids—must be given supplemental oral or IV glucocorticoids at times of severe stress. Failure to do so can prove fatal.)
22. b
23. c
24. c
25. a
26. b
27. d
28. a
29. b
30. c (The most severe adverse effects of omalizumab are malignancy and anaphylaxis. Perioral edema is symptomatic of anaphylaxis.)
31. d (Smoking cigarettes [one to two packs a day] accelerates metabolism and decreases the half-life by about 50%.)
32. a (Patients with peanut allergy should avoid two ipratropium products: Atrovent HFA [ipratropium alone] and Combivent [ipratropium/albuterol]. Both products contain soya lecithin as a carrier. Soya is in the same plant family as peanuts, and about 10% of people with peanut allergy are cross-allergic to soya.)
33. c
34. c
35. d
36. 1.6 mL/dose
37. 1.2 mL at 2 subcutaneous sites (total 2.4 mL)

CHAPTER 77

1. c
2. g

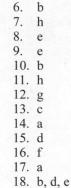

3. a
4. f
5. d
6. b
7. h
8. e
9. e
10. b
11. h
12. g
13. c
14. a
15. d
16. f
17. a
18. b, d, e
19. b
20. c
21. b
22. c
23. a
24. d
25. b (By activating alpha$_1$-adrenergic receptors on systemic blood vessels, sympathomimetics can cause widespread vasoconstriction; for individuals with cardiovascular disorders—hypertension, coronary artery disease, cardiac dysrhythmias, cerebrovascular disease—widespread vasoconstriction can be hazardous.)
26. c
27. b
28. b
29. b
30. d
31. b (If benzonatate is sucked or chewed, rather than swallowed, the drug can cause laryngospasm, bronchospasm, and circulatory collapse.)
32. a, b
33. 2 capsules
34. 8 capsules

CHAPTER 78

1. h
2. a
3. e
4. g
5. b
6. f
7. c
8. d
9. T
10. F
11. T
12. F
13. T

14. F
15. T
16. T
17. F
18. c (Smoking delays ulcer healing and increases the risk of recurrence.)
19. d
20. b
21. c
22. a (Bismuth can impart a harmless black coloration to the tongue and stool. Patients should be forewarned. However, stool discoloration may confound interpretation of gastric bleeding. Therefore, an abdominal assessment is a priority.)
23. a
24. b
25. b, d, e
26. c
27. b
28. a (PPIs have been associated with a dose-related increase in the risk of infection with *C. difficile*, a bacterium that can cause severe diarrhea. Patients experiencing diarrhea while taking omeprazole or other PPIs should report immediately to their health care provider for testing.)
29. d
30. b, e
31. a, b, c, e
32. a
33. c
34. d
35. b
36. 10 mL
37. 16-17 drops per 15 seconds

CHAPTER 79

1. c
2. d
3. a
4. b
5. d
6. c (The Rome III criteria determines constipation more by stool consistency [degree of hardness] than by how often bowel movements occur.)
7. a
8. a
9. d
10. c (Laxatives should not be used in patients with fecal impaction or obstruction of the bowel, because increased peristalsis could cause bowel perforation. High-pitched, tinkling sounds are a sign of early intestinal obstruction.)
11. b
12. c
13. d
14. a (Lactulose can enhance intestinal excretion of ammonia. This property has been exploited to lower blood ammonia content in patients with portal hypertension and hepatic encephalopathy secondary to chronic liver disease. Normal ammonia levels range from 15-110 mcg/dL [this number may vary dependent upon lab].)
15. b
16. d
17. b
18. d
19. a (Easy bruising and mucosal bleeding can occur when medications interfere with vitamin K absorption.)
20. b
21. 30 mL
22. 1 capsule

CHAPTER 80

1. medulla oblongata
2. reflexive (or reflex)
3. chemoreceptor trigger zone
4. vagus
5. before (or prior to) chemotherapy
6. serotonin (or 5-HT3)
7. dexamethasone
8. doxylamine; vitamin B$_6$
9. prolong
10. Irritable bowel syndrome
11. b (A patient with prolonged vomiting and diarrhea will show a decrease in sodium and potassium [electrolytes] and an elevated BUN.)
12. a
13. b, d, e
14. d (Patients should be advised to report local burning or pain immediately when receiving promethazine IV. Extravasation of IV promethazine can cause abscess formation, tissue necrosis, and gangrene that requires amputation. Therefore, the priority action is to stop the IV infusion.)
15. c
16. c (Cannabinoids can cause tachycardia and hypotension. Normal blood pressure is less than 120/80 mm Hg. Symptoms of hypotension are not typically present unless BP is less than 90/60 mm Hg. Tachycardia is a resting heart rate greater than 100 bpm. Therefore, the priority for this patient is a pulse increase.)
17. b
18. c
19. c
20. a
21. d
22. d
23. d
24. c
25. d (Postmarketing data indicate that tegaserod can cause serious cardiovascular events, namely, myocardial infarction (MI), unstable angina, and stroke. Because of the potential for cardiovascular harm, access to tegaserod is restricted.)
26. b, f
27. a
28. c (The most common adverse effect of olsalazine is watery diarrhea, which occurs in 17% of patients. The electrolyte imbalance and fluid loss associated with diarrhea, combined with diuretic use, makes Fluid volume deficit the priority nursing diagnosis.)
29. a, b
30. b
31. d (Tuberculosis and opportunistic infections are of particular concern in patients receiving infliximab. Therefore, a productive cough would be a priority nursing concern.)
32. a
33. d
34. b
35. c
36. a
37. Yes. The recommended dose calculates to 5.5 mg, so a 5-mg capsule is safe and effective.
38. 377 mg

CHAPTER 81

1. d
2. a
3. b
4. e

5. c
6. b
7. a
8. d, e
9. a (In high doses, vitamin A can cause liver injury.)
10. b
11. a
12. c
13. a (Vitamin A has been used for skin conditions, including acne; it has also been used to treat heavy menstrual periods and premenstrual syndrome.)
14. b
15. d
16. d
17. b
18. c
19. b
20. a
21. 1 1/2 tablets
22. 0.25 mL

CHAPTER 82

1. c
2. b
3. a
4. b
5. a
6. d
7. d
8. c (By reducing fat absorption, orlistat can reduce absorption of fat-soluble vitamins [vitamins A, D, E, and K]. Vitamin K deficiency can intensify the effects of warfarin, an anticoagulant. In patients taking warfarin, anticoagulant effects should be monitored closely.)
9. a
10. a
11. a, d
12. 2 capsules
13. 0.5 (1/2) tablet

CHAPTER 83

1. T
2. F
3. T
4. F
5. T
6. T
7. F
8. F
9. T
10. T
11. F
12. T
13. F

14. T
15. F
16. F
17. T
18. F
19. F
20. b (Unasyn is a broad-spectrum antibiotic. Narrow-spectrum antibiotics are active against only a few species of micro-organisms. In contrast, broad-spectrum antibiotics are active against a wide variety of microbes. Narrow-spectrum drugs are generally preferred to broad-spectrum drugs.)
21. c
22. a
23. c, d
24. c (As a rule, patients with a history of allergy to penicillins should not receive them again. The exception is treatment of a life-threatening infection for which no suitable alternative is available. For emergency treatment, people typically receive epinephrine; antihistamines and corticosteroids may also be ordered.)
25. b (Tetracycline has been assigned to pregnancy category D by the FDA.)
26. d
27. c
28. a, c, d
29. a

CHAPTER 84

1. F
2. T
3. F
4. T
5. F
6. F
7. T
8. T
9. T
10. F
11. T
12. F
13. T
14. a (All patients who are candidates for penicillin therapy should be asked if they have penicillin allergy.)
15. c
16. b
17. d
18. c (Anaphylaxis [laryngeal edema, bronchoconstriction,

severe hypotension] is an immediate hypersensitivity reaction, mediated by IgE. Anaphylactic reactions occur more frequently with penicillins than with any other drugs.)
19. a
20. c
21. a, e
22. d
23. d
24. c (Ticarcillin interferes with platelet function and can thereby promote bleeding.)
25. c
26. No. Dose is 500 mg/day. 7.5 kg × 20 mg = 150 mg/day; 7.55 kg × 40 mg = 300 mg/day.
27. 200 mL/hr

CHAPTER 85

1. beta-lactamases
2. positive
3. Methicillin-resistant *Staphylococcus aureus* (MRSA)
4. increased
5. negative
6. Ceftaroline (Teflaro)
7. good
8. c (In patients with renal insufficiency, dosages of most cephalosporins must be reduced [to prevent accumulation to toxic levels].)
9. c (Ceftriaxone can cause bleeding tendencies.)
10. b (Hypersensitivity reactions are the most frequent adverse events. Maculopapular rash that develops several days after the onset of treatment is most common. Prior to any other action, since a rash is not a severe reaction requiring administration of epinephrine, the assessment must be completed in order to have all relevant information available for the prescriber.)
11. c, d
12. b
13. a
14. c (Because of structural similarities between penicillins and cephalosporins, a few patients allergic to one type of drug may experience cross-reactivity with the other. For patients with mild penicillin allergy, cephalosporins can be used with minimal concern. However, because of the potential for fatal

anaphylaxis, cephalosporins should not be given to patients with a history of severe reactions to penicillins.)

15. a
16. a
17. c
18. a
19. b
20. b
21. c (Imipenem can reduce blood levels of valproate, a drug used to control seizures. Breakthrough seizures have occurred. The patient is a safety risk due to the possibility of seizures.)
22. d
23. b
24. a
25. d
26. No. 750 mg is higher than the 10 mg/kg recommended for persons with normal renal function.
27. 254 mg. Yes, this is a safe dose.

CHAPTER 86

1. F
2. T
3. T
4. F
5. F
6. T
7. F
8. F
9. T
10. F
11. b, c, e
12. d
13. a
14. c
15. c
16. d (Tetracyclines irritate the GI tract. As a result, oral therapy is frequently associated with epigastric burning, cramps, nausea, vomiting, and diarrhea. Because diarrhea may result from superinfection of the bowel [in addition to nonspecific irritation], it is important that the cause of diarrhea be determined.)
17. a
18. a, c, d
19. c
20. c
21. b
22. d
23. c
24. a
25. c
26. d

27. c (Linezolid can cause reversible myelosuppression, manifesting as anemia, leukopenia, thrombocytopenia, or even pancytopenia. Complete blood counts should be done weekly.)
28. a
29. c
30. d (Telithromycin can cause severe liver injury [fulminant hepatitis, hepatic necrosis] and acute hepatic failure. If liver injury is diagnosed, telithromycin should be discontinued and never used again.)
31. a
32. c (Chloramphenicol is a broad-spectrum antibiotic with the potential for causing fatal aplastic anemia and other blood dyscrasias. Anemia is one of the most common causes of pallor.)
33. b
34. a
35. 4 mL
36. No. The safe dose is 837.5 mg every 6 hours.

CHAPTER 87

1. bactericidal
2. CSF (cerebrospinal fluid)
3. kidneys
4. narrow
5. negative
6. kidneys; inner ear
7. hours
8. concentration-dependent
9. enzymes; aminoglycosides
10. anaerobes
11. a, c, f
12. b
13. a (Patients on aminoglycoside therapy should be monitored for ototoxicity. The first sign of impending vestibular damage is headache, which may last for 1 or 2 days. A complete assessment must be performed prior to notifying the prescriber, in order for him/her to determine whether the headache is related to tobramycin. Therefore, assessment is the priority action.)
14. d
15. d
16. c (Aminoglycosides can inhibit neuromuscular transmission, causing flaccid paralysis and potentially fatal respiratory depression. Most episodes of neuromuscular blockade have

occurred following intraperitoneal or intrapleural instillation of aminoglycosides. However, neuromuscular blockade has also occurred with IV, IM, and oral dosing.)
17. b
18. d (Comparing the eGFR to the dosing recommendations provided in the package insert or IV drug book, in concert with trough drug level, will enable the nurse to determine if the dosing is appropriate.)
19. c
20. b
21. a (In patients with normal renal function, half-lives of the aminoglycosides range from 2-3 hours. However, because elimination is almost exclusively renal, half-lives increase dramatically in patients with renal impairment. Accordingly, to avoid serious toxicity, dosage must be reduced or the dosing interval increased in patients with kidney disease.)
22. c
23. 100-166 mg every 8 hours. Calculating 1.7 mg/kg equals 170 mg per dose, but that exceeds 5 mg/day.
24. An appropriate dose is 325 mg every 8 hours; the prescribed dose is too low.

CHAPTER 88

1. T
2. F
3. T
4. T
5. F
6. F
7. T
8. F
9. T
10. F
11. T
12. T
13. d
14. b (To minimize the risk of renal damage, adults should maintain a daily urine output of 1200 mL. This can be accomplished by consuming 8 to 10 glasses of water each day. Because the solubility of sulfonamides is highest at elevated pH, alkalinization of the urine can

further decrease the chances of crystalluria.)

15. c (In addition to hemolytic anemia, sulfonamides can cause agranulocytosis, leukopenia, thrombocytopenia, and very rarely, aplastic anemia; red cell distribution width [RDW] may be elevated in persons with hemolytic anemia.)
16. a
17. b
18. a
19. c (Local application of mafenide is frequently painful.)
20. c
21. a, d
22. b (People with hyperkalemia may report symptoms such as muscle weakness, tiredness, tingling sensations, or nausea.)
23. a
24. c
25. a
26. d
27. 9 mL/dose

CHAPTER 89
1. c
2. f
3. b
4. a
5. e
6. d
7. b
8. b (Prevention of repeat UTIs in women includes wiping front to back.)
9. a, b, c, d
10. d (If treatment is to succeed, the identity and drug sensitivity of the causative organism must be determined. To do so, urine for microbiologic testing should be obtained before giving any antibiotics.)
11. c
12. b
13. a
14. a, b, c, e
15. c (For two reasons, nitrofurantoin should not be administered to individuals with renal impairment [creatinine clearance less than 40 mL/min]. First, in the absence of good renal function, levels of nitrofurantoin in the urine are too low to be effective. Second, renal impairment reduces nitrofurantoin excretion, causing plasma levels of

the drug to rise, thereby posing a risk of systemic toxicity.)
16. a
17. 2 capsules
18. 0.5 tablet

CHAPTER 90
1. T
2. F
3. F
4. F
5. T
6. F
7. F
8. T
9. F
10. T
11. T
12. b, c, d
13. a
14. d
15. b
16. d (Isoniazid can cause hepatocellular injury and multilobular necrosis. Patients should be informed about signs of hepatitis [anorexia, malaise, fatigue, nausea, yellowing of the skin or eyes] and instructed to notify the prescriber immediately if these develop.)
17. b
18. a, c, e
19. c
20. b
21. a
22. b
23. c
24. b
25. a, d
26. b (Ethambutol can produce dose-related optic neuritis, resulting in blurred vision, constriction of the visual field, and disturbance of color discrimination.)
27. a
28. c
29. a
30. c (GI symptoms [nausea, vomiting, cramping, diarrhea] are common but mild. The drug frequently imparts a harmless red color to feces, urine, sweat, tears, and saliva. Deposition of clofazimine in the small intestine produces the most serious effects: intestinal obstruction, pain, and bleeding.)
31. 507 mL divided by 3 = 169 mL/hr

32. Yes. Safe dose range is 400-800 mg/day = 200-400 mg/dose.

CHAPTER 91
1. tendon
2. *Neisseria gonorrhoeae*
3. anaerobes
4. phototoxicity (or severe sunburn)
5. Achilles tendon
6. a (If treatment is to succeed and drug resistance reduced, the identity and drug sensitivity of the causative organism must be determined.)
7. b (Ciprofloxacin can induce a variety of mild adverse effects, including GI reactions [nausea, vomiting, diarrhea, abdominal pain]; vomiting and diarrhea put the child at increased risk of electrolyte imbalance.)
8. a, d, e
9. d
10. c
11. c
12. d
13. b
14. b, c
15. c
16. a
17. c
18. a
19. d
20. a, b, c
21. 494 mg is the recommended dose. This is safe.
22. Yes, it is safe. 1.2 g is the recommended dose.

CHAPTER 92
1. mycosis
2. external (or outside)
3. throughout the body
4. T
5. T
6. F
7. T
8. F
9. T
10. T
11. F
12. T
13. b
14. d
15. c
16. a
17. c
18. c
19. b
20. d

21. a (Amphotericin is toxic to cells of the kidney. Renal impairment occurs in practically all patients.)
22. c
23. a
24. b
25. c
26. b
27. d
28. c
29. b (Treatment with fluconazole has been associated with hepatic necrosis, Stevens-Johnson syndrome, and anaphylaxis. Fever, along with mucocutaneous lesions, are early symptoms of Stevens-Johnson syndrome.)
30. d
31. b
32. b (Posaconazole inhibits CYP3A4, and can thereby increase levels of many other drugs. Combined use of posaconazole with ergot alkaloids is contraindicated, because raising their levels can lead to ergotism.)
33. a
34. c
35. d
36. d
37. a
38. c
39. 86 or 87 mL/hr; total volume is 130 mL over 90 minutes.
40. 12.5 mg; yes, 12 mg is safe.

CHAPTER 93
1. T
2. F
3. T
4. T
5. T
6. F
7. T
8. T
9. F
10. F
11. d
12. c
13. a (Intravenous acyclovir is generally well-tolerated. The most common reactions are phlebitis and inflammation at the infusion site.)
14. c (Reversible nephrotoxicity, indicated by elevations in serum creatinine and blood urea nitrogen, occurs in some patients. The risk of renal injury

is increased by dehydration and use of other nephrotoxic drugs. Dry mucous membranes are indicative of dehydration. To avoid nephrotoxicity, hydrating the patient is priority.)
15. a (For herpes simplex genitalis, valacyclovir is indicated for treatment of initial and recurrent episodes for immunocompetent patients; however, for suppressive therapy, this drug is approved for management in immunocompetent and HIV-infected adults with a CD4+ cell count of at least 100 cells/mm³.)
16. a
17. b
18. d
19. c
20. c
21. d
22. c
23. a
24. a (Lactic acidosis, pancreatitis, and severe hepatomegaly are rare but dangerous complications. If one of these conditions develops, lamivudine should be discontinued. A sign of lactic acidosis is deep, rapid breathing.)
25. a
26. c
27. b
28. a, b, c, d, e
29. c
30. d
31. 300-400 mg in three divided doses (100-133 mg)
32. 600 mL

CHAPTER 94
1. d
2. b
3. a
4. e
5. f
6. c
7. c
8. a
9. b, c (Trimethoprim-sulfamethoxazole has been associated with thrombocytopenia, leukopenia, and neutropenia; it has also been associated with kidney failure, and elevated BUN/creatinine.)
10. b
11. d

12. b (Rilpivirine can cause depression. Instruct patients to contact the provider immediately if they start feeling sad, hopeless, or suicidal.)
13. a
14. c
15. d (The most common adverse effect is rash; for most patients, the rash is benign. However, if the patient experiences severe rash or rash associated with fever, blistering, oral lesions, conjunctivitis, muscle pain, or joint pain, nevirapine should be withdrawn, because these symptoms may indicate development of erythema multiforme or Stevens-Johnson syndrome.)
16. c
17. d
18. d (Use of PIs has been associated with redistribution of body fat, sometimes referred to as *lipodystrophy syndrome* or *pseudo-Cushing's syndrome*. Fat accumulates in the abdomen ["protease paunch"] in the breasts of men and women, and between the shoulder blades ["buffalo hump"]. Fat is lost from the face, arms, buttocks, and legs. Leg and arm veins become prominent.)
19. d
20. a
21. c
22. d
23. d
24. a, b, d
25. d (Enfuvirtide has also been associated with Guillain-Barré syndrome.)
26. a
27. d
28. a
29. a, b
30. d
31. c
32. c
33. 30 mL
34. 40 mg

CHAPTER 95
1. T
2. T
3. a
4. d (About half of the infants born to women with cervical *C. trachomatis* acquire the infection

during delivery, putting them at risk for pneumonia.)
5. a
6. c
7. b
8. c (Among preadolescent children, the most common cause of gonococcal infection is sexual abuse. Vaginal, anorectal, and pharyngeal infections are most common.)
9. a
10. b
11. d (Neonatal gonococcal infection is acquired through contact with infected cervical exudates during delivery. Infection can be limited to the eyes or it may be disseminated. Gonococcal neonatal ophthalmia is a serious infection. The initial symptom is conjunctivitis.)
12. b
13. d
14. a
15. c
16. b
17. 40 mg every 6 hours; 160 mg total per day.
18. 100 mL/hr

CHAPTER 96
1. e
2. b
3. c
4. d
5. f
6. a
7. g
8. F
9. F
10. T
11. T
12. F
13. T
14. F
15. T
16. F
17. a
18. a
19. b
20. a (Isopropanol promotes local vasodilation and can thereby increase bleeding from needle punctures and incisions.)
21. a, b
22. b
23. a, c
24. b
25. a (Because BAC is inactivated by soap, all soap must be removed by rinsing with water and 70% alcohol prior to BAC application.)
26. b
27. c

CHAPTER 97
1. T
2. T
3. F
4. T
5. F
6. T
7. T
8. T
9. F
10. b
11. d
12. c
13. b, c, d, f, g
14. c (Limited experience with mebendazole in pregnant women has shown no increase in spontaneous abortion or fetal malformation. Nonetheless, pregnant women should avoid this drug, especially during the first trimester.)
15. a
16. a
17. d (Indirect effects of diethylcarbamazine, occurring secondary to death of the parasites, can be more serious. These include rashes, intense itching, encephalitis, fever, tachycardia, lymphadenitis, leucocytosis, and proteinuria.)
18. 5 chewable tablets
19. 202.5 mg (200-mg tablet)

CHAPTER 98
1. young
2. resistant
3. *Anopheles* mosquito
4. tuberculosis
5. hepatocytes (or liver cells)
6. erythrocytes
7. Vivax
8. relapse
9. Black water fever
10. c
11. b
12. a
13. c
14. c
15. b
16. a (Falciparum malaria can produce serious complications, including pulmonary edema.)
17. a (Symptoms of hypoglycemia include sweating, chills, and clamminess.)
18. d
19. b
20. a (The most serious and frequent effect from primaquine is hemolysis, which can develop in patients with glucose-6-phosphate dehydrogenase [G6PD] deficiency. During primaquine therapy, the urine should be monitored [darkening indicates the presence of hemoglobin].)
21. c (Quinine has quinidine-like effects on the heart and must be used cautiously in patients with atrial fibrillation. By enhancing atrioventricular conduction, quinine can increase passage of atrial impulses to the ventricles, thereby causing a dangerous increase in ventricular rate.)
22. b
23. b
24. a (Intravenous quinidine is more cardiotoxic than quinine. Accordingly, patients require continuous electrocardiographic monitoring and frequent monitoring of blood pressure.)
25. c
26. a
27. c
28. 5.6 mL/hr
29. 166 (or 165) mg every 8 hours

CHAPTER 99
1. c
2. b
3. f
4. e
5. a
6. d
7. c (Cryptosporidiosis is characterized by diarrhea, abdominal cramps, anorexia, low-grade fever, nausea, and vomiting. For immunocompromised individuals the disease can be prolonged and life-threatening, with diarrhea volume up to 20 L/day. For this person on prednisone for chronic illness, fluid volume deficit would be a priority as he/she is immunocompromised and could potentially have life-threatening diarrhea.)
8. b
9. d

10. a
11. c
12. a
13. a (Suramin concentrates in the kidneys and can cause local damage, resulting in the appearance of protein, blood cells, and casts in the urine. If urinary casts are observed, treatment should cease.)
14. b
15. b
16. d (In people with a deficiency of glucose-6-phosphate dehydrogenase, nifurtimox can cause hemolysis.)
17. 254.5 mg; dose is safe and therapeutic.
18. Yes, the dose is safe. It falls between the 30-40 mg/kg/day in 3 divided doses recommended for children (295 mg to 394 mg every 8 hours).

CHAPTER 100

1. P
2. S
3. S
4. B
5. P
6. S
7. B
8. B
9. P
10. B
11. c
12. d
13. a
14. c, d
15. 30-lb child: None, because the child weighs 13.6 kg (less than 15 kg). 44-lb child: 4-8 mg.
16. 3 tablets

CHAPTER 101

1. heart disease
2. 30; 74
3. Prostate
4. surgery
5. Cytotoxic
6. divide indefinitely
7. d
8. b, d
9. c
10. d
11. a
12. b
13. a
14. c
15. a
16. b

17. c (The major concern with hyperuricemia is injury to the kidneys secondary to deposition of uric acid crystals in renal tubules.)
18. b

CHAPTER 102

1. T
2. F
3. T
4. F
5. T
6. T
7. F
8. F
9. T
10. F
11. d
12. a (Bone marrow suppression [neutropenia, thrombocytopenia] is the usual dose-limiting toxicity for patients receiving cytotoxic drugs.)
13. b
14. a
15. b
16. d
17. c (Other adverse effects of cisplatin include ototoxicity, which manifests as tinnitus and high-frequency hearing loss.)
18. b
19. d
20. c (High doses can directly injure the kidneys. To promote drug excretion, and thereby minimize renal damage, the urine should be alkalinized and adequate hydration maintained.)
21. b (It should be noted that leucovorin rescue is potentially dangerous: Failure to administer leucovorin in the right dose at the right time can be fatal.)
22. a
23. c
24. b
25. a, c, e
26. d (Bone marrow suppression [neutropenia, thrombocytopenia, anemia] is the principal dose-limiting toxicity. Petechiae often occur in the setting of thrombocytopenia.)
27. d
28. d
29. c (Bleomycin can cause severe injury to the lungs.)
30. a (For adolescents, hair loss secondary to chemotherapy can

be devastating; nurses must assist the adolescent to find ways to cope with this problem.)
31. b (Severe hypersensitivity reactions [hypotension, dyspnea, angioedema, urticaria] have occurred during infusion of Taxol.)
32. c
33. d
34. 300 micrograms
35. 1237.5 mg

CHAPTER 103

1. F
2. T
3. T
4. F
5. F
6. F
7. c
8. d (Perhaps the biggest concern with tamoxifen is endometrial cancer. In postmenopausal women, endometrial cancer is usually caught early, due to abnormal menstrual bleeding.)
9. b
10. a (Because of its estrogen agonist actions, tamoxifen poses a small risk of thromboembolic events, including deep vein thrombosis, pulmonary embolism, and stroke.)
11. b
12. c (Toremifene prolongs the QT interval, and thereby poses a risk of potentially fatal dysrhythmias. To reduce risk, toremifene should be avoided in patients with hypokalemia or hypomagnesemia. A potassium level of 2.7 is low; a magnesium level of 2.2 is acceptable.)
13. d
14. a
15. d
16. a, d
17. c
18. d
19. b
20. c
21. d
22. c
23. a
24. b (Side effects of ketoconazole include nausea and vomiting. These may lead to electrolyte imbalance.)
25. a, c
26. a

27. d
28. b
29. b, d, e
30. a (Fluid retention occurs in 52% to 68% of patients taking imatinib, and may lead to pleural effusion, pericardial effusion, pulmonary edema, or ascites.)
31. d
32. b
33. c
34. a
35. c
36. a
37. d
38. a
39. a
40. c
41. c
42. c
43. d (In patients taking interferon alfa-2b, neuropsychiatric effects—especially depression—are a serious concern, owing to a risk of death by suicide. Therefore, preventing injury is the priority.)
44. 125 seconds = 2 minutes plus 5 seconds. It is acceptable. Even though it is taking 5 seconds longer than 2 minutes, it is safe. Because of the setup of a clock (watch), it is easier to time a drug every 5 seconds than every 3 or 4 seconds.
45. Yes. The patient's BSA = 2 m². 2 × 400 mg = 800 mg.

CHAPTER 104

1. c
2. m
3. f
4. d
5. a
6. n
7. e
8. g
9. i
10. j
11. k
12. l
13. b
14. h
15. central
16. Drusen
17. dry; wet
18. anemia
19. b (Since POAG has no symptoms [until significant and irreversible optic nerve injury has occurred], regular testing for early POAG is important among individuals at high risk. With early detection and treatment, blindness can usually be prevented.)
20. d (Angle-closure glaucoma develops suddenly and is extremely painful. In the absence of treatment, irreversible loss of vision occurs in 1 to 2 days.)
21. a, e
22. a
23. c
24. b
25. a, d
26. c
27. b (Osmotic agents cause fluid to move from the eye into the plasma, thereby causing a rapid and marked reduction of IOP. However, osmotic agents must be used with caution in persons with CKD and compromised cardiac function. Urine output must be monitored to ensure fluid is not retained.)
28. c, e
29. c
30. d (The biggest concern is endophthalmitis, an inflammation inside the eye caused by bacterial, viral, or fungal infection. Patients who experience symptoms [e.g., redness, light sensitivity, pain] should seek immediate medical attention.)
31. a
32. b
33. 2 tablets
34. 18.75 grams

CHAPTER 105

1. epidermis
2. stratum germinativum or basal layer
3. keratin
4. corneum
5. Melanin
6. dermis
7. sebum
8. fat
9. Open comedones
10. Closed comedones or whiteheads
11. androgens
12. scrubbing; foods
13. a
14. d
15. a (Salicylic acid is readily absorbed through the skin, so systemic toxicity [salicylism] can result when large amounts are used for a prolonged period. Symptoms of salicylism include tinnitus.)
16. c
17. a (Some formulations of benzoyl peroxide contain sulfites, which can cause potentially serious allergic reactions. The incidence of reactions is highest in patients with asthma.)
18. a
19. a, c, e
20. a, b, c
21. d, e, f, g
22. d
23. a
24. b
25. a
26. d
27. b
28. d
29. c
30. b
31. d
32. a (Sunscreens alone cannot completely protect against sun damage. Accordingly, to further reduce risk, sunglasses, protective clothing, and a wide-brimmed hat should be worn. In addition, avoid sun exposure in the middle of the day, especially between 10:00 AM and 4:00 PM. If you must be outside at these times, try to stay in the shade as much as possible. All of these work together to reduce chronic exposure of the skin to sunlight.)
33. c
34. a
35. b
36. d
37. b
38. 83 to 84 mL/hr
39. 1 mL

CHAPTER 106

1. auricle; pinna
2. external ear
3. eardrum; inner
4. auditory (eustachian) tube
5. semicircular canals
6. F
7. T
8. F
9. T
10. F
11. c
12. d

13. a
14. d
15. a, b, d
16. d
17. d
18. Yes, the dose is safe; it falls between 80-90 mg/kg/d in 2 divided doses. 0.8 mL
19. No, the dose is too low; should administer 1000 mg per dose (the maximum dose); 15 mL

CHAPTER 107

1. c
2. e
3. b
4. a
5. f
6. d
7. a (More importantly, in persons taking iloprost, peripheral vasodilation may result in orthostatic hypotension and syncope.)
8. d
9. c
10. b
11. c
12. c (These are symptoms of hyperglycemia; glucose level is the priority.)
13. a (Surfactant therapy lowers the surface tension forces that cause alveolar collapse, and thereby rapidly improves oxygenation and lung compliance and reduces the need for supplemental oxygen and mechanical ventilation. Based on these factors, Ineffective airway clearance is the highest priority in a neonate receiving beractant.)
14. c
15. b
16. c
17. a
18. d
19. a
20. a
21. c
22. b (Recall that both depression and suicidality are common in HD. Tetrabenazine increases the risk of both. Accordingly, all patients using the drug should be watched closely for new or worsening depression, and for expression of suicidal thoughts or behavior.)
23. b
24. a, b, d
25. 625 mg

26. 15 mg; 100 mL/hr

CHAPTER 108

1. i
2. d
3. h
4. f
5. c
6. e
7. a
8. b
9. j
10. g
11. F
12. T
13. F
14. T
15. T
16. T
17. F
18. T
19. a
20. c (Rather than wait for implementation of CGMPs, four private organizations—the U.S. Pharmacopeia [USP], ConsumerLab, the Natural Products Association, and NSF International—have already begun testing dietary supplements for quality. A "seal of approval" is given to products that meet their standards, which are very similar to the CGMPs described previously. The USP standards are enforceable by the FDA.)
21. a (Herbal products and other dietary supplements can interact with conventional drugs, sometimes with significant harmful results. The principal concerns are increased toxicity and decreased therapeutic effects. Clinicians and consumers should be alert to these possibilities.)
22. b
23. c (CoQ-10 is structurally similar to vitamin K_2, and hence may antagonize the effects of warfarin.)
24. c
25. b
26. d
27. a, b, c
28. a
29. c
30. d (Symptoms of hypoglycemia include pounding heart, sweating, chills, and clamminess.)
31. d (There is concern that ginkgo may promote seizures.

Accordingly, the herb should be avoided by patients at risk for seizures, including those taking drugs that can lower the seizure threshold, including antipsychotics, antidepressants, cholinesterase inhibitors, decongestants, first-generation antihistamines, and systemic glucocorticoids.)
32. a
33. a (St. John's wort is known to interact adversely with many drugs—and the list continues to grow. Three mechanisms are involved: induction of cytochrome P450 enzymes, induction of P-glycoprotein, and intensification of serotonin effects.)
34. c
35. b (Ma huang [ephedra] contains ephedrine, a compound that can elevate blood pressure and stimulate the heart and CNS.)

CHAPTER 109

1. b, e, f
2. e, f
3. d
4. b, e
5. a, e
6. b, c, e, f
7. b, e, f
8. b (Supportive care is the most important element in managing acute poisoning. Support is based on the clinical status and requires no knowledge specific to the poison involved. Maintenance of respiration and circulation are primary concerns.)
9. b, e
10. a
11. d
12. c
13. b
14. d
15. a
16. a
17. b
18. c
19. d
20. a
21. d
22. c
23. c
24. a
25. 2 1/2 mL
26. 333 mL/hr

CHAPTER 110

1. T
2. T
3. F
4. F
5. F
6. T
7. F
8. T
9. T
10. T
11. F
12. d (Initial symptoms of anthrax include fever, cough, malaise, and weakness. They may be relatively mild.)

13. a
14. d
15. a
16. b
17. b
18. b
19. a
20. c
21. a (Supportive care, which may be needed for several months, includes mechanical assistance of ventilation; hence, effective breathing is the highest nursing priority.)

22. c
23. d
24. c
25. c
26. 1/2 tablet
27. 0.25 mL every 10 seconds × 200 seconds = 5 mL